STRUCTURE–ACTIVITY CORRELATION AS A PREDICTIVE TOOL IN TOXICOLOGY

CHEMICAL INDUSTRY INSTITUTE OF TOXICOLOGY SERIES

STRUCTURE–ACTIVITY CORRELATION AS A PREDICTIVE TOOL IN TOXICOLOGY

Fundamentals, Methods, and Applications

Edited by

Leon Golberg

Chemical Industry Institute of Toxicology

⬤ HEMISPHERE PUBLISHING CORPORATION

Washington New York London

DISTRIBUTION OUTSIDE THE UNITED STATES
McGRAW–HILL INTERNATIONAL BOOK COMPANY

Auckland Bogotá Guatemala Hamburg Johannesburg Lisbon
London Madrid Mexico Montreal New Delhi Panama Paris
San Juan São Paulo Singapore Sydney Tokyo Toronto

This book was set in Press Roman by Hemisphere Publishing Corporation. The editors were Christine Flint and Sandra J. King; the production supervisor was Miriam Gonzalez; and the typesetter was Frederick B. Wright.
Braun-Brumfield, Inc., was printer and binder.

STRUCTURE-ACTIVITY CORRELATION AS A PREDICTIVE TOOL
IN TOXICOLOGY: Fundamentals, Methods, and Applications

1 2 3 4 5 6 7 8 9 0 B R B R 8 9 8 7 6 5 4 3

Library of Congress Cataloging in Publication Data
Main entry under title:

Structure activity correlation as a predictive tool in
    toxicology.

   (Chemical Industry Institute of Toxicology series)
   Papers from a symposium held in Raleigh, N.C.,
Feb. 10–12, 1981, cosponsored by the Chemical Industry
Institute of Toxicology, and others.
   Includes bibliographical references and index.
   1. Toxicology—Congresses. 2. Structure-activity
relationship (Pharmacology)—Congresses. I. Golberg,
Leon. II. Chemical Industry Institute of Toxicology.
III. Series.
RA1216.S78 1983   615.9′07   82-3007
ISBN 0-89116-276-3   AACR2
ISSN 0278-6265

Contents

PART 2: FUNDAMENTALS

PART 3: CORRELATIVE METHODS

Contributors

ANN H. AKLAND
U.S. Environmental Protection Agency
Research Triangle Park, North Carolina

MARSHALL W. ANDERSON, Ph.D.
National Institute of Environmental
   Health Sciences
Research Triangle Park, North Carolina

HOWARD C. BAILEY
SRI International, Life Sciences
   Division
Research Triangle Park, North Carolina

LESLIE BERNSTEIN
University of Southern California
Los Angeles, California

M. BOROUJERDI
U.S. Environmental Protection Agency
Research Triangle Park, North Carolina

JAMES S. BUS, Ph.D.
Chemical Industry Institute
   of Toxicology
Research Triangle Park, North Carolina

COLIN F. CHIGNELL, Ph.D.
National Institute of Environmental
   Health Sciences
Research Triangle Park, North Carolina

J. T. CHOU
Spectra-Physics
Santa Clara, California

PAUL N. CRAIG, Ph.D.
National Library of Medicine/National
  Toxicology Program
Bethesda, Maryland

CHRISTOPHER W. CRANDELL
Stanford University
Stanford, California

WILLIAM J. DUNN, Ph.D.
University of Illinois Medical Center
Chicago, Illinois

KURT ENSLEIN, Ph.D.
Health Designs, Inc.
Rochester, New York

JAMES FERRELL
SRI International, Life Sciences
  Division
Menlo Park, California

RALPH GINGELL
University of Nebraska Medical Center
Omaha, Nebraska

LEON GOLBERG, M.B., D.Sc., D. Phil.
Chemical Industry Institute
  of Toxicology
Research Triangle Park, North Carolina

STEPHEN S. HECHT, Ph.D.
American Health Foundation
Naylor Dana Institute for Disease
  Prevention
Valhalla, New York

C. TUCKER HELMES
SRI International, Life Sciences
  Division
Research Triangle Park, North Carolina

DIETRICH HOFFMAN
American Health Foundation
Naylor Dana Institute for Disease
  Prevention
Valhalla, New York

LAURA HORN
Lawrence Berkeley Laboratory
Berkeley, California

Y. M. IOANNOU
U.S. Environmental Protection Agency
Research Triangle Park, North Carolina

HOWARD L. JOHNSON, Ph.D.
SRI International, Life Sciences
  Division
Research Triangle Park, North Carolina

PETER C. JURS, Ph.D.
The Pennsylvania State University
University Park, Pennsylvania

JOHN KALDOR
Lawrence Berkeley Laboratory
Berkeley, California

JOYCE J. KAUFMAN, Ph.D.
The Johns Hopkins University
Baltimore, Maryland

KARL KUHLMAN
SRI International, Life Sciences
  Division
Research Triangle Park, North Carolina

HSIAO–CHIA KUNG
U.S. Environmental Protection Agency
Research Triangle Park, North Carolina

CHARLES KUSZYNSKI
University of Nebraska Medical Center
Omaha, Nebraska

ROBERT LANGENBACH, Ph.D.
U.S. Environmental Protection Agency
Research Triangle Park, North Carolina

EDMOND J. LAVOIE, Ph.D.
American Health Foundation
Naylor Dana Institute for Disease
  Prevention
Valhalla, New York

TERRY LAWSON
University of Nebraska Medical Center
Omaha, Nebraska

GERRY LITTON
Lawrence Berkeley Laboratory
Berkeley, California

GILDA H. LOEW, Ph.D.
SRI International, Life Sciences
    Division
Menlo Park, California

JOYCE McCANN, Ph.D.
Lawrence Berkeley Laboratory
Berkeley, California

RENAE MAGAW
Lawrence Berkeley Laboratory
Berkeley, California

YVONNE MARTIN, Ph.D.
Abbott Laboratories
North Chicago, Illinois

DONALD NAGEL
University of Nebraska Medical Center
Omaha, Nebraska

STEPHEN C. NESNOW, Ph.D.
U.S. Environmental Protection Agency
Research Triangle Park, North Carolina

JAMES G. NOURSE
Stanford University
Stanford, California

GLENN I. OUCHI
University of California
Santa Cruz, California

MALCOLM PIKE
University of Southern California
Los Angeles, California

JAMES A. POPP. D.V.M., Ph.D.
Chemical Industry Institute
    of Toxicology
Research Triangle Park, North Carolina

MICHAEL POULSEN
SRI International, Life Sciences
    Division
Menlo Park, California

PARVITZ POUR
University of Nebraska Medical Center
Omaha, Nebraska

WILLIAM P. PURCELL, Ph.D.
University of Tennessee Center
    for the Health Sciences
Memphis, Tennessee

CAROLINE C. SIGMAN, Ph.D.
SRI International, Life Sciences
    Division
Menlo Park, California

DENNIS H. SMITH, Ph.D.
Stanford University
Stanford, California

JOHN F. TINKER
Eastman Kodak Company
Rochester, New York

KAROL L. THOMPSON
SRI International, Life Sciences
    Division
Research Triangle Park, North Carolina

MICHAEL D. WATERS, Ph.D.
U.S. Environmental Protection Agency
Research Triangle Park, North Carolina

A. G. E. WILSON
U.S. Environmental Protection Agency
Research Triangle Park, North Carolina

W. TODD WIPKE, Ph.D.
University of California
Santa Cruz, California

SVANTE WOLD
Umea University
Umea, Sweden

Preface

This volume is based on a symposium held in Raleigh, North Carolina, February 10-12, 1981. The symposium was cosponsored by the Chemical Industry Institute of Toxicology (CIIT), the United States Environmental Protection Agency (EPA), the National Institute of Environmental Health Sciences (NIEHS), and the Burroughs Wellcome Company (BW). It broke new ground as a joint endeavor by four neighboring organizations located in Research Triangle Park, North Carolina sharing a common interest in toxicology.

It is thus appropriate to acknowledge with deep appreciation the contributions made by the following scientific colleagues to the planning of the meeting: Dr. Michael Cory, BW; Dr. James E. Gibson, CIIT; Dr. Peter C. Jurs, The Pennsylvania State University; Dr. Stephen C. Nesnow, EPA; and Dr. Michael D. Waters, EPA.

The organization of the meeting was in the capable hands of the following members of the CIIT administrative staff, to whom we are all most grateful: Ms. Willanna Griffin, Mrs. Elizabeth Barnhill, Mrs. Edna Mangum, Ms. Sena Taylor, Dr. Donald A. Hart, Mr. Lanny Bynum, Mr. Charles Overton, and Mr. Sterling Isom. In addition, Ms. Willanna Griffin worked tirelessly and effectively to organize the manuscript for publication. Ms. Linda Smith and Ms. Joanne Quate were responsible for word processing.

Leon Golberg

Introduction

The subject of structure-activity relationships is seldom far from the toxicologist's consciousness when exploring the biological properties of new compounds or examining those of existing materials whose potential hazards are under further investigation. The attributes observed in the test materials inevitably invite an intuitive comparison with the structures of compounds sharing the same, or similar, toxicological properties. The volume of literature on which these comparisons are based has grown to such an extent as to defy the ability of any individual to recall an adequate expanse of data. Simultaneously, the toxicologist is called on to deal with more and more complex mixtures of environmental or industrial origin. Thus, for instance, in the development of synthetic fuels, the old, familiar, and seemingly innocuous materials like shale or coal are transformed into liquids containing hundreds of characterized or identifiable mutagens and carcinogens. It is time for new approaches.

The correlation of biological properties with chemical structure has its roots in the study of pharmacological action in animals and therapeutic efficacy in humans. Such comparisons were drawn early in the nineteenth century, even before chemical structures could be accurately assigned to many of the medicinal agents under investigation (1). Early enthusiasm for the predictive power of such correlations, and the possibility of beneficial practical applications for clinical purposes, is illustrated by Thomas Huxley's forecast—a century ago—of a radiant future:

> ... there surely can be no ground for doubting that, sooner or later, the pharmacologist will supply the physician with the means of affecting, in any desired sense, the functions of any physiological element of the body. It will, in short, become possible to introduce into the economy a molecular mechanism which, like a cunningly contrived torpedo, shall find its way to some particular group of living elements, and cause an explosion among them, leaving the rest untouched [2].

All this has a familiar ring, especially when applied to the advances and achievements in chemotherapy and other branches of therapeutics. At the time, however, the passing years brought initial disillusion that the brave new world promised by Huxley had not materialized (3). Nevertheless, belief in the importance of structure-activity correlation remained strong. Spurred on by the work of Hansch (4) and others, drug development began to utilize the new techniques involving quantitative structure-activity relationships (QSAR). Toxicology entered the picture with the application of quantum chemistry by the Pullmans (5) to account for carcinogenic activity of polycyclic aromatic hydrocarbons. The advent of the computer has transformed the situation in the field of QSAR, making possible applications of a wide variety of techniques to an ever-widening range of biological properties, from psychotropic agents to olfactory stimulants (6).

In the belief that QSAR is a powerful instrument with whose vast potentialities toxicologists should become familiar, a symposium was convened that forms the basis of this book. Its purpose was twofold: to develop tools to be used in setting priorities for toxicological testing of chemicals and to foster discussions and collaborative interactions in this important area of research between those in a position to develop and perfect the methods and those seeking to utilize them.

The term "predictive tool" was introduced into the title of the symposium to stress the distinction between judgment and computation. The toxicologist's experience, perspective, understanding of, and intuitive feeling for biological phenomena are essential parts of the judgment that he or she brings to bear on findings labeled as statistically significant. There is a parallel with clinical judgment and the breadth of comprehension that it requires, vis à vis the role of computers as adjuncts to decision-making in the handling of clinical laboratory and dosage data (7).

Enthusiasm for the application of QSAR methodologies needs to be tempered by a realization of the weaknesses of existing biological data bases. Equally, one should take note of the multitude of variables that influence the toxicological end-results—animal species, strains, experimental conditions, and other factors. For this reason, care should be exercised in selecting data that may be considered valid. Even when this is done, one is faced with the complexities, not to say the vagaries, of metabolic transformation and the multitude of modulating factors that help to determine the biological outcome in any given situation. Two further confounding factors are the often unique susceptibilities of individuals in animal, and especially human populations, dependent on complex genetic, environmental, and lifestyle factors; also, the effects of simultaneous exposures to a variety of toxicants such as alcohol and tobacco smoke can exercise a striking influence on the toxic manifestations of a test material (8).

These considerations need to be borne in mind lest we be carried away by an excess of euphoria as great as Huxley's. Until an Einstein appears on the scene to rationalize the present state of confusion and provide some standard criteria by which to foretell the range of individual human responses to various types of chemical exposure, the role of QSAR is to warn and to predict. "Double, double toil and trouble" (9) surely continues ahead for toxicologists; but we should learn from Macbeth's experience and not take predictions too literally, even when they come from a computer rather than a Witch.

REFERENCES

1 Bynum, W. F. Chemical structure and pharmacological action: A chapter in the history of 19th century molecular pharmacology. *Bull. Hist. Med.* 44:518 (1970).

2 Huxley, T. The connection of the biological sciences with medicine. *Nature* 24:346 (1881). [Cited by Parascandola, J. Structure-activity relationships— the early mirage. *Pharmacy in History* 13:3 (1971).]

3 Parascandola, J. Early efforts to relate structure and activity. *Trends Pharmacol. Sci.* 1:417 (1980).

4 Hansch, C., and S. M. Anderson. The structure-activity relationship in barbiturates and its similarity to that in other narcotics. *J. Med. Chem.* 10:745 (1967).

5 Pullman, A., and B. Pullman. Electronic structure and carcinogenic activity of aromatic molecules. *Adv. Cancer Res.* 3:117 (1955).

6 Stuper, A. J., W. E. Brügger, and P. C. Jurs. *Computer Assisted Studies of Chemical Structure and Biological Function.* New York: Wiley (1979).

7 Blois, M. S. Clinical judgment and computers. *N. Engl. J. Med.* 303:192 (1980).

8 Golberg, L. Toxicology: Has a new era dawned? *Pharmacol. Rev.* 30:351 (1979).

9 Shakespeare, W. Macbeth, act iv, scene I. In *The Complete Works of William Shakespeare.* New York: Avenel Books (1975).

Leon Golberg

Part One

Biological Activities

Chapter 1

Types of Toxic Response

James A. Popp

How a toxic response is perceived by the experimental toxicologist is dependent on the parameter or methodology used to identify and describe the toxic response. A toxic response may be described in clinical terms (e.g., depression, decreased food consumption, reduced weight gain), clinical pathological terms [e.g., elevated serum glutamic pyruvate transaminase (SGPT), depressed hemoglobin (Hgb)], biochemical terms (e.g., altered cytochrome P-450 levels), physiological terms (e.g., altered respiratory rate), or morphological terms (e.g., centrilobular hepatic necrosis). Frequently, several or all of these approaches are utilized to describe the toxic response induced by a single toxic agent.

The description of a single toxic response is probably never complete, as new technology and methodology continue to evolve and become available. The toxic response is frequently studied by multiple independent groups, each with a particular expertise in training or approach. All too frequently the description of a toxic response is fragmented and poorly correlated. A special need exists for an integrated multidisciplinary approach to the study of toxic responses.

Toxic responses may involve either a single organ or multiple organs. Organ specificity of a toxic response can be dependent on many factors, including the route of entry, the dose, the blood supply, and, perhaps most importantly, the preferential metabolic activation of the toxin by the target organ. The experimental toxicologist should always be careful that assumption of a localized toxic response is not based on the lack of information on other organs. Historically, carbon tetrachloride was described as a hepatotoxin and was first used to study mechanisms of fatty liver formation. When other organs were subsequently studied, toxic responses also were described in the kidney (1), lung (2), and pancreas (3). The most simple and easily understood examples of single organ localized toxic responses occur with either ingestion or inhalation of irritants or caustic substances that fail to be distributed throughout the body. Anthracosis in coal miners (black lung disease) is an example of a localized toxic response, since the initiating particulate material is largely restricted to the pulmonary tissues.

A localized toxic response may involve only part of an organ, as demonstrated by the sublobular distribution of necrosis induced by a variety of hepatotoxins. Using carbon tetrachloride liver injury as an example, the necrogenic lesion is restricted to the centrilobular area (4). This localized necrogenic response is due to increased metabolism, reflecting the high centrilobular cytochrome P-450-associated enzymes (5), and perhaps to a reduced glutathione level (6) relative to other lobular areas.

Toxic chemicals may produce multiorgan effects. The potent carcinogen dimethylnitrosamine (DMN) has been shown to induce neoplasia in multiple organ sites, such as liver, kidney, lung, and nasal sinus (7). It should be stressed that multiple sites may be affected under the same conditions or the organ site specificity may be altered due to changes in the experimental protocol. For example DMN, a potent carcinogen, is primarily a hepatocarcinogen when given at low doses that allow animal survival for 30 weeks or more. However DMN is a primary kidney carcinogen when given at higher doses for a shorter period of time or as a single dose (8). Toxic responses may also have generalized effects involving many body organs rather than being limited to a specific target organ or group of target organs. Ethylene glycol has a whole body effect due to the induced metabolic acidosis (9).

In experimental toxicology, one should always be cautious to distinguish between a direct action of the toxin and an indirect secondary response to the toxin. A *secondary response* is defined as a structural or functional alteration resulting from a primary toxic response induced in a different organ of the body. This point is exemplified by toxins that affect endocrine organs. Streptozotocin causes destruction of pancreatic islets, resulting in diabetes mellitus (10). Glycogen and lipid accumulation in the liver is a secondary response induced by an alteration in physiological function and should not be misinterpreted to indicate a direct hepatotoxic effect of streptozotocin.

Mineralization of various parenchymal organs secondary to uremia induced by any chronic nephrotoxin would be another example of a secondary toxic response.

Toxin-induced injury is frequently categorized as acute or chronic responses. Acute responses occur shortly after exposure to the toxin. An acute response can occur within minutes, as demonstrated by the rapid onset of methemoglobinemia after exposure to a variety of toxic agents, including sodium nitrate (11). In contrast, acute necrosis induced by DMN appears several days after toxin administration (12).

In contrast to an acute response, a chronic toxic response is one that has been present for a prolonged period of time or has taken a long time to produce. A strict definition is impossible because of differing usage in the literature, but in general a response must be present at least several weeks for it to be termed chronic. However, one should not be overly concerned with categorizing morphological lesions or other toxic responses into acute and chronic phases. It is much more important to remember that a toxic response is a dynamic process that has different characteristics at each stage. A toxic response is rarely static. It is also important to recognize that a toxin may have a cumulative tissue effect leading to progressive lesion development. Feeding of α-naphthylisothiocyanate causes progressive bile duct proliferation (13). The chronic development of alcoholic fibrosis first described in humans and subsequently in baboons (14) is also an excellent example of progressive lesion development. Progressive lesion development has been extensively studied in hepatocarcinogenesis systems (15-17). In this example, several intermediate stages have been identified in the process of tumor formation. The neoplasm is the result of the cumulative effect of prior carcinogen exposures.

The consequence of a toxic response is dependent on multiple factors. The severity of the lesion affects the consequence. Severity, however, is not only related to the number of cells affected or destroyed but is also dependent on alterations of the vascular supply and supporting structure of the tissue. The consequence of a toxic response is dependent on the organ affected. For example, destruction of 50 percent of the hepatocytes is compatible with life while destruction of a small number of neurons at strategic locations may be lethal. The location of a lesion within the organ will alter the consequence of the response. The ultimate consequence of a toxic response is frequently dependent on the ability of the damaged tissue to repair at both a functional and structural level. The toxic response may be completely and rapidly reversed, such as occurs with methemoglobinemia induced by sodium nitrate. In this case, repair is complete and involves only biochemical alterations. Repair of morphological lesions may be complete and rapid, with the tissue or cell returning to a normal structure as demonstrated by the repair of carbon tetrachloride-induced balloon cells to morphologically normal hepatocytes (18). In contrast, repair may never occur, as exemplified in chemical carcinogenesis in which initiated cells retain a selective susceptibility to promotion and never become normal cells again (16). Although the altered cells may appear normal and even function normally by most criteria, the cell retains the potential for neoplastic development indefinitely.

Repair at the tissue level can occur by different routes and may result in complete or only partial repair. Repair may occur by regeneration of the tissue to replace the lost cells. In the liver, regeneration results in the duplication of hepatocytes, with the new hepatocyte population being normal by both biochemical and structural methods of evaluation (2, 3, 10). In other tissues, however, regenerative repair may result in a metaplastic change to another cell type. In the nasal mucosa, destruction of the epithelium with continued exposure to the damaging agent results in repair by a metaplastic change of normal respiratory epithelium to squamous epithelium (19). Although regeneration with metaplasia results in a repaired tissue, it has certainly not returned to its normal structural, biochemical, or functional state.

Two types of toxic responses based on mechanism of action deserve brief mention since they are not traditionally considered in toxicology. First, inflammatory lesions are frequently viewed by the toxicologist as a response to infectious agents and therefore outside the realm of toxicology. However, primary inflammatory responses may be the result of chemical toxicity. Glucan has recently been shown to induce hepatic granulomas (20, 21), and we have recently induced comparable hepatic granulomas by feeding β-naphthylisothiocyanate (22). Second, alterations of the immune system have been extensively studied only in recent years (23). A developing body of knowledge indicates that a wide range of chemicals and metals are immunosuppressive. In the future, greater attention will be focused on identifying immunotoxic effects as well as developing an understanding of the mechanism of immunotoxicity.

Problems exist with the traditional biochemical and morphological approaches for the assessment of cellular toxic responses. Although toxic responses have been studied for many years by increasingly sophisticated techniques, our attempts to interpret the data back to a biological system have been less than adequate. Traditionally, biochemical approaches have been used to quantitate a biochemical toxic response but have been deficient in qualifying the tissue and cellular distribution of the toxic response. By contrast, morphological techniques specify the exact location and cell type involved in a toxic response but usually fail to provide a quantitative assessment. Fortunately, these respective deficiencies of biochemical and morphological approaches are being overcome. In the study of liver, new techniques (24) allow separation of the specific cell types for detailed biochemical study. This approach has been utilized in elegant experiments that demonstrate differences in DNA repair as measured by O^6 methylguanine removal in hepatocytes compared to nonparenchymal cells (25). Morphological studies are becoming quantitative through the use of stereologic procedures (26-28). The application of cell separation techniques for biochemical studies and the use of stereologic techniques for pathologic studies have been slow in development. However, the trend toward these approaches will enhance our basic understanding of cellular toxic responses.

REFERENCES

1   Stricker, G. E., E. A. Smuckler, P. W. Kohnen, and R. B. Nagle. Structural and functional changes in rat kidney during CCl$_4$ intoxication. *Am. J. Pathol.* 53:767-778 (1968).

2   Chen, W. J., E. Y. Chi, and E. A. Smuckler. Carbon tetrachloride-induced changes in mixed function oxidases and microsomal cytochromes in the rat lung. *Lab. Invest.* 36:388-394 (1977).

3   de Castro, C. R., A. S. Bernacchi, E. C. de Ferreyra, O. M. de Fenos, and J. A. Castro. Carbon tetrachloride induced ultrastructural alterations in pancreatic acinar cells and in the hepatocytes. Similarities and differences. *Toxicology* 11:289-296 (1978).

4   Morrison, G. R., F. E. Brock, I. E. Karl, and R. E. Shank. Quantitative analysis of regenerating and degenerating areas within the lobule of the carbon tetrachloride-injured liver. *Arch. Biochem. Biophys.* 111:448-460 (1965).

5   Gooding, P. E., J. Chayen, B. Sawyer, and T. F. Slater. Cytochrome P-450 distribution in rat liver and the effect of sodium phenobarbitone administration. *Chem. Biol. Interact.* 20:299-310 (1978).

6   Smith, M. T., N. Loveridge, E. D. Wills, and J. Chayen. The distribution of glutathione in rat liver lobule. *Biochem. J.* 182:103-108 (1979).

7   Magee, P. N., and J. M. Barnes. Carcinogenic nitroso compounds. *Adv. Cancer Res.* 10:163-246 (1967).

8   Magee, P. N., and J. M. Barnes. Induction of kidney tumors in the rat with dimethylnitrosamine. *J. Pathol. Bacteriol.* 84:19-31 (1962).

9   Borden, T. A., and C. D. Bidwell. Treatment of acute ethylene glycol poisoning in rats. *Invest. Urol.* 6:205-210 (1968).

10 Ganda, O. P., A. A. Rossini, and A. A. Like. Studies on streptozotocin diabetes. *Diabetes* 25:595-603 (1976).

11 Kiese, J. *Methemoglobinemia: A Comprehensive Treatise.* Cleveland: CRC (1974).

12 Barnes, J. M., and P. N. Magee. Some toxic properties of dimethylnitrosamine. *Br. J. Ind. Med.* 11:167 (1954).

13 McLean, M. R., and K. R. Rees. Hyperplasia of bile ducts induced by alpha-naphthol-iso-thiocyanate: Experimental biliary cirrhosis free from biliary obstruction. *J. Pathol. Bacteriol.* 76:175-189 (1958).

14 Popper, H., and C. S. Lieber, Histogenesis of alcoholic fibrosis and cirrhosis in the baboon. *Am. J. Pathol.* 98:695-716 (1980).

15 Farber, E., D. S. R. Sarma, S. Rajalakshimi, and H. Shinozuka. Liver carcinogenesis: A unifying hypothesis. In F. F. Becker (ed.), *The Liver: Normal and Abnormal Functions*, part B, pp. 755–820. New York: Marcel Dekker (1975).

16 Farber, E. Reversible and irreversible lesions in processes of cancer development. In R. Montesano, H. Bartsch, and L. Tomatis (eds.), *Molecular and Cellular Aspects of Carcinogen Screening Tests*, pp. 143–151. Lyon: IARC Scientific Publication No 27 (1980).

17 Frith, C. H., K. P. Bactcke, C. J. Nelson, and G. Schieferstein. Sequential morphogenesis of liver tumors in mice given benzidine dihydrochloride. *Eur. J. Cancer* 16:1205–1216 (1980).

18 Popp, J. A., H. Shinozuka, and E. Farber. The protective effect of diethyldithiocarbonate and cycloheximide on the multiple hepatic lesions induced by carbon tetrachloride in the rat. *Toxicol. Appl. Pharmacol.* 45:549–564 (1978).

19 Swenberg, J. A., W. D. Kerns, R. I. Mitchell, E. J. Gralla, and K. L. Pavkov. Induction of squamous cell carcinomas of the rat nasal cavity by inhalation exposure to formaldehyde vapor. *Cancer Res.* 40:3398–3402 (1980).

20 Deimann, W., and H. D. Fahimi. Hepatic granulomas induced by glucan. An ultrastructural and peroxidase-cytochemical study. *Lab. Invest.* 43:172–181 (1980).

21 DiLuzio, N. R. Influence of glucan on hepatic macrophage structure and function: Relation to inhibition of hepatic metastases. In E. Wisse and D. L. Knook (eds.), *Kupffer Cells and Other Liver Sinusoidal Cells*, pp. 397–406. Amsterdam: Elsevier/North-Holland (1977).

22 Leonard, T. B., J. A. Popp, M. E. Graichen, and J. G. Dent. β-Naphthylisothiocyanate induced alterations in hepatic drug metabolism and liver morphology. *Toxicol. Appl. Pharmacol.* (in press).

23 Vos, J. G. Immune suppression as related to toxicology. *CRC Crit. Rev. Toxicol.* 5:67–101 (1977).

24 Knook, D. L., and E. Ch. Sleyster. Separation of Kupffer and endothelial cells of the rat liver by centrifugal elutriation. *Exp. Cell Res.* 99:444–449 (1976).

25 Lewis, J. G., and J. A. Swenberg. Differential repair of O^6-methylguanine in DNA of rat hepatocytes and nonparenchymal cells. *Nature* 228:185–187 (1980).

26 Massey, E. D., and W. H. Butler. Zonal changes in the rat liver after chronic administration of phenobarbitone: An ultrastructural, morphometric and biochemical correlation. *Chem. Biol. Interact.* 24:329–344 (1979).

27 Bolendar, R. P. Morphometric analysis in the assessment of the response of the liver to drugs. *Pharmacol. Rev.* 30:429–443 (1979).

28 Fowler, B. A., and J. S. Woods. The effects of prolonged oral arsenate exposure on liver mitochondria of mice: Morphometric and biochemical studies. *Toxicol. Appl. Pharmacol.* 50:177–187 (1979).

Chapter 2

Modifying Factors Affecting Toxic Responses: Example-Inhibitors of Carcinogenesis

M. W. Anderson, M. Boroujerdi,
Y. M. Ioannou, Hsiao-Chia Kung,
and A. G. E. Wilson

Many toxic agents require activation to highly reactive intermediates in order to exert their toxicity. For carcinogens such as polycyclic aromatic hydrocarbons, nitrosamines, and aromatic amines, reaction of such intermediates with DNA, particularly the amount of specific or critical carcinogen-DNA adduct(s) formed, is usually considered to be a necessary event in the initiation of tumorigenesis. Expression of carcinogenesis is dependent on the balance between metabolic activation and detoxification, which is determined by a variety of factors influencing the activities of enzyme systems involved. For example the induction of experimental tumors by a variety of chemical

The authors wish to thank Ms. Catherine White and Ms. Julie Angerman-Stewart for their excellent technical assistance, Drs. J. R. Bend and R. M. Philpot for their helpful suggestions, and Ms. Nancy Mitchell, who typed the manuscript.

The abbreviations used are: BP, benzo[a]pyrene; HPLC, high-pressure liquid chromatography; 3-MC, 3-methylcholanthrene; BPDEI, (±)-7β, 8α-dihydroxy-9α, 10α-epoxy-7,8,9,10-tetrahydrobenzo(a)pyrene; BPDEII, (±)-7β,8α-dihydroxy-9β, 10β-epoxy-7,8,9,10-tetrahydrobenzo(a)pyrene; BPDE, BPDEI and BPDEII; TCDD, 2,3,7,8,-tetrachlorodibenzo-*p*-dioxin; PAH, polycyclic aromatic hydrocarbons; AHH, aryl hydrocarbon hydroxylase; βNF, β-naphthoflavone; BHA, butylated hydroxyanisole; DMN, dimethylnitrosamine; BHT, butylated hydroxytoluene.

carcinogens can be inhibited by administration of certain chemicals prior to, or simultaneously with, the carcinogen. Antioxidants such as BHA, BHT, and ethoxyquin can inhibit the induction of tumors in rodents by a variety of carcinogens including several PAH (1, 2). BP-induced neoplasia of the forestomach and lung in mice is inhibited by BHA in the diet as well as by a single oral dose of BHA (2-4). The initiation of papilloma formation in the skin of mice is inhibited by prior administration of BHA (5). As another example, inducers of microsomal AHH protect against the carcinogenic effects of compounds such as BP (1, 6); βNF has been shown to inhibit pulmonary adenoma formation in A/HeJ mice and BP tumorigenesis in mouse skin (7); and TCDD has been shown to be an effective inhibitor of BP-induced papillomas in mouse skin (8, 9). There have been numerous suggestions as to the mechanism(s) by which these antioxidants and AHH inducers inhibit BP-induced neoplasia (1-17). The proposed mechanisms suggest that treatment with antioxidants and AHH inducers affects the types and amounts of the various oxidative and conjugating enzyme systems, such that the amount of reactive metabolite(s) of the carcinogen available for interaction with DNA is decreased. Thus, implicit in all of these suggested mechanisms of anticarcinogenic action of antioxidants and AHH inducers is a resulting decreased level of carcinogen metabolites-DNA adduct formation.

In this report, we will discuss the results from our investigations of BP metabolite-DNA adduct formation under conditions known to inhibit BP-induced neoplasia by BHA and AHH inducers. In addition, we will discuss the possibility that the amount of carcinogen metabolite-DNA adduct(s) formed in the target tissue can be used as a predictive tool in carcinogenesis.

EFFECT OF THE ANTIOXIDANT BHA ON *IN VIVO* FORMATION OF BP METABOLITE-DNA ADDUCTS: CORRELATION WITH INHIBITION OF BP-INDUCED NEOPLASIA BY BHA

We have investigated BP metabolite-DNA adduct formation in lung and forestomach of female A/HeJ mice under conditions known to result in inhibition of BP-induced neoplasia by BHA. In one study, the experimental protocol followed was that used by Wattenberg (4), which resulted in 53 percent inhibition of BP-induced pulmonary adenoma formation in female A/HeJ mice by BHA feeding, 0.5 percent of diet for 21 days. BP was administered orally (6 mg/mouse) on the fourth and eighteenth days of the diet. This BHA treatment regimen resulted in a 53 percent reduction of BP-induced pulmonary adenomas. In our study, ^{3}H-BP (6 mg/mouse) was administered to one group (A) of animals, both BHA-treated and control, on the fourth day of the diet (11). To another group (B) of mice, BHA-treated and control, unlabeled BP (6 mg/mouse) was given on the fourth day of the diet and ³H-BP (6 mg/mouse) was administered on the eighteenth day of the diet. Animals were returned to control diets after administration of ³H-BP and sacrificed 48 h later. DNA isolated from lung and liver was enzymatically digested and the deoxyribonucleosides were chromatographed on HPLC (11). The major adduct in lung, as well as liver, was the BPDEI-deoxyguanosine adduct (peak II, Fig. 1). The BPDEII-deoxyguanosine adduct (peak III, Fig. 1) was 10–15 percent of the BPDEI adduct in both lung and liver, and the unidentified peak I (Fig. 1) was 10–20 percent of BPDEI adduct (11, 12). A discussion of the identification of these adducts is given in Wilson et al. (12) and Anderson et al. (11).

As seen in Fig. 1, BHA treatment significantly inhibited the formation of the BP-DNA adducts in the lungs of group B animals. Table 1 gives the percentage decrease in BPDE-DNA adduct formation in the lung of BHA-treated mice for group A and group B animals. The decrease in the amount of the BPDE-DNA adduct in the lung (53–62 percent) appears to correlate with the inhibition of pulmonary adenoma formation (53 percent) (4, 11). BHA treatment also inhibited the formation of the BPDE-DNA adducts in the liver

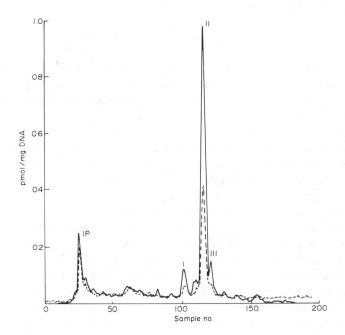

Figure 1 HPLC of BP metabolites-deoxyribonucleoside adducts in lung of untreated (—) and BHA-treated (— — —) mice. Untreated or BHA-treated mice (group B) were killed 48 h after an oral dose of ³H-BP (6 mg/mouse). DNA isolated from lung was enzymatically digested and the deoxyribonucleosides were chromatographed on HPLC. The observed peaks are discussed in the text. Abscissas, fraction number, and each fraction represents 0.5 min; ordinate, specific activity (pmole/mg DNA).

Table 1 Effect of Dietary BHA on *In Vivo* Formation of BPDE–DNA
Adducts in Lung and Liver of A/HeJ Mice

Treatment	Tissue	% Decrease in specific activity (pmoles/mg DNA) of BPDE–DNA adducts in BHA-treated mice[†]
4-d BHA[*]	Lung	53
(group A)	Liver	74
18-d BHA[*]	Lung	55
(group B, exp. 1)	Liver	75
18-d BHA[*]	Lung	62
(group B, exp. 2)	Liver	74

Untreated or BHA-treated female A/HeJ mice were killed 48 h after an oral dose of ^{3}H-BP (6 mg/mouse). DNA isolated from tissue was enzymatically digested and the deoxyribonucleosides were chromatographed on HPLC. The specific activity (pmoles/mg DNA) of the BPDE–DNA adducts was calculated from an HPLC chromatogram.

[*]Dietary BHA treatment regimens for 4-day BHA (group A) and 18-day BHA (group B) animals are detailed in text and Anderson, M. W., et al. (11).

[†]Data from Anderson, M. W., et al. (11).

(Table 1). The inhibition in the liver was approximately 75 percent in both group A and group B animals.

The effect of BHA on the *in vivo* formation of BP metabolite-DNA adducts in the forestomach of female A/HeJ mice was examined. In this study, mice were fed BHA, 0.5 percent of diet, for 14 days. ^{3}H-BP (6 mg/mouse) was administered and the animals were sacrificed 48 h later. As in lung and liver, the BPDEI-deoxyguanosine adduct was the predominant adduct formed in the forestomach. BHA treatment inhibited the formation of BPDE-DNA adducts in the forestomach by 50–55 percent. Wattenberg (2) has shown that BHA treatment inhibits BP-induced forestomach tumors by approximately 90 percent. Although our protocol for administration of BP was not identical to that used in the tumorigenicity studies, we can still see a definite trend between BHA inhibition of BPDE-DNA adduct formation in the forestomach of A/HeJ mice and reduction in tumor formation.

We have also studied the effect of dietary BHA on the *in vivo* formation of BP metabolite-DNA adducts in the lung, forestomach, and liver of ICR/Ha mice. BHA inhibits BP-induced forestomach neoplasia in this mouse strain, whereas dietary BHA was reported to have no effect on BP-induced pulmonary neoplasia in this same strain of mice (2, 10, 17). As in the A/HeJ strain of mice, the major adduct formed in lung, liver, and forestomach was the BPDEI-deoxyguanosine adduct (Y. M. Ioannou et al., unpublished data). Table 2 shows that BHA significantly inhibited the formation of BPDE-DNA adducts in the forestomach and liver, whereas there was only a marginal effect in the lung. In the forestomach, BPDE-DNA adduct formation was inhibited by 59 percent, while in tumorigenicity studies, dietary BHA reduced tumors in the forestomach by 50–90 percent (2, 10, 17). Thus, although our protocol for BP administration was not identical to those used in the tumorigenicity studies, we can see a correlation between BHA inhibition of BPDE-DNA adduct formation in the forestomach of ICR/Ha mice and reduction in tumor formation. These results on BHA effect on adduct formation in the lung of ICR/Ha mice (Table 2) are also in agreement with the tumor data obtained by Wattenberg et al. (10), which showed that dietary BHA had no effect on BP-induced pulmonary adenoma formation in ICR/Ha mice. There is a definite difference between the ICR/Ha and A/HeJ strains of mice as far as the pulmonary action of BHA is concerned. BPDE-DNA adduct formation was inhibited in the liver of both strains of mice to the same extent, being 75 and 60 percent in the A/HeJ and ICR/Ha mice, respectively (Tables 1 and 2).

In summary, BHA appears to inhibit BP-induced neoplasia in the lung and forestomach of mice by inhibiting the amount of the BPDE-DNA adducts formed in the target tissue. The mechanism(s) by which BHA treatment inhibits the formation of BPDE-DNA adducts is not fully understood (11). It is possible that induction of glutathione transferase and distinct forms of cytochrome P-450 by BHA as well as a direct action of BHA or its metabolites could all play a role in the inhibition of the formation of BPDE-DNA adducts by BHA.

EFFECT OF ARYL HYDROCARBON HYDROXYLASE INDUCERS ON *IN VIVO* FORMATION OF BP METABOLITE-DNA ADDUCTS: CORRELATION WITH INHIBITION OF BP-INDUCED NEOPLASIA BY AHH INDUCERS

We have investigated the effect of AHH inducers on BP metabolite-DNA adduct formation in lung, liver, and forestomach of mice. In one study,

Table 2   Effect of Dietary BHA on *In Vivo* Formation
of BPDE–DNA Adducts in ICR/Ha Mice

Tissue	% Decrease in specific activity (pmoles/mg DNA) of BPDE–DNA adducts in BHA-treated mice
Forestmach	59[*]
Lung	14
Liver	65

Untreated or BHA-treated (0.5% diet for 16 days) female IRC/Ha mice were killed 48 h after an oral dose of ^{3}H-BP (6 mg/mouse). DNA isolated from tissue was enzymatically digested and the deoxyribonucleosides were chromatographed on HPLC. The specific activity (pmoles/mg DNA) of the BPDE–DNA adducts was calculated from an HPLC chromatogram.
[*]Average of two experiments (30 mice per experiment).

adducts were determined under conditions known to result in inhibition of BP-induced pulmonary neoplasia by βNF (7). Female A/HeJ mice were fed either βNF diet (0.3 percent of diet) or control diet for 16 days and then BP (6 mg/mouse) was administered. Animals were returned to control diet for 2 weeks and then placed on either βNF diet or control diet for another 16 days. This βNF treatment regimen resulted in a 94 percent reduction of BP-induced pulmonary adenomas (7). In our study, ^{3}H-BP (6 mg/mouse) was administered to one group (A) of animals, both control and βNF-treated, on the sixteenth day of the first βNF feeding (12). To another group (B) of mice, control and βNF-treated, unlabeled BP (6 mg/mouse) was given on the sixteenth day of the first βNF feeding, and ^{3}H-BP (6 mg/mouse) was administered on the sixteenth day of the second βNF feeding. Animals in both groups, A and B, were returned to control diets after administration of ^{3}H-BP and sacrificed 48 h later.

As seen in Fig. 2, βNF treatment almost completely inhibited the formation of the BPDE-DNA adducts in the lungs of group B animals. Table 3 gives the percentage decrease in BPDE-DNA adducts formation in the lung and

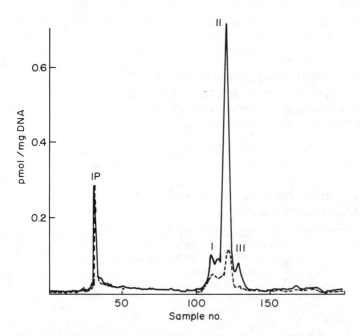

Figure 2 HPLC of BP metabolites-deoxyribonucleoside adducts in lung of untreated (—) and βNF-treated (— — —) mice. Untreated or βNF-treated mice (group B) were killed 48 h after an oral dose of ^{3}H-BP (6 mg/mouse). DNA isolated from lung was enzymatically digested and the deoxyribonucleosides were chromatographed on HPLC. The observed peaks are discussed in the text. Abscissas, fraction number, and each fraction represents 0.5 min; ordinate, specific activity (pmole/mg DNA).

Table 3 Effect of Dietary βNF on *In Vivo* Formation of BPDE-DNA Adducts in Lung and Liver of A/HeJ Mice

Treatment	Tissue	% Decrease in specific Activity (pmoles/mg DNA) of BPDE-DNA adducts in βNF-treated mice[†]
Group A[*]	Lung	86
	Liver	100[‡]
Group B[*]	Lung	93
	Liver	100[‡]

Untreated or βNF-treated female A/HeJ mice were killed 48 h after an oral dose of ^{3}H-BP (6 mg/mouse). DNA isolated from tissue was enzymatically digested and the deoxyribonucleosides were chromatographed on HPLC. The specific activity (pmoles/mg DNA) of the BPDE-DNA adducts was calculated from an HPLC chromatogram.

[*]Dietary βNF treatment regimens for group A and B animals are detailed in text and Wilson, A.G.E., et al. (12).

[†]Data from Wilson, A.G.E., et al. (12).

[‡]100 means that the adducts were not detected in treated animals.

liver of βNF-treated mice for groups A and B animals. The decrease in the amount of BPDE-DNA adducts in the lung (86–93 percent), appears to correlate with the inhibition of pulmonary adenoma formation (94 percent) (7, 12). No BPDE-DNA adducts were detected in the liver of βNF-treated mice.

The AHH inducer TCDD has been shown to be an effective inhibitor of BP-induced papillomas in mouse skin (8, 9). Cohen et al. (8) recently reported that treatment with TCDD inhibits the formation of the BPDE-DNA adduct in mouse skin, an inhibition that appears to correlate with TCDD's inhibitory effect on BP-induced papilloma formation. Our results together with those of Cohen et al. (8) suggest that AHH inducers inhibit BP-induced neoplasia by reducing the amount of the BPDE-DNA adducts formed in the target tissue.

We also examined the effects of two other AHH inducers, TCDD and Aroclor 1254, on BP-DNA adduct formation in A/HeJ mice (12). These inducers, like βNF, markedly decreased the formation of the BPDE adducts (Table 4). We have also shown that βNF treatment of ICR/Ha mice results in a 80–90 percent reduction in the amount of BPDE-DNA adduct in lung, liver, and forestomach. Thus, AHH inducers inhibit BPDE-DNA adduct formation in every tissue of every mouse strain examined. The effects of AHH inducers on the binding of BP to DNA *in vivo* markedly contrast with their effect *in vitro* [see Wilson et al. (12) for discussion]. The reason for the difference between the *in vivo* results and those predicted from *in vitro* studies is unclear. In particular, the relationship between induction of AHH and decreased *in vivo* adduct formation is not understood.

Table 4 Effect of TCDD and Aroclor 1254 Pretreatment on *In Vivo* Formation of BPDE-DNA Adducts in Lung and Liver of A/HeJ MICE

Treatment	Tissue	% Decrease in specific activity (pmoles/mg DNA) of BPDE-DNA adducts in treated-mice[†]
TCDD[*]	Lung	96
	Liver	100[‡]
Aroclor 1254[*]	Lung	92
	Liver	100[‡]

Untreated or TCDD-treated or Aroclor 1254-treated female A/HeJ mice were killed 48 h after an oral dose of ^{3}H-BP (6 mg/mouse). DNA isolated from tissue was enzymatically digested and the deoxyribonucleosides were chromatographed on HPLC. The specific activity (pmole/mg DNA) of the BPDE-DNA adducts was calculated from an HPLC chromatogram.

[*]Treatment regimens for TCDD and Aroclor 1254 are detailed in Wilson, A.G.E., et al. (12).

[†]Data from Wilson, A.G.E., et al. (12).

[‡]100 means that the adducts were not detected in treated animals.

AMOUNT OF CRITICAL CARCINOGEN–DNA ADDUCT AS A PREDICTIVE TOOL IN CARCINOGENESIS

It has been suggested that the amount of carcinogen-DNA binding is a measure of the effective dose of a carcinogen (18). This proposal is consistent with the somatic mutation theory of tumor initiation by chemical carcinogens. Although the extent of carcinogen-DNA binding has been successfully used to rank order the carcinogenic potency of a series of carcinogens such as PAH and alkylating agents (19–21), there have been few, if any, serious attempts to use the amount of carcinogen-DNA adducts formed in the target tissue as a predictive tool in the low-dose extrapolation problem in carcinogenesis. Anderson et al. (22) and Gehring and Blau (23) suggested a general scheme for the incorporation of pharmacokinetics in low-dose risk estimation for chemical carcinogenesis.

Recent studies have suggested that levels of specific carcinogen-DNA adducts should be used as a measure of effective dose instead of total DNA binding. For example, for the nitrosamines and nitrosamides, correlation between carcinogenicity and nucleic acid alkylation has only been observed with O^6 alkylation of guanine and not with N^7 alkylation of guanine, even though the latter alkylation is approximately ten times greater than the former (24–26). Current evidence suggests that the bay-region diol epoxides such as BPDE are the ultimate carcinogenic forms for most PAH (27). The BPDE adducts are the predominant, and in many cases the only, ones observed *in vivo* in the target tissues of animals known to be susceptible to

BP-induced neoplasia (8, 9, 11, 12, 28–30). The lack of formation of substantial amounts of BPDE adducts in Sprague-Dawley rat lung may explain the apparent lack of induction of pulmonary tumors in this species by BP (31).

Most *in vivo* studies of carcinogen-DNA adduct formation have used total DNA content in the organ to calculate the specific acitivity (pmole/mg DNA) of the adducts. However, it is likely that the amounts of adducts formed in different cell types vary considerably. This possibility has the greatest implication for organs, such as the lung, that contain a multitude of cell types and where the cytochrome P-450 dependent monooxygenase enzymes are localized in a few cell types (32–34). Obviously, the specific activities of carcinogen-DNA adducts in individual cell populations would be a better measure of the effective dose of a carcinogen than the values based on the total DNA content of the organ.

In spite of these limitations in the interpretation of *in vivo* specific activities of carcinogen-DNA adducts, results from several investigations suggest that the use of carcinogen-DNA adduct levels in low-dose risk estimation for chemical carcinogenesis will prove to be fruitful. Our studies (11, 12), as well as those of Cohen et al. (8), with inhibitors of carcinogenesis show that tumor response changes quantitatively with BPDE-DNA adduct levels. In a similar type of study, Swann et al. (35) show that changes in DMN-induced kidney tumor incidence produced by changes in the diet and by treatment with BP correspond to the changes these treatments produce in the alkylation of the target tissue DNA by DMN. In addition, several studies have shown that although the time for appearance of the first tumor was not necessarily dose dependent, the average time between the administration of a single dose of the carcinogen and the appearance of each tumor was definitely dose dependent. This measure in the average time for the development of tumors as the dose is lowered has led Swann et al. (35) to suggest that the time needed to achieve full malignancy is a function of the amount of the initial preneoplastic lesion, i.e., the formation of carcinogen-DNA adducts.

In addition to the extent of carcinogen-induced DNA damage, the capacity of cells to repair such damage and the degree of cell replication represent critical events in the initiation of carcinogenesis. Like the measurements of specific activities of carcinogen-DNA adducts, most *in vivo* studies of repair of carcinogen-induced DNA damage have been based on the total cell population and thus represent average cellular values. Lewis and Swenberg (36) did study the differential repair of O^6-methylguanine in the DNA of rat hepatocytes and nonparenchymal cells (NPCs) after administration of 1,2-dimethylhydrazine. The NPCs are the target cells in 1,2-dimethylhydrazine-induced liver neoplasia. Although the initial alkylation was similar in both cell types, the NPCs repair O^6-methylguanine slower than the hepatocytes. This leads to a much greater accumulation of the promutagenic lesion in the target cells (NPCs). Also, the rate of cell division may be higher in the target cells. Thus in this model system, there is a definite correlation between carcinogen-DNA adduct levels, as well as cell division rates, with target cell susceptibility.

Carcinogen-DNA adducts, their rates of removal, or both may not explain the difference in organ susceptibility and species susceptibility to chemical-induced neoplasia. For example, the amount of BPDE-DNA adducts formed and their rates of disappearance were not that dissimilar in the lungs and liver of A/HeJ mice (11, 12). The lungs of these mice are susceptible to BP-induced neoplasia whereas the liver is resistant. The amounts of BPDE-DNA adducts formed and their removal rates were similar in the lungs of A/HeJ and C57BL/6J mice (37). These data also do not explain the strain difference in susceptibility to BP-induced pulmonary neoplasia (38). Phillips et al. (30) examined the covalent binding of PAH to DNA in the skin of mice of different strains. Neither the level of DNA binding nor the removal rates of the DNA adducts showed a correlation with the reported susceptibilities of the strains to PAH carcinogenesis. In contrast, Eastman and Bresnick (28) suggest that the persistent binding of 3-MC to mouse lung DNA correlates with strain susceptibility to pulmonary neoplasia. Whether or not adduct formation, its removal rate, or both can explain strain (or species) and organ difference in susceptibility to BP-induced neoplasia awaits more detailed examination of *in vivo* adduct formation and removal in individual cell types, such as the study by Lewis and Swenberg (36).

Even if adduct levels or their removal rates do not explain organ and species difference to chemical-induced neoplasia, this does not distract from the ability of carcinogen-DNA adduct levels to predict low-dose response to carcinogens in known target tissues. This use of the amount of critical carcinogen-DNA adducts as a predictive tool in carcinogenesis is of practical significance since levels of adducts can usually be measured at dosages much lower than those used in bioassay studies.

REFERENCES

1 Wattenberg, L. W. Inhibitors of carcinogenesis. In A. C. Griffin and C. R. Shaw (eds.), *Carcinogens: Identification and Mechanisms of Action*, pp. 229–316. New York: Raven Press (1979).

2 Wattenberg, L. W. Inhibition of carcinogenic and toxic effects of polycyclic hydrocarbons by phenolic antioxidants and ethoxyquin. *J. Natl. Cancer Inst.* 48:1425–1430 (1972).

3 Speier, J. L., L. K. Lam, and L. W. Wattenberg. Effects of administration to mice of butylated hydroxyanisole by oral intubation on benzo(a)-pyrene-induced pulmonary adenoma formation and metabolism of benzo-(a)pyrene. *J. Natl. Cancer Inst.* 60:605–609 (1978).

4 Wattenberg, L. W. Inhibition of chemical-carcinogen-induced pulmonary neoplasia by butylated hydroxyanisole. *J. Natl. Cancer Inst.* 50:1541–1544 (1973).

5   Slaga, T. J., and W. M. Bracken. The effects of antioxidants on skin tumor initiation and aryl hydrocarbon hydroxylase. *Cancer Res.* 37:1631–1635 (1977).

6   Wattenberg, L. W. Inhibition of chemical carcinogenesis. *J. Natl. Cancer Inst.* 60:11–18 (1978).

7   Wattenberg, L. W., and J. L. Leong. Inhibition of the carcinogenic action of benzo(a)pyrene by flavones. *Cancer Res.* 30:1922–1925 (1970).

8   Cohen, G. M., W. M. Bracken, R. P. Iyer, D. L. Berry, J. K. Selkirk, and T. J. Slaga. Anticarcinogenic effects of 2,3,7,8-tetrachlorodibenzo-p-dioxin on benzo(a)pyrene and 7,12-dimethylbenz(a)anthracene tumor initiation and its relationship to DNA binding. *Cancer Res.* 39:4027–4033 (1979).

9   DiGiovanni, J., D. L. Berry, G. L. Gleason, G. S. Kishore, and T. J. Slaga. Time-dependent inhibition by 2,3,7.8-tetrachlorodibenzo-p-dioxin of skin tumorigenesis with polycyclic hydrocarbons. *Cancer Res.* 40:1580–1587 (1980).

10 Wattenberg, L. W., D. M. Jerina, L. K. T. Lam, and H. Yagi. Neoplastic effects of oral administration of (±)-trans-7,8-dihydroxy-7,8-dihydrobenzo(a)pyrene and their inhibition by butylated hydroxyanisole. *J. Natl. Cancer Inst.* 62:1103–1106 (1979).

11 Anderson, M. W., M. Boroujerdi, and A. G. E. Wilson. Inhibition *in vivo* of the formation of adducts between metabolites of benzo(a)pyrene and DNA by butylated hydroxyanisole. *Cancer Res.* 41:4309–4315 (1981).

12 Wilson, A. G. E., H. C. Kung, M. Boroujerdi, and M. W. Anderson. Inhibition *in vivo* of the formation of adducts between metabolites of benzo(a)pyrene and DNA by aryl hydrocarbon hydroxylase inducers: *Cancer Res.* 41:3453–3460 (1981).

13 Kahl, R., and U. Wulf. Induction of rat hepatic epoxide hydrotase by dietary antioxidants. *Toxicol. Appl. Pharmacol.* 47:217–227 (1979).

14 Lam, L. K., and L. W. Wattenberg. Effects of butylated hydroxyanisole on the metabolism of benzo(a)pyrene by mouse liver microsomes. *J. Natl. Cancer Inst.* 58:413–417 (1977).

15 Speier, J. L., and L. W. Wattenberg. Alterations in microsomal metabolism of benzo(a)pyrene in mice fed butylated hydroxyanisole. *J. Natl. Cancer Inst.* 55:469–472 (1975).

16 Wiebel, F. J., and H. L. Waters. Effect of butylated hydroxytoluene and hydroxyanisole on benzo(a)pyrene metabolism and binding. In J. R. Fouts and I. Gut (eds.), *Industrial and Environmental Xenobiotics*, pp. 258–260. Amsterdam: Excerpta Medica (1978).

17 Lam, L. K., R. P. Pai, and L. W. Wattenberg. Synthesis and chemical carcinogen inhibitory activity of 2-tert-butyl-4-hydroxyanisole. *J. Med. Chem.* 22:569–571 (1979).

18 Lawley, P. D. Approaches to chemical dosimetry in mutagenesis and carcinogenesis: The relevance of reactions of chemical mutagens and carcinogens with DNA. In P. L. Grover (ed.), *Chemical Carcinogens and DNA*, vol. 1, pp. 1–36. Boca Raton, Fla: CRC (1979).

19 Brookes, P., and Lawley, P. D. Evidence for the binding of polynuclear aromatic hydrocarbons to the nucleic acids of mouse skin: Relation

between carcinogenic power of hydrocarbons and their binding to deoxyribonucleic acid. *Nature* 202:781-784 (1964).

20 Huberman, E., and L. Sachs. DNA binding and its relationship to carcinogenesis by different polycyclic hydrocarbons. *Int. J. Cancer* 19:122-127 (1977).

21 Colburn, N. H., and R. K. Boutwell. The binding of β-propiolactone and some related alkylating agents to DNA, RNA, and protein of mouse skin: Relation between tumor-initiating power of alkylating agents and their binding to DNA. *Cancer Res.* 28:653-660 (1968).

22 Anderson, M. W., D. G. Hoel, and N. L. Kaplan. A general scheme for the incorporation of pharmacokinetics in low-dose risk estimation for chemical carcinogenesis: Example—vinyl chloride. *Toxicol. Appl. Pharmacol.* 55:154-161 (1980).

23 Gehring, P. J., and G. E. Blau. Mechanisms of carcinogenesis: Dose response. *J. Environ. Pathol. Toxicol.* 1:163-179 (1977).

24 Loveless, A. Possible relevance of 0-6 alkylation of deoxyguanosine to the mutagenicity and carcinogenicity of nitrosamines and nitrosamides. *Nature* 223:206-207 (1969).

25 Pegg, A. E. Formation and metabolism of alkylated nucleosides: Possible role in carcinogenesis by nitroso-compounds and alkylating agents. *Adv. Cancer Res.* 25:195-269 (1977).

26 Margison, G. P., and P. J. O'Connor. Nucleic acid modification by N-nitroso compounds. In P. L. Grover (ed.), *Chemical Carcinogens and DNA*, vol. 1, pp. 111-159. Boca Raton, Fla.: CRC (1979).

27 Lehr, R. E., H. Yagi, D. R. Thakker, W. Levin, A. W. Wood, A. H. Conney, and D. M. Jerina. The bay region theory of polycyclic aromatic hydrocarbon-induced carcinogenicity. In P. W. Jones and R. I. Freudenthal (eds.), *Polynuclear Aromatic Hydrocarbons: Analysis, Chemistry, and Biology*, vol. 3, pp. 231-241. New York: Raven Press (1978).

28 Eastman, A., and E. Bresnick. Persistent binding of 3-methylcholanthrene to mouse lung DNA and its correlation with susceptibility to pulmonary neoplasia. *Cancer Res.* 39:2400-2405 (1979).

29 Eastman, A., J. Sweetenham, and E. Bresnick. Comparison of *in vivo* and *in vitro* binding of polycyclic hydrocarbons to DNA. *Chem.-Biol. Interact.* 23:345-353 (1978).

30 Phillips, D. H., P. L. Grover, and P. Sims. The covalent binding of polycyclic hydrocarbons to DNA in the skin of mice of different strains. *Int. J. Cancer* 22:487-494 (1978).

31 Boroujerdi, M., H. C. Kung, A. G. E. Wilson, and M. W. Anderson. Metabolism and DNA binding of benzo(a)pyrene *in vivo* in the rat. *Cancer Res.* 41:951-957 (1981).

32 Dees, J. H., L. D. Coe, Y. Yasukochi, and B. S. Masters. Immunofluorescence of NADPH-cytochrome c (P-450) reductase in rat and minipig tissues injected with phenobarbital. *Science* 208:1473-1475 (1980).

33 Serabit-Singh, C. J., T. R. Devereux, J. R. Fouts, and R. M. Philpot. Rabbit pulmonary monooxygenase enzymes in tissue section and in

isolated cell fraction. In J. A. Sustafsson, J. Carlstedt-Duke, A. Mode, and J. Rafter (eds.) *Biochemistry, Biophysics, and Regulation of Cytochrome P-450*, pp. 451–454. Amsterdam: Elsevier/North Holland (1980).

34 Serabjit-Singh, C. J., C. R. Wolf, R. M. Philpot, and C. G. Plopper. Cytochrome P-450; localization in rabbit lung. *Science* 207:1469–1470 (1980).

35 Swann, P. F., D. G. Kaufman, P. N. Magee, and R. Mace. Induction of kidney tumours by a single dose of dimethylnitrosamine: Dose response and influence of diet and benzo(a)pyrene pretreatment. *Br. J. Cancer* 41:285 (1980).

36 Lewis, J. G., and J. A. Swenberg. Differential repair of 0^6-methylguanine in DNA of rat hepatocytes and nonparenchymal cells. *Nature* 288:185–187 (1980).

37 Anderson, M. W., and A. G. E. Wilson. Formation and disappearance *in vivo* of benzo(a)pyrene (BP)-DNA adducts in lung and liver of A/HeJ and C57BL/6J mice. AACR, Abstract No. 0351, Washington, D.C. (1981).

38 Shimkin, M. B., and G. D. Stoner. Lung tumors in mice: Application to carcinogenesis bioassay. *Adv. Cancer Res.* 21:2–58 (1975).

Chapter 3

Chemical and Toxicological Data Bases for Assessment of Structure-Activity Relationships

Ann H. Akland
and Michael D. Waters

INTRODUCTION

This report is an attempt to catalog the major sources that can provide information for assessing structure-activity relationships. No attempt is made to present details of the various data bases. Rather, contacts are provided to enable the interested reader to obtain further information (see Appendix).

Several types of existing computerized and noncomputerized data bases can be useful:

1 Biological Research Results Data Bases: These data bases contain qualitative and quantitative results of laboratory experiments. The information may or may not have been evaluated by experts in the field.

2 Information Data Bases: These data bases contain information about individual chemical compounds, such as chemical or physical properties, molecular formula, structure, Chemical Abstracts Service (CAS) Registry Number, synonyms, and toxicity values.

3 Literature/Citation Data Bases: These data bases contain references to the published literature or ongoing research projects. Abstracts are sometimes included.

BIOLOGICAL RESEARCH RESULTS DATA BASES

Probably of greatest interest to structure-activity researchers are the data bases that contain actual results of biological experimentation. This category includes both manual and automated data bases. The results may be qualitative or quantitative in nature and may or may not have been evaluated by experts in the field.

Unfortunately, there are few computerized sources of such data. Although several scientists and government agencies are at various stages in establishing computerized bases, the information is, in most cases, available only to the researchers themselves and their institutions (1). However, one data base that should prove extremely valuable for this application is GENE-TOX.

GENE-TOX (2) is a two-phase evaluation of selected short-term bioassays for detecting mutagenicity and presumptive carcinogenicity. Sponsored and directed by the Office of Testing and Evaluation within EPA's Office of Pesticides and Toxic Substances, GENE-TOX aids EPA in establishing standard genetic testing and evaluation procedures for the regulation of toxic substances. GENE-TOX also helps to determine the direction of research and development in the field of genetic toxicology.

In the first phase of GENE-TOX evaluation, groups of 5-10 scientists use the existing literature to prepare reports on the applicability and performance of each selected bioassay. The data are edited and placed in a computer file. To date, information on approximately 2800 different chemicals has been entered.

In the second phase, another panel of scientists critically evaluates the reports on the bioassays, comparing them on a chemical-by-chemical and class-by-class basis, to determine which groups of tests are most useful for particular purposes.

Pertinent Data Elements:
Identification
    Chemical name of agent tested
    CAS Registry Number (chemical)
    Authors of published article
    CAS Registry Number (article)
    Citation of published article
    Comments by reviewer or Environmental Mutagen Information Center (EMIC) representative
    EMIC Accession Number

Title of published article
Endpoint assayed
Evaluation
    Author's evaluation
    Reviewer's evaluation
    Reviewer's name
    Lowest effective dose
    Percent survival
    Expression time
    Background (spontaneous) mutation frequency $\times 10^6$ survivors
    Mutant frequency
Materials and methods
    Agent concentration
    Controls (positive and negative)
    Purity of agent
    Source of agent
    Solvent
    Test organism, species/strain
    Cell type
    Metabolic activation used in treatment protocol
    Metabolic activation: inducer used
    Metabolic activation: organ used to obtain the microsomal fraction
    Metabolic activation: sex of animal donating organ
    Metabolic activation: species of animal donating organ
    Metabolic activation: strain of animal donating organ
    Metabolic activation comments
    Exposure time
    Number treated
    Number of cells plated per vessel or plate
    Age of animals tested
    Buffer
    Interval between doses
    Interval between treatment and mating
    Plant material used for test
    Number assayed
    pH of agent solution administered
    Route of administration of agent
    Germ cell stage sampled
    Sex of animal
    Species of plants tested

In addition to GENE-TOX two other sources of biological information are accessible via computer.

Registry of Toxic Effects of Chemical Substances (RTECS) is the result of a continuing effort by the National Institute of Occupational Safety and Health (NIOSH) to collect, collate, and disseminate toxic effects information for "all known toxic substances." For purposes of inclusion in this list, "toxic substances" are interpreted to include all mined, manufactured, processed, synthesized, and naturally occurring inorganic and organic compounds having the potential to cause or induce any of a number of abnormal biological effects. Specifically excluded from the list are tradename products representing commercially available compounded or formulated proprietary mixtures.

Pertinent Data Elements:
  Prime name
  CAS Registry Number
  Molecular formula
  Wisswesser Line Notation
  Synonyms
  Measured toxicity data
  Cited references
  Aquatic toxicity ratings
  Reviews
  Applicable U.S. occupational standards
  Applicable NIOSH criteria documents

Since the inception of this effort in 1970, the primary means of information dissemination has been the annual publication of *Registry of Toxic Effects of Chemical Substances* (3), which is available through the U.S. Government Printing Office. Each edition of this publication supersedes the previous edition (i.e., each edition contains all of the information in the previous volume as well as all new material). With the 1977 edition, the RTECS data base also became available on microfiche and computer magnetic tape. The microfiche is available from the U.S. Government Printing Office; arrangements are being completed to make the magnetic tape available through the National Technical Information Service (NTIS).

The RTECS data base is also fully searchable and displayable in the RTECS component of the Chemical Information System (CIS) and National Library of Medicine (NLM) computer systems. Access is obtained through general subscription to CIS or NLM. An example of an interactive search of the RTECS data base is included as Fig. 1.

Quantitatively Analyzed Results from Short-Term Tests (McCann) is a computerized data base that is in the first year of development at Lawrence Berkeley Laboratory. This data base will cover results from the major short-term tests for carcinogenesis and mutagenesis; it is now completely

```
RTECS SEARCH SYSTEM (VERSION 3.1/3.2 APRIL, 1980) ($36/HR)

LATEST NEWS FOR RTECS . . .
  7 SEPT 80; TOXIC EFFECT OF "MUT" NO LONGER ACCEPTED AS SEARCH CRITERIA
OPTION? TSHOW 82-68-8

CAS RN 82-68-8          NIOSH NUMBER DA6650000

BENZENE, PENTACHLORONITRO-
C6-CL5-N-O2

TOXICITY DATA:                               CODEN:
ORL-RAT LD50:1650 MG/KG                      WRPCA2 9,119,70
ORL-MUS TDLO:2500 MG/KG/(7-11D PREG) TFX:TER TXAPA9 35,239,76
ORL-MUS TDLO:135 GM/KG/77W-C TFX:CAR         JNCIAM 42,1101,69
SKN-MUS TDLO:576 MG/KG/12W-I TFX:NEO         CNREA8 26,12,66
UNK-MAM LD50:1650 MG/KG                      30ZDA9 -,82,71

DATA REFERENCES:
CARCINOGENIC DETERMINATION:ANIMAL POSITIVE   IARC** 5,211,74
TOXICOLOGY REVIEW                            RREVAH 56,107,75
TOXICOLOGY REVIEW                            85CVA2 5,250,70
TOXICOLOGY REVIEW                            27ZTAP 3,139,69
NCI CARCINOGENESIS BIOASSAY COMPLETED;RESULTS NCITR*
    NEGATIVE                                 NCI-CG-TR-61,78
SELECTED BY NCI FOR CARCINOGENESIS BIOASSAY AS OF FEBRUARY 1980
REPORTED IN EPA TSCA INVENTORY, JULY 1979
```

Figure 1 Example of a CIS RTECS information display. Compound: parathion.

operational for data from the *Salmonella* (Ames) assay. Other test methods to be incorporated into the data base in 1981 include mammalian cell mutagenesis assays, *in vitro* transformation assays, and tests for sister chromatid exchange. Thus far, data for approximately 300 different chemicals have been entered.

The data base is limited to reports in the published literature that include sufficient quantitative information to satisfy minimum criteria for calculation of a potency. Included are results, both quantitative and qualitative, that are relevant to quantitative analysis; bibliographic information; and results of the developers' own statistical analysis of the data. These data elements are displayed in a summary printout that permits direct visual comparison of results.

Pertinent Data Elements:
   Results relevant to quantitative analysis
      Quantitative
      Qualitative
   Bibliographic information
   Results of statistical analysis
      Potency value
      Confidence limits of potency value
      Probability that the results are positive or negative

Published reference works are another valuable source of biological research results. Some of these reference works are described below; others are listed in Table 1.

Survey of Compounds which Have Been Tested for Carcinogenic Activity (formerly U.S. Public Health Service Publication 149) (4) is a National Institutes of Health (NIH) series developed by identifying relevant material in the open scientific literature. Data extracted from published information are presented in a stylized display matrix, with entries organized by tested material. A preferred name and alternate names are provided for each material (usually a particular chemical compound). In most cases, the CAS Registry Number and a structural diagram are also provided. Sequential acquisition numbers are assigned to the materials in the order in which they are entered in the volume. Some conditions and results of each experiment performed on that material are then cited. No attempt is made to evaluate the design and conduct of the experiments or the data presented by the various authors.

Pertinent Data Elements:
  Author/citation
  Chemical
    Nomenclature
    CAS Registry Number
    Molecular formula
    Wisswesser Line Notation
  Biological
    Species/strain used
    Vehicle for the test material
    Site or route of application of the test material
    Site of induced tumor

There are currently eight volumes in the series; each volume covers the literature for a particular time period, with the general style of the original edition being maintained throughout. The first three volumes were published by the U.S. Public Health Service; thereafter, responsibility for publication was assumed by the Carcinogenesis Area, Division of Cancer Cause and Prevention, National Cancer Institute (NCI). All volumes are available through the U.S. Government Printing Office and NTIS.

International Agency for Research on Cancer (IARC) Monographs on the Evaluation of the Carcinogenic Risk of Chemicals to Humans (5) seek to provide government authorities with expert, independent scientific opinion on environmental carcinogenesis. The objective of the IARC program is to elaborate and publish, in the form of monographs, critical reviews of

Table 1   Examples of Toxicological Reference Works

Topic	Reference work	Comments
Chemical carcinogens	Searle, C. E. (ed.). *Chemical Carcinogens*, ACS Monograph 173. Washington, D.C.: American Chemical Society (1976).	Contains 75 structural formulas
Pesticides	Wisswesser, W. J. *Pesticide Index*, 5th ed. College Park, MD: Entomological Society of America (1976).	Contains 1600 main and 1460 cross-indexed entries; indexes: numeric (5), Wisswesser Line Notation, molecular formula, CAS nomenclature
Industrial hazardous materials	Sax, N. I. *Dangerous Properties of Industrial Materials*, 5th ed. New York: Van Nostrand-Reinhold (1979).	Hazardous analysis information for nearly 15,000 common industrial laboratory materials
Environmental effects of organic chemicals	Verschveren, K. *Handbook of Environmental Data on Organic Chemicals*. New York: Van Nostrand-Reinhold (1977).	Considers the effects of less toxic chemicals in the environment; information categories: properties, air pollution factors, water pollution factors, biological effects
Industrial hygiene and toxicology	*Patty's Industrial Hygiene and Toxicology, Toxicology*, 3rd revised ed. Vol. I, General Principles; Vol. II, Toxicology; Vol. III, Theory and Rationale of Industrial Hygiene Practice. New York: Wiley (1978).	
Chemical carcinogen testing	Carcinogenesis Testing Program, Division of Cancer Cause and Prevention, National Cancer Institute. *NCI Reports on Bioassays of Chemicals for Possible Carcinogenicity*. Washington, D.C.: National Cancer Institute.	
Correlation analysis	Hansh and Leo. *Substituent Constants for Correlation Analysis in Chemistry and Biology*. New York: Wiley (1979).	Includes substituents partition coefficients, linear free energy relationship, and structure-activity relationships

carcinogenicity and related data in light of the present state of knowledge. The final aims are to evaluate possible human risk and to target areas for additional research. Publication is partially funded by NCI.

The IARC monographs summarize the evidence for the carcinogenicity of individual chemicals and other relevant information on the basis of data compiled, reviewed, and evaluated by a working group of experts. Priority is given mainly to chemicals belonging to particular groups and for which there is at least some suggestion of carcinogenicity from observations in animals or humans and evidence of human exposure. However, the inclusion of a particular compound in a volume does not necessarily mean that it is considered to be carcinogenic. Equally, the fact that a substance has not yet been considered does not imply the absence of carcinogenic hazard. No recommendations are given concerning preventive measures or legislation, since these matters involve risk-benefit evaluations that are best made by individual governments, international agencies, or both. As new data on chemicals for which monographs have already been prepared and new principles for evaluation become available, reevaluations are made at subsequent meetings, and revised monographs are published as necessary.

The IARC monographs are distributed to international and governmental agencies, made available to industries and scientists dealing with these chemicals, and offered to any interested reader through worldwide distribution as World Health Organization (WHO) publications. The monographs also form the basis of IARC advice on the carcinogenicity of these substances.

The Merck Index (6) is designed to serve a variety of scientists and to fulfill a multitude of functions. The nearly 10,000 indexed monographs contain approximately 8000 structural displays or line formulas and over 50,000 synonyms. These monographs address the most important chemicals, drugs, pesticides, and biologically active substances known. Compounds selected for inclusion in the *Index* are generally limited to single substances; with few exceptions, synthetic mixtures are deliberately omitted. The information contained in each monograph has been carefully extracted from the published literature.

Pertinent Data Elements:
  Monograph number and title
  CAS names (both 8th and 9th *Collective Index* names are provided where available)
  Alternate names (other chemical names, trivial names, experimental drug codes, and trademarks)
  Empirical formula, molecular weight, and percent composition
  Literature references
  Structure (two-dimensional image with modern stereochemical and spatial representations)
  Physical data (melting point, boiling point, color, solubility, stability, optical rotations, etc.; special effort made to include toxicity data in the form of LD50, LC50, etc., as well as the source of these data)
  Derivatives (data cited as for parent compound)
  Use, therapeutic categories

Monographs are organized simply by monograph number. Cross indexes are provided for both chemical names and molecular formula. An index relating the chemical names to CAS Registry Numbers is also provided.

INFORMATION DATA BASES

Data bases that aid in the identification and characterization of specific chemical substances represent a second major category.

CHEMLINE (CHEMical Dictionary on-LINE) is NLM's on-line, interactive chemical dictionary file created in collaboration with CAS. Over 550,000 chemical substance names representing over 248 unique substances can be searched and retrieved on-line.

Pertinent Data Elements:
  CAS Registry Number
  Molecular formula
  Preferred chemical index nomenclature
  Generic and trivial names derived from the CAS Registry Nomenclature File
  Locator designation (such as TOXLINE), which points to other files in the
  NLM system containing information on the substance

The user searches CHEMLINE by entering a chemical name, trivial name, company identification name, or molecular formula. If the exact name of a chemical substance is unknown, a search may be conducted using the Boolean operator "and" to connect those fragments of the name, ring analysis terms, and/or molecular formula, which are known. Figure 2 is an example of an on-line retrieval from CHEMLINE.

CHEMLINE is available through the NLM system. Other literature retrieval services offer their own versions of an on-line chemical dictionary file similar to CHEMLINE. The DIALOG system offers data bases called CHEMNAME, CHEMSEARCH, and CHEMSIS, while the System Development Corporation (SDC) ORBIT offers a data base called CHEMDEX.

Toxicology Data Bank (TDB) is an on-line, interactive file of biological, chemical, pharmacological, toxicological, and environmental information on selected chemical substances that are potentially hazardous to humans or the environment.

TDB consists of data selected from sources such as TOXLINE and from secondary sources that include standard reference books, handbooks, criteria documents, and monographs. The data extracted from secondary sources are reviewed on a quarterly basis by a panel of experts from the Toxicology Study Section, NIH. Information from TOXLINE is incorporated by Peer

```
RN  -  111-40-0
ON  -  8076-55-9 (CAS)
ON  -  26915-78-6 (CAS)
ON  -  53303-76-7 (CAS)
ON  -  54018-92-7 (CAS)
ON  -  59135-90-9 (CAS)
MF  -  C4-H13-N3
NI  -  Diethylenetriamine (8CI)
NI  -  1,2-Ethanediamine, N-(2-aminoethyl)- (9CI)
SY  -  3-Azapentane-1,5-diamine
SY  -  Bis(beta-aminoethyl)amine
SY  -  2,2'-Diaminodiethylamine
SY  -  Bis(2-aminoethyl)amine
SY  -  N,N-Bis(2-aminoethyl)amine
SY  -  1,4,7-Triazaheptane
LO  -  TOXLINE
LO  -  RTECS
LO  -  TDB
LO  -  TOXBACK
LO  -  TSCAINV
```

Figure 2 Example of an interactive search of CHEMLINE.

Review Committee members to assure that TDB contains the most relevant theories and correct information.

Pertinent Data Elements:
  Synonyms
  Chemical and physical properties
  Molecular formula
  CAS Registry Number
  Human toxicity
  Nonhuman toxicity
  Aquatic toxicity
  Analytical laboratory methods
  Interactions
  Poisoning potential
  Radiation hazards
  Threshold limit values
  Pharmacology and toxicology
  Absorption, distribution, and excretion
  Metabolism
  Antidote and treatment
  Modes of action
  Consumption pattern
  Safety and health precautions

Disposal methods
Environmental pollution potential
Manufacturing information

TDB is accessible on-line or off-line through the NLM system. An example of the results of an interactive search appears in Fig. 3.

NAME OF SUBSTANCE	SODIUM CACODYLATE
MOLECULAR FORMULA	C2-H6-AS-NA-02
CAS REGISTRY NUMBER	124-65-2
TDB NUMBER	0731
MOLECULAR WEIGHT	159.98
WISWESSER LINE NOTATION	Q-AS-Q&1&1 & NA
SYNONYMS	ARSINE OXIDE, HYDROXYDIMETHYL-, SODIUM
SYNONYMS	ANSAR 160
MAJOR USE	MERCK INDEX 8TH ED 956 HAS BEEN USED IN CHRONIC SKIN DISEASES, LEUKEMIA
MELTING POINT	APPROX 60 DEG C
BOILING POINT	120 DEG C
ANTIDOTE & TREATMENT	GOSSELIN. CTCP 4TH ED II-91 DIAGNOSIS: STRONG GARLIC ODOR IS IMPARTED TO BREATH, SWEAT & URINE.
COLOR/FORM	WHITE
SPECTRAL & OTHER PROPS	SUNSHINE. HDBK ANALY TOX 1969 323 INDICES OF REFRACTION: 1.478 (ALPHA), 1.485 (BETA), 1.503 (GAMMA)
TOXICITY VALUES	NIOSH. REG TOX EFFECT CHEM SUB 1975 128 LD50 RATS ORAL 2600 MG/KG /ANHYDROUS/
TOXICITY VALUES	NIOSH. TOXIC SUBSTANCE LIST 1973 207 LDLO RABBITS SUBCUTANEOUS 500 MG/KG
MANUFACTURING INFO	MERCK INDEX 8TH ED 956 PREPARATION: ...DISTILLATION OF MIXT OF ARSENIC TRIOXIDE& POTASSIUM ACETATE...YIELDS CADET'S LIQ, CONTAINING...DIMETHYLARSINE OXIDE.../OXIDIZE/ WITH MERCURIC OXIDE YIELDING CRYSTALS OF CACODYLIC ACID.../NEUTRALIZE/ WITH NA2CO3 OR NAOH: ...VALEUR, GAILLOT, COMPT REND 185, 956 (1927).
POISONING POTENTIAL	MERCK INDEX 8TH ED 956 TOXICITY: SEE ARSENIC. MOST FORMS OF ARSENIC ARE HIGHLY TOXIC. /ARSENIC/

Figure 3   Example (edited) of an interactive search of TDB.

```
ABSORP/DISTRIB/EXCRETE    MERCK INDEX 8TH ED     956 /IT IS AN/ ORG
                          COMPD OF ARSENIC YIELDING INORGANIC,
                          TRIVALENT ARSENIC IN BODY (IS EXCRETED PARTLY
                          UNCHANGED, ALSO YIELDS DIMETHYLARSINE OXIDE).
METABOLISM                KEARNEY, HERBICIDES 2ND ED     755
                          .../RESEARCHER/ REPORTED ON FORMATION OF
                          TRIMETHYLARSINEFROM SODIUM CACODYLATE BY MOLD
                          PENICILLIUM BREVICAULE.
STATUS                    080178COMPLETE WITH PEER REVIEW COMMENTS
                          INCORPORATED
ANIMAL TOXICITY EXCERPT   GARNER'S VET TOX 3RD ED     48
                          ...INTOXICATION OF A HORSE /WAS SEEN/
                          FOLLOWING INJECTION OF SODIUM CACODYLATE...
CONTINUE PRINTING? (YES/NO)

USER:
YY
PROG:


ANIMAL TOXICITY KEYWORDS  ACUTE;HORSES;;INJECTIONS;ND;POISONING


HUMAN TOXICITY EXCERPT    MERCK INDEX 8TH ED     956 SEE ARSENIC. ACUTE
                          SYMPTOMS FOLLOWING INGESTION RELATE TO
                          IRRITATION OF GI TRACT: NAUSEA, VOMITING,
                          DIARRHEA WHICH CAN PROGRESS TO SHOCK & DEATH.
                          CHRONIC POISONING CAN RESULT IN EXFOLIATION &
                          PIGMENTATION OF SKIN, HERPES, POLYNEURITIS,
                          ALTERED HEMATOPOIESIS, DEGENERATION OF LIVER,
                          KIDNEYS. /ARSENIC/
HUMAN TOXICITY KEYWORDS   ACUTE;;;ND;ORAL;DIGESTIVE SYSTEM;NAUSEA
                          VOMITING;DIARRHEA;GASTROENTERITIS
                          ACUTE;;;ND;ORAL;CARDIOVASCULAR SYSTEM
                          SHOCK
                          ACUTE;;;ND;ORAL;ND;DEATHCHRONIC;;;ND;ND;ND
                          POISONING
                          CHRONIC;;;ND;ND;NERVOUS SYSTEM
                          POLYNEURITIS
                          CHRONIC;;;ND;ND;HEMIC AND LYMPHATIC SYSTEMS
                          HEMATOPOIESIS;HEMATOLOGIC DISEASES
                          CHRONIC;;;ND;ND;LIVER;LIVER DISEASES
                          CHRONIC;;;ND;ND;KIDNEY;KIDNEY
                          DISEASES
                          CHRONIC;;;ND;ND;SKIN;PIGMENTATION DISORDERS
                          SKIN DISEASES;DERMATITIS EXFOLIATIVA
                          CHRONIC;;;ND;ND;IMMUNE SYSTEM;HERPESVIRUS
                          INFECTIONS




LAB METHODS EXCERPT       PRC SILVER DIETHYLDITHIOCARBONATE IODINE
                          (GUTZCIT)
LAB METHODS KEYWORDS      ND;

SS 2 /C?
USER:
SSTOPP  YY
```

Figure 3 Example (edited) of an interactive search of TDB. (*Continued*)

Chemical Abstracts Service (CAS) ONLINE is a new service that was scheduled to begin on November 1, 1980 (7). Initially, CAS ONLINE will have access to those substances cited in the literature since 1977 (nearly 2 million substances). Also, 6000 newly registered substances will be added weekly, and substances registered before 1977 will be added regularly so that the file should be complete by the end of 1981.

An important feature of CAS ONLINE is the capacity for substructural searches.

Chemical Information System (CIS) Structure and Nomenclature Search System (SANSS), a data base within the NIH/EPA Chemical Information System is designed to locate chemical compounds on the basis of structural characteristics. CIS SANSS can also search on the basis of molecular formula, systematic chemical name, name fragment, common or trade name, or other synonym.

A large number of collections make up the CIS SANSS data base. Some of these collections are associated with regulatory activities or categories of chemicals, while others are associated with certain classes of compounds (such as those contained in the *Merck Index*). The user can focus on a specific collection of chemical data or search the entire data base. Figure 4 lists the collections available to be searched. Figure 5 describes one of these collections.

1. EPA TSCA Inventory List (43,277)
2. CIS EI Mass Spectrometry (33,898)
3. CIS Carbon 13 NMR Spectrometry (7,565)
4. EPA Pesticides Registered Active Ingredients (2,103/380)
5. EPA OHM/TADS: Oil and Hazardous Materials -
    Technical Assistance Data System (1,005/19)
6. Cambridge X-Ray Crystallography (14,673)
7. Merck Index (8,979)
8. EPA Pesticides Analytical Reference Standards (473)
9. EPA STORET Water Quality Data Base (234)
10. EPA Chemical Spills (577)
11. EPA AEROS SOTDAT (572)
12. NIMH Psychotropic Activity (2,036)
13. EPA AEROS SAROAD (65)
14. NBS/NIH Proton Affinity Data Base (439)
15. CPSC CHEMRIC (890)
16. EPA Pesticides Registered Inert Ingredients (779/353)
17. NBS - NIH Ionization Potential Data Base (3,136)
18. NFPA - Hazardous Chemical Data (395)
19. EPA/FDA Pesticides Reference Standards (612)
20. U.S. International Trade Commission Production Statistics (9,144)
21. NBS Crystal Data File (18,169)
22. EPA Effluent Guidelines Priority Pollutants (128/1)

Figure 4 Chemical data resources in CIS SANSS.

23. EPA Organic Chemical Producers Data Base Program (375)
24. IPC Chemical Product Data (104)
25. IPC Chemical Plant Data (103)
26. NSF Hazardous Chemicals List (224)
27. EROICA (Estimation and Retrieval of Organic Properties) (4,488)
28. PNS-149 Carcinogenic Activity (4,416)
29. NIOSH Registry of Toxic Effects of Chemical Substances (26,974/2,197)
30. NIOSH National Occupational Hazards Survey (NOHS) (4,556)
31. Environmental Mutagen Information Center (6,851)
32. Environmental Teratology Information Center (3,244)
33. IERL Noncriteria Pollutant Emissions (253/54)
34. Section 111(d) of the Clean Air Act (1/2)
35. EPA Chemical Indicators of Industrial Contamination (49/13)
36. EPA Selected Organic Air Pollutants by the Pollutant Strategic Branch (591/37)
37. Section 112 of the Clean Air Act (5)
38. EPA Carcinogen Assessment Group List of Chemicals (41/4)
39. Comprehensive Index of API 44-TRC Selected Data on Thermodynamics and Spectroscopy 1974 (3,298/8,013)
40. FAO/WHO-Pesticide Data Sheets (20)
41. Potential Industrial Carcinogens and Mutagens (86/13)
42. Assessment of the Contribution of Environmental Carcinogens to Cancer Incidences in the General Population (27/3)
43. DHEW, National Cancer Institute (NCI) Laboratory Chemicals (55/7)
44. EPA/NSF, Economic and Toxicologic Data for Commercially Significant Chemicals (499/149)
45. EPA, Restricted Use Pesticides (23)
46. Compounds for Mutagenicity Evaluation (25)
47. Study of Potential Carcinogenicity of Selected Chemicals based on Structure Activity Analysis (409/5)
48. Chemical Industry Institute of Technology (CIIT) Priority Chemicals (27)
49. JCPDS Powder Diffraction File (24,130/1973)
51. Potential Industrial Carcinogens and Mutagens (1,444/292)
52. TOX-TIPS (472/4)
53. CHEMLINE (31,176)
54. Fish Control Lab Data Base (91/97)
55. National Marine Fisheries Service Survey of Trace Elements in the Fishery Resource (15)
56. Military Entomology Information Service (MEIS) (123/25)
57. Summary of Testing Rcommendations by the TSCA Interagency Testing Committee (4/6)
58. Environmental Determinants of Cancer (74/9)
59. EPA, Quality Criteria for Water (37/9)
60. 1976 OHSA Concentration Limits for Gases and Varpos (257/25)
61. NFPA 491M - Manual of Hazardous Chemical Reactions (899/762)
62. NFPA 325M Fire Hazard Properties of Flammable Liquids, Gases, and Volatile Solids (1150/484)
63. FAO/WHO - Joint Meetings on Pesticide Residues in Food (86/12)
64. EPA, Office of Research and Development Interim Procedures for the Control of Toxic Substances Inventories (21)
65. Distribution Register of Organic Pollutants in Water (WaterDROP) (859/840)
66. CIS CI Mass Spectrometry (1,147)

Figure 4 Chemical data resources in CIS SANSS. (*Continued*)

Pertinent Data Elements:
  CAS Registry Number
  Names of collectors and identifiers
  Molecular formula
  Systematic chemical name

```
              1 - EPA TSCA INVENTORY (43,277)
75 LINES LEFT.  CONTINUE WITH DETAILED EXPLANATION (Y/N)  (Y)?Y

    IN ACCORDANCE WITH SECTION 8 OF THE TOXIC SUBSTANCES
CONTROL ACT (PUBLIC LAW 94-469), THE U.S. ENVIRONMENTAL
PROTECTION AGENCY HAS COMPILED AND PUBLISHED AN INVENTORY OF
CHEMICAL SUBSTANCES MANUFACTURED, IMPORTED, OR PROCESSED FOR
A COMMERCIAL PURPOSE IN THE UNITED STATES SINCE JANUARY 1,
1975.  THIS INVENTORY DEFINES THOSE CHEMICAL SUBSTANCES
"EXISTING" IN U.S. COMMERCE FOR PURPOSES OF IMPLEMENTING THE
TOXIC SUBSTANCES CONTROL ACT.  SUBSTANCES NOT INCLUDED ON
THE INVENTORY ARE CONSIDERED "NEW", AND THUS SUBJECT TO THE
PREMANUFACTURE NOTIFICATION REQUIREMENTS OF SECTION 5 OF THE
TSCA.  IT SHOULD BE EMPHASIZED, HOWEVER, THAT THE INVENTORY
DOES NOT PURPORT TO IDENTIFY ALL CHEMICAL SUBSTANCES
CURRENTLY IN U.S. COMMERCE, SINCE SOME SUCH SUBSTANCES ARE
SPECIFICALLY EXCLUDED FROM THE INVENTORY BY REGULATION.
FURTHERMORE, THE INVENTORY IS NOT INTENDED TO BE A LIST OF
TOXIC CHEMICALS; TOXICITY WAS NOT A CRITERION IN DETERMINING
THE ELIGIBILITY OF SUBSTANCES FOR INCLUSION ON THE
INVENTORY.
    56 LINES LEFT.  CONTINUE WITH DETAILED EXPLANATION (Y/N)  (Y)?Y

    THIS COLLECTION IN THE SANSS DATA BASE CURRENTLY
CORRESPONDS TO THE INITIAL INVENTORY PUBLISHED BY EPA IN
MAY, 1979 ("TOXIC SUBSTANCES CONTROL ACT CHEMICAL SUBSTANCES
INVENTORY - INITIAL INVENTORY", U.S. GOVERNMENT PRINTING
OFFICE:  1979, 261-699/6179).  ALL CHEMICAL SUBSTANCES ON
THIS INITIAL INVENTORY, WITH THE EXCEPTION OF AUTOMATICALLY
INCLUDED "NATURALLY OCCURRING SUBSTANCES", HAVE BEEN
IDENTIFIED FROM REPORTS SUBMITTED TO EPA BY MANUFACTURERS
AND IMPORTERS IN RESPONSE TO THE TSCA INVENTORY REPORTING
REGULATIONS (40 CFR PART 710). THE INITIAL INVENTORY DOES
NOT, HOWEVER, INCLUDE ALL SUBSTANCES CITED ON THE
AFOREMENTIONED MANUFACTURER AND IMPORTER SUBMITTED REPORTS.
SUBSTANCES WHICH WERE MANUFACTURED OR IMPORTED FOR THE FIRST
TIME SINCE MAY 1, 1978 MAY HAVE BEEN REPORTED TOO LATE TO BE
INCLUDED IN THE PUBLISHED LIST.  OTHER REPORTED SUBSTANCES
WERE INADEQUATELY IDENTIFIED, AND PUBLICATION OF THESE
SUBSTANCES HAS BEEN DELAYED PENDING RESOLUTION OF THESE
IDENTITY PROBLEMS.  A SUPPLEMENT TO THE INITIAL INVENTORY,
PUBLISHED BY EPA IN OCTOBER, 1979, (U.S. G.P.O.: 1979
0-303-431) INCLUDES SUBSTANCES WHICH WERE REPORTED FOR THE
INITIAL INVENTORY, BUT WERE NOT INCLUDED IN THE MAY, 1979
PUBLICATION FOR THE REASONS STATED ABOVE.
    33 LINES LEFT.  CONTINUE WITH DETAILED EXPLANATION (Y/N)  (Y)?Y
```

Figure 5 Example (edited) of the background information that is available for each collection of chemical data in CIS SANSS.

```
      THE INVENTORY IS INTENDED TO BE DYNAMIC, AND WILL CHANGE
FOR OTHER REASONS AS WELL.  FOR EXAMPLE, CHEMICAL SUBSTANCES
WHICH ARE NOT ON THE INITIAL INVENTORY, BUT WHICH HAVE BEEN
PROCESSED OR IMPORTED AS PART OF MIXTURES OR ARTICLES SINCE
JANUARY L, 1975, MAY BE REPORTED BY PROCESSORS OR IMPORTERS
WITHIN 210 DAYS OF THE PUBLICATION OF THE INITIAL INVENTORY.
IN ADDITION, CHEMICAL SUBSTANCES THAT COMPLETE
PREMANUFACTURE REVIEW WILL BE ADDED TO THE INVENTORY WHEN
THEY BEGIN TO BE MANUFACTURED OR IMPORTED FOR COMMERCIAL
PURPOSES.  EPA WILL REPUBLISH THE INVENTORY SOMETIME IN 1980
TO INCORPORATE THE MAJOR ADDITIONS TO THE INITIAL
PUBLICATION, AND WILL THEREAFTER PERIODICALLY PUBLISH
SUPPLEMENTS TO KEEP THE PRINTED INVENTORY AS CURRENT AS
POSSIBLE.  CORRESPONDING ADDITIONS WILL BE MADE TO THE SANSS
DATA BASE PERIODICALLY TO MAINTAIN CURRENCY WITH RESPECT TO
THE EPA PUBLICATION.
    16 LINES LEFT.  CONTINUE WITH DETAILED EXPLANATION (Y/N)  (Y)?Y

      THE INVENTORY PUBLICATION ITSELF CONSISTS OF FOUR
VOLUMES. THE FIRST OF THESE IS THE INVENTORY AND LISTS
SUBSTANCES BY A PREFERRED NAME AND MOLECULAR FORMULA IN
ORDER OF INCREASING CAS REGISTRY NUMBER.  THE SECOND AND
THIRD VOLUMES PROVIDE AN INDEX TO THE INVENTORY BY
SYNONYMOUS NAMES. THE FOURTH VOLUME THEN PROVIDES AN INDEX
TO THE INVENTORY BY MOLECULAR FORMULA, AND A UVCB INDEX FOR
CHEMICAL SUBSTANCES OF "UNKNOWN OR VARIABLE COMPOSITION,
COMPLEX REACTION PRODUCTS, AND BIOLOGICAL MATERIALS".

      FOR A MORE DETAILED EXPLANATION OF THE NATURE AND
LIMITATIONS OF TSCA INVENTORY DATA AND MATERIALS, YOU MAY
CONTACT THE INDUSTRY ASSISTANCE OFFICE BY TELEPHONING
TOLL-FREE 800-424-9065 OR, IF IN WASHINGTON, 544-1404 OR BY
WRITING TO THE INDUSTRY ASSISTANCE OFFICE, OFFICE OF TOXIC
SUBSTANCES (TS-799), U.S.  E.P.A., WASHINGTON, D.C. 20460.
```

Figure 5 Example (edited) of the background information that is available for each collection of chemical data in CIS SANSS. (*Continued*)

Synonyms
Structural image

The structural image for each substance is derived from a connection table obtained from CAS and stored in the data base.

Two general search strategies are available. First, to identify a specific compound the user can search for a substance on the basis of a chemical or common name or by specifying its structure, or a known CAS Registry Number may be used to obtain the best systematic chemical name or a list of synonyms. This procedure is termed an "identity search."

Another strategy is employed to identify all substances in the data base that have certain substructural features. For example, CIS SANSS may be used to locate all substances that have a certain nucleus (set of contiguous rings) and a certain set of substituents to those rings. This is called a "characteristic search." Figure 6 presents the results of an interactive search of CIS SANSS.

```
OPTION? SSHOW 82-68-8

CAS RN 82-68-8             IN FILE

CIS SOURCES OF INFORMATION

    CIS, EI MASS SPECTROMETRY
    CIS, CAMBRIDGE X-RAY CRYSTALLOGRAPHY: 82-68-8.01
    NIOSH/CIS, RTECS: DA66500
    JCPDS/CIS, POWDER DIFFRACTION PATTERNS: 251598
    CIS, CI MASS SPECTROMETRY

19 NON-CIS REFERENCES AVAILABLE
                                              C6CL5NO2
```

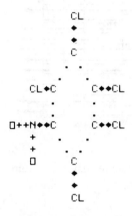

```
BENZENE, PENTACHLORONITRO- (8CI9CI)
AVICOL (PESTICIDE) (VAN)
BATRILEX
BOTRILEX
BRASSICOL
  25 MORE NAMES AVAILABLE
```

Figure 6 Example of a CIS SANSS information display. Compound: parathion. + = double bond; ♦ = single bond; ■ = ring alternate bond.

Access to the CIS SANSS data base is available through general subscription to CIS.

LITERATURE/CITATION DATA BASES

The limited availability of data bases containing biological research results means that researchers usually must resort to the literature searches to obtain the data necessary for structure-activity analyses.

Data bases that contain citations to published literature or ongoing research projects are by far the largest group. These data bases encompass research reported in thousands of journals over the time period of 1963 to the

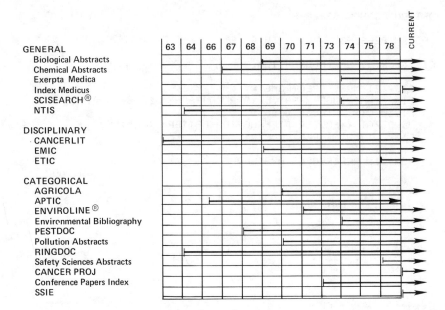

Figure 7 Time periods covered by bibliographic data bases.

present (Fig. 7). Following are brief descriptions of some major literature/ citation data bases relevant to structure-activity analysis.

General Citation Systems (Manual and Computerized)

Biological Abstracts covers worldwide research in the life sciences. Information is taken from approximately 8000 journals and other sources such as symposia, reviews, reports, and other research communications.

    Supplier: Biosciences Information Service
    Computer Networks: BRS, ORBIT, DIALOG, NLM (TOXLINE)
    Coverage: 1969 to present

Chemical Abstracts covers worldwide research in the chemical sciences. Information is taken from over 12,000 journals, patents, books, conference proceedings, and government research reports. This data base can be searched by CAS Registry Number or Molecular Formula Fragment.

    Supplier: Chemical Abstracts Service of the American Chemical Association
    Computer Networks: BRS, ORBIT, DIALOG, NLM (TOXLINE)
    Coverage: 1967 to present

Excerpta Medica covers the entire field of human medicine and such related disciplines as environmental health, pollution control, and pharmacology. Information is taken from over 3500 biomedical journals published throughout the world.

    Supplier: Excerpta Medica, Amsterdam, the Netherlands
    Computer Network: DIALOG
    Coverage: 1974 to present

Index Medicus (MEDLINE) contains references to biomedical journal articles published in the current and two preceding years. The articles are from 3000 journals published in the United States and 70 foreign countries.

    Supplier: National Library of Medicine
    Computer Network: NLM
    Coverage: Current and two preceding years; previous years to 1966 are covered in back files

The National Technical Information Service (NTIS) covers government-sponsored research, development, and engineering.

    Supplier: National Technical Information Service of the U.S. Department of Commerce
    Computer Networks: DIALOG, ORBIT, BRS
    Coverage: 1964 to present

SCISEARCH covers the multidisciplinary fields of science and technology. Included are all records published in *Science Citation Index* (SCI) and additional records from the *Current Contents* series.

    Supplier: Institute for Scientific Information
    Computer Network: DIALOG
    Coverage: 1974 to present

**Disciplinary Citation Systems
(Manual and Computerized)**

CANCERLIT (Cancer Literature) covers both carcinogenesis and cancer therapy publications. Over 3000 U.S. and foreign journals as well as monographs, conference proceedings, reports, and dissertations are abstracted for inclusion.

Supplier: National Library of Medicine, sponsored by the National Cancer Institute
Computer Network: NLM
Coverage: 1963 to present

The Environmental Mutagen Information Center (EMIC) data base contains information gathered from the open literature on mutagenicity testing of chemical agents. Currently the data base consists of 28,000 records published primarily since 1969 in approximately 2350 publication sources. Each record includes bibliographic details and key words for the chemicals, organisms, and assay systems studied. To permit simplified information retrieval, chemicals are associated with CAS Registry Numbers.

Supplier: Environmental Mutagen Information Center, Oak Ridge National Laboratory
Computer Networks: NLM (TOXLINE), RECON
Coverage: 1969 to present

The Environmental Teratology Information Center (ETIC) data base contains information gathered from the open literature on the testing and evaluation for teratogenic activity of environmental factors such as chemical, biological, and physical agents. The main emphasis is on the administration of an agent to pregnant animals and examination of the offspring at or near birth for structural or functional anomalies. The ETIC data base currently has over 18,000 entries. Each record contains bibliographic details and key words for the chemicals, organisms, and assay systems studied. Chemicals are associated with CAS Registry Numbers.

Supplier: Environmental Teratology Information Center, Oak Ridge National Laboratory
Computer Networks: NLM (TOXLINE), RECON
Coverage: 1975 to present

Categorical Citation Data Bases (Computerized)

AGRICOLA covers worldwide journal and monographic literature on agriculture and related disciplines. AGRICOLA represents the actual holdings of the National Agricultural Library.

Supplier: National Agricultural Library
Computer Networks: ORBIT, DIALOG, BRS
Coverage: 1970 to present

The **Air Pollution Technical Information Center (APTIC)** covers the field of air pollution. Components of this data base include effects on human health, materials, plants, and livestock; atmospheric interactions; control methods; economic aspects; emission sources; government participation; measurement methods; pollution data; and social aspects.

Supplier: U.S. Environmental Protection Agency, Research Triangle Park, North Carolina
Computer Network: DIALOG
Coverage: 1966 to 1978

ENVIROLINE covers the world's environmental information. This data base includes the subjects of management, technology, planning, law, political science, economics, geology, biology, and chemistry as each relates to environmental issues. More than 5000 publications are abstracted and indexed for inclusion.

Supplier: Environment Information Center
Computer Networks: DIALOG, ORBIT
Coverage: 1971 to present

Environmental Bibliography covers the fields of general human ecology, atmospheric studies, energy, land resources, water resources, nutrition, and health. Approximately 325 periodicals are indexed.

Supplier: Environmental Studies Institute
Computer Network: DIALOG
Coverage: 1974 to present

PESTDOC provides journal literature coverage of agricultural chemicals.

Supplier: Derrvent Publications, Ltd., London, England
Computer Network: ORBIT
Coverage: 1968 to present

Pollution Abstracts is a leading resource for reference to environmentally related literature on pollution, its sources, and control. Coverage includes some 2500 journals, conference proceedings, government documents, and monographs. Subjects include air pollution, water pollution, solid waste, noise, pesticides, radiation, and general environmental quality.

Supplier: Data Courier, Inc.
Computer Networks: DIALOG, ORBIT, BRS
Coverage: 1970 to present

RINGDOC provides extensive coverage of the pharmaceutical literature. Over 400 scientific journals are included.

>   Supplier: Derrvent Publications, Ltd., London, England
>   Computer Network: ORBIT
>   Coverage: 1964 to present

Safety Sciences Abstracts provides broad, interdisciplinary coverage of literature related to the science of safety.

>   Supplier: Cambridge Scientific Abstracts
>   Computer Network: ORBIT
>   Coverage: 1975 to present

Research in Progress Data Bases

CANCERPROJ (Cancer Research Projects) contains 20,000 descriptions of ongoing cancer research projects. The descriptions are provided by cancer researchers in many countries and are collected for NCI by the Smithsonian Science Information Exchange (SSIE).

>   Supplier: National Library of Medicine, sponsored by the National Cancer Institute
>   Computer Network: NLM
>   Coverage: Current and two previous years

Conference Papers Index provides access to records of scientific and technical papers presented at conferences. Primary subject areas include the life sciences, chemistry, physical sciences, geosciences, and engineering. Because new findings may be reported at conferences a year or more in advance of journal publication, users of this data base are able to keep abreast of the very latest research and development in science and technology.

>   Supplier: Data Courier, Inc.
>   Computer Networks: DIALOG, ORBIT
>   Coverage: 1973 to present

The Smithsonian Science Information Exchange (SSIE) covers ongoing and recently completed research in the agricultural sciences, behavioral sciences, biological sciences, earth sciences, chemistry and chemical engineering, electronics, engineering, materials, mathematics, medical sciences, physics, and social sciences. Project descriptions are received from over 1300 organizations that fund research. However, almost 90 percent of the information in the data base is provided by agencies of the Federal Government.

Supplier: Smithsonian Science Information Exchange
Computer Networks: BRS, DIALOG, ORBIT, NLM (TOXLINE)
Coverage: Two previous years

CONCLUSIONS

All of the information and literature/citation data bases discussed are
accessible via commercial or governmental computer networks. The major
networks are as follows:

National Library of Medicine (NLM)
RECON
ORBIT
Bibliographic Retrieval Service, Inc. (BRS)
Chemical Information System (CIS)
DIALOG Information Retrieval Service

Addresses for these networks are given in the Appendix.

Figures 8-13 display the various biological, toxicological, chemical, and
related data bases that reside in the major computer networks. Some of the
same data bases are available from several networks (Fig. 14). For example,
the EMIC and ETIC files are available from both NLM (through TOXLINE)
and RECON. *Biological Abstracts* is available through four of the networks:
DIALOG, BRS, ORBIT, and NLM. The RTECS data base resides in both the
NLM and CIS systems.

The NLM system contains several subsystems, some of which contain
several data bases. For example, TOXLINE is the subdivision in the NLM
system that consolidates the toxicity portions of EMIC, ETIC, *Biological
Abstracts, Chemical Abstracts, Pesticides Abstracts, Index Medicus,* and
Research Projects in Progress (SSIE).

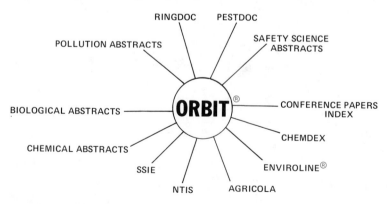

Figure 8 Relevant ORBIT data bases.

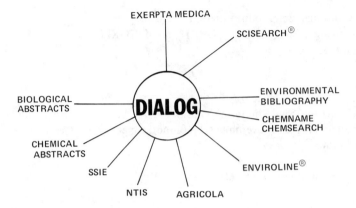

Figure 9   Relevant DIALOG data bases.

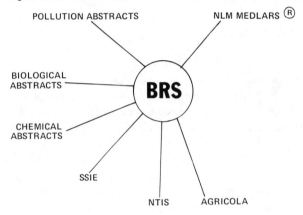

Figure 10   Relevant BRS data bases.

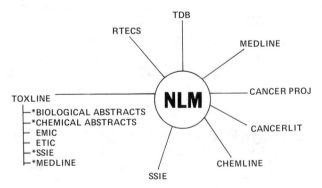

*TOXICITY PORTION

Figure 11   Relevant NLM data bases.

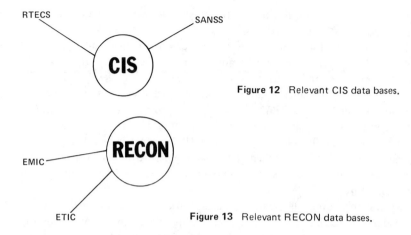

Figure 12 Relevant CIS data bases.

Figure 13 Relevant RECON data bases.

The direct on-line availability of these information resources facilitates the acquisition of bibliographic, physical/chemical, substance identification, and toxicity data. However, since the various data bases reside in different computer networks, the user must learn several vastly different search procedures. Also, most computer networks contain no analysis capabilities. (CIS does contain a statistical analysis component, MLAB). And, with the

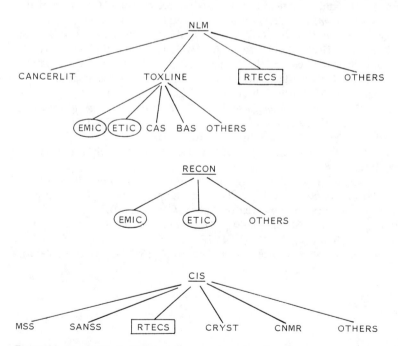

Figure 14 Examples of data bases in computer networks.

exception of toxicity data, not one of the existing networks offers a data base containing biological research results.

Clearly, a computer network able to provide coordinated on-line chemical substance data would be of great value to structure-activity analysts. The Chemical Substances Information Network (CSIN) being developed by the Interagency Toxic Substances Data Committee (cochaired by the Council on Environmental Quality and EPA) is expected to provide such a service. Most of the computerized data bases discussed in this paper are projected components of CSIN. In addition, the PROPHET system, which has powerful analytical capabilities, is a scheduled component. Although CSIN is not presently operational, some system components are expected to be operational in the near future.

Unfortunately, even the creation of a sophisticated computer network will not "produce" data bases containing the biological research results requisite for assessing structure-activity relationships. Only painstaking effort by researchers will fulfill this need.

REFERENCES

1 Ames, B. N., et al. Carcinogenic potency: A progress report. *Ethylene Dichloride: A Potential Health Risk?* Banbury Report 5, 1980.

2 Waters, M. D., and A. Auletta. The GENE–TOX program: Genetic activity evaluation. *J. Chem. Inf. Comput. Sci.* (in press).

3 *Registry of Toxic Effects of Chemical Substances,* 1977 ed., 2 vols. U.S. Department of Health, Education, and Welfare Publication (NIOSH)78-104-A and B. (Prepared for the National Institute of Occupational Safety and Health by Tracor Jitco, Inc., Rockville, Maryland.) Washington, D.C.: U.S. Department of Health, Education, and Welfare (1978).

4 *Survey of Compounds Which Have Been Tested for Carcinogenic Activity,* 1978 ed. National Institutes of Health Publication 80-453. (Prepared for the National Cancer Institute by Franklin Research Center, Philadelphia, Pennsylvania.) Washington, D.C.: U.S. Department of Health, Education, and Welfare (1978).

5 *IARC Monographs on the Evaluation of the Carcinogenic Risk of Chemicals to Humans,* vols. 1–24 and supplements. Lyons, France: International Agency for Research on Cancer (1972–1980).

6 Windholz, M. (ed.). *Merck Index: An Encyclopedia of Chemicals and Drugs,* 9th ed. Rahway, NJ: Merck (1976).

7 CAS offers new online service. *Chem. Eng. News* 58:34–35 (Oct. 6, 1980).

Part Two

Fundamentals

Chapter 4

Biochemical Mechanisms Underlying the Toxic Actions of Chemicals

James S. Bus

INTRODUCTION

Literally hundreds, and perhaps thousands, of biochemical mechanisms responsible for chemical toxicity have been described in the literature. Thus, a complete discussion of biochemical mechanisms responsible for the toxic actions of chemicals is far beyond scope of this review. The purpose of this presentation, therefore, is to outline several fundamental mechanisms that serve as a foundation for a general overview of mechanisms of xenobiotic-induced toxicity.

Several of the important biochemical mechanisms of toxicity, which will be the focus of this review, are summarized in Fig. 1 (1). Following exposure and subsequent absorption, a chemical is distributed to various body tissues. The distribution of a chemical to various tissues is not always uniform, however, and may be influenced by specific transport mechanisms or solubility and binding factors unique to that tissue. Thus, an organ-specific uptake or retention of a chemical or its metabolite(s) in a tissue is an important factor in many target organ-directed toxicities. After distribution of

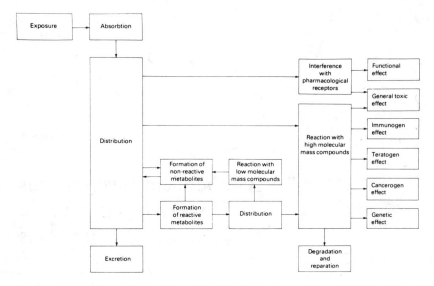

Figure 1 Interaction of chemicals with biological systems. *From Malmfors (1), with permission.*

a chemical to a tissue, it may directly react with various pharmacological receptors, producing functional or general toxic effects. In many instances, however, the parent chemical is metabolized to electrophilic products that may readily react with cellular macromolecules such as proteins, nucleic acids, and lipids. A wide spectrum of potential toxic responses, as listed in Fig. 1, can result from these reactions. It should be noted that formation of reactive metabolites will not always result in toxicity, since several biochemical defense mechanisms, such as further metabolism to nonreactive products, reaction with low molecular weight compounds, and degradation or repair of the damaged cellular macromolecules, may modulate the toxic response.

TISSUE-SPECIFIC DISTRIBUTION

The toxicity of many chemicals is not always characterized by a nonspecific organ toxicity but often is limited to one or more specific target organs. An example of such an agent is the bipyridylium herbicide paraquat, which is highly toxic to the lung following systemic absorption (2). An important component of the lung-directed toxicity of paraquat is the ability of the lung to accumulate paraquat via an active transport system that is relatively specific for several amines (3). The importance of the transport mechanism in mediating the pulmonary toxicity of paraquat is readily seen by comparison to a structural analog of paraquat, diquat, which is considerably less toxic to the lung. Diquat, whose molecular mechanism of toxicity may be similar to that of paraquat but is not a substrate for the transport system, does not accumulate in lung (3). Thus, it is clear from examples such as paraquat that an organ-specific localization of a chemical may play an important mechanistic role in the development of target organ toxicity.

METABOLIC ACTIVATION OF CHEMICALS

Following distribution to tissues, many chemicals are metabolized to electrophilic products that are capable of covalently binding to cellular macromolecules. Among the most well-characterized metabolic activation reactions are those leading to the formation of epoxides. Epoxides are formed by the addition of oxygen across a carbon-carbon unsaturated bond, in a reaction catalyzed by the microsomal mixed function oxidase system enzymes (Fig. 2). Many epoxides are sufficiently electrophilic to react with tissue macromolecules and are thus capable of producing several toxic endpoints (e.g., general toxicity, carcinogenicity, etc.).

The potential toxic reactions of epoxides are controlled, however, by several important enzymatic and nonenzymatic detoxification mechanisms. First, epoxides may spontaneously rearrange to phenols, which are readily conjugated with sulfate or glucuronide and subsequently excreted. Second, epoxides may be enzymatically converted to dihydrodiols via epoxide hydrolase or glutathione conjugates by glutathione-S-transferases. The products of both of these reactions are generally less toxic than the epoxide intermediates and are readily excreted. Finally, alkylation or arylation of cellular macromolecules by epoxides does not necessarily insure a toxic response, since the damaged macromolecule may be repaired or degraded with nontoxic consequences.

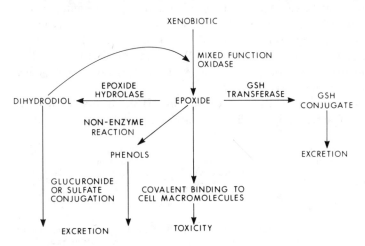

Figure 2   Metabolic activation and detoxification reactions of epoxides.

Thus, the potential for an epoxide to produce toxicity is dependent on several factors, including the rate of epoxide formation, the stability and reactivity of the epoxide formed, and the capability of the various defense mechanisms to cope with the epoxide formed (4).

An extensively studied class of agents whose toxicity is mediated by formation of epoxides is the polycyclic aromatic hydrocarbons (PAH). The metabolism of PAH has been well characterized, particularly by evaluation of a typical PAH, benzo[a]pyrene (BP) (Fig. 3). The initial metabolic events leading to formation of the carcinogenic metabolite are oxidation of BP by the mixed function oxidases to the 7,8-epoxide, and subsequent metabolism to the 7,8-dihydrodiol. This metabolite is sufficiently lipophilic so as to be further metabolized by the mixed function oxidase to the *anti*-7,8-dihydrodiol-9,10-epoxide, which is thought to be the final activated carcinogen of BP(5).

The PAH are also a good example of compounds that have the capability to modify their own metabolism and, as a result, their subsequent toxicity. Administration of PAH to animals selectively induces microsomal cytochrome P-448, resulting in enhanced formation of toxic metabolites (5). The importance of the cytochrome P-448 induction in the production of toxicity is further supported from studies in which mice that are resistant to PAH-induced carcinogenicity were resistant to PAH induction of cytochrome P-448 (5).

Not all metabolic activation reactions, however, involve the formation of epoxides. Acetaminophen, a widely used analgesic, produces liver toxicity in animals and humans following administration of a high dose of the compound (6). The hepatotoxicity of acetaminophen is thought to be mediated by mixed function oxidase-catalyzed generation of a reactive quinoneimine, which readily arylates critical macromolecules (6). Recently, it has been proposed that acetaminophen may also be oxidized to a semiquinone radical that is even more reactive than the quinoneimine (7). In addition, further oxidation of the semiquinone forms not only the quinoneimine but also the potentially toxic superoxide anion (O_2^-·).

An elegant study by Potter and co-workers (6) demonstrated that the hepatotoxicity of acetaminophen directly correlated with the capacity of an

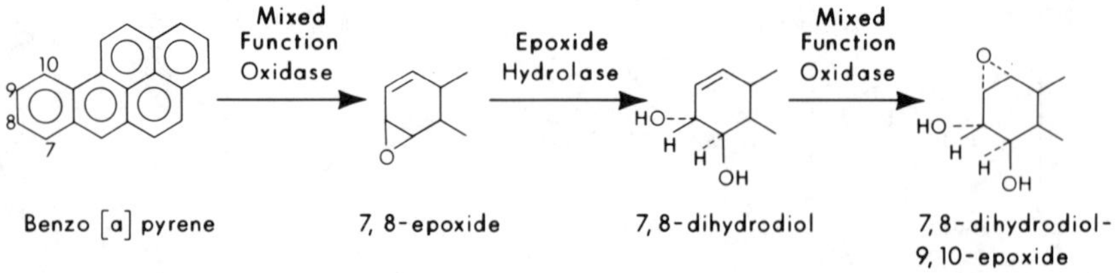

| Benzo [a] pyrene | 7, 8-epoxide | 7, 8-dihydrodiol | 7,8-dihydrodiol-9,10-epoxide |

Figure 3 Metabolic activation of the polycyclic aromatic hydrocarbon benzo[a]pyrene.

important defense mechanism, reduced glutathione (GSH), to detoxify the reactive metabolites of acetaminophen. As the dose of acetaminophen in hamsters was increased, liver GSH steadily declined, presumably due to a nonenzymatic conjugation of GSH with the reactive intermediate. However, covalent binding of ^{3}H-acetaminophen and associated hepatotoxicity did not dramatically increase until GSH was reduced approximately 70 percent. Thus, these studies suggested that as long as the dose of acetaminophen was insufficient to overwhelm the GSH detoxification mechanism, toxicity would not ensue.

Metabolic activation catalyzed by the microsomal mixed function oxidase system is not the only mechanism whereby reactive intermediates may be generated. The metabolism of aromatic amines, as typified by the carcinogen 2-acetylaminofluorene (2-AAF), is an example of such an activation mechanism. The initial activation step for 2-AAF is an N-hydroxylation catalyzed by the mixed function oxidase enzyme system. However, further metabolism of the N-hydroxymetabolite to acetate, sulfate, or glucuronide esters of the N-hydroxy amide is required before covalent binding to cellular macromolecules occurs (5). These conjugation reactions are carried out by acyltransferase, sulfotransferase, and glucuronyl transferase. It is interesting to note that in the example of 2-AAF, hydroxylation of the aromatic ring by the mixed function oxidase system is a metabolic detoxification pathway (5).

Another area of metabolic activation reactions that has attracted increasing attention in recent years is the production of "activated oxygen" as a result of xenobiotic metabolism. The primary form of activated oxygen generated in these reactions is the single electron reduction product of molecular oxygen, superoxide anion (O_2^-). Although O_2^- is both an oxidant and reductant, it is likely that O_2^- *per se* does not mediate the toxic endpoints associated with O_2^-. In 1934, Haber and Weiss (8) proposed formation of the hydroxyl radical (OH$^\bullet$), which is an extremely potent oxidant, from O_2^- in the following reaction:

$$O_2^- + H_2O_2 \rightarrow OH^\bullet + OH^- + O_2$$

Subsequent studies have shown that although the above reaction does not directly proceed in biological tissues, it does appear to occur in the presence of chelated iron as follows (9):

$$O_2^- + ADP\text{-}Fe^{+3} \rightarrow O_2 + ADP\text{-}Fe^{+2}$$

$$ADP\text{-}Fe^{+2} + H_2O_2 \rightarrow ADP\text{-}Fe^{+3} + OH^\bullet + OH^-$$

The generation of OH$^\bullet$ has many potential toxic consequences to the cell, since it will readily react with nucleic acids, proteins, and lipids. The results of these reactions may be DNA strand breakage, protein crosslinking, and initiation of lipid peroxidation.

Superoxide anion is primarily generated from two types of metabolic processes, single electron redox cycling reactions and autoxidation reactions. The pulmonary toxin paraquat is an example of a chemical generating $O_2 \cdot \bar{}$ via redox cycling (Fig. 4). Paraquat undergoes a single electron reaction catalyzed by NADPH cytochrome P-450 reductase, forming the paraquat radical. Under aerobic conditions, however, reduced paraquat is immediately reoxidized to the paraquat parent compound, with resultant formation of $O_2 \cdot \bar{}$ (10). Other classes of chemicals capable of undergoing redox cycling are quinones and aromatic nitro compounds. Examples of agents that generate $O_2 \cdot \bar{}$ via spontaneous autoxidation are the neurotoxin 6-hydroxydopamine (11) and the pancreatic β-cell toxin dialuric acid (12).

Since biochemical defense mechanisms exist to combat the toxic effects of epoxide or other electrophilic metabolite formation, it is not surprising that the cell also possesses several defense mechanisms to prevent the toxic effects of $O_2 \cdot \bar{}$. The first level of defense against a chemical-generated flux of $O_2 \cdot \bar{}$ is the enzyme superoxide dismutase (SOD), which detoxifies $O_2 \cdot \bar{}$ as follows (13):

$$O_2 \cdot \bar{} + O_2 \cdot \bar{} + 2H^+ \xrightarrow{\text{SOD}} O_2 + H_2O_2$$

The potentially toxic hydrogen peroxide formed as a product of the reaction is subsequently detoxified by cellular catalase or peroxidases or both. The importance of SOD in modulating the toxic effects of $O_2 \cdot \bar{}$ has been convincingly demonstrated in studies of paraquat toxicity in *Escherichia coli.* Aerobic incubation of *E. coli* with paraquat in nutrient-rich media markedly increased the intracellular activity of SOD, presumably a response to enable the *E. coli* to better withstand the increased flux of $O_2 \cdot \bar{}$ generated from paraquat redox cycling (14). When protein synthesis was inhibited in *E. coli* cultures, which prevented the synthesis of additional SOD, paraquat had a significantly greater bacterial toxicity (15). In addition, *E. coli* containing high

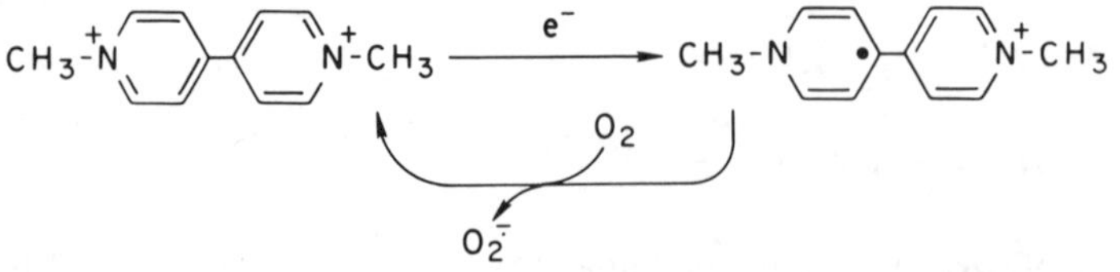

Figure 4 Paraquat redox cycling resulting in superoxide anion generation.

activities of SOD were found to be more resistant to the toxic effects of paraquat than those with low enzyme activity.

An additional level of defense also exists to prevent the membrane-damaging process of lipid peroxidation, which can be readily initiated by activated oxygen. The lipid-soluble antioxidant vitamin E serves to terminate the chain reaction process, while the enzyme GSH peroxidase consumes lipid hydroperoxides, which are otherwise a source of additional lipid radicals (16). The significance of these defense mechanisms in controlling the toxic effects of activated oxygen can again be seen from the example of paraquat. Mice fed a selenium-deficient diet (which decreases the activity of GSH peroxidase, a selenium-dependent enzyme) or a vitamin E-deficient diet were markedly more susceptible to paraquat toxicity (17).

TOXICITY ASSOCIATED WITH SPECIFIC DISRUPTION OF CELLULAR METABOLISM

The biochemical mechanisms described to this point are all somewhat nonselective in their cellular targets, i.e., the reactive intermediates produced by the various metabolic activation pathways can potentially damage a spectrum of critical macromolecules (nucleic acids, proteins, lipids). The toxicity of several chemicals, however, is a result of a relatively specific interference with a critical metabolic process (e.g., energy production).

One example of such a phenomenon is the inhibition of acetylcholinesterase by organophosphate pesticides such as parathion. Parathion is metabolized by the mixed function oxidase system to paraoxon, which selectively phosphorylates the esteratic site of acetylcholinesterase (18). The toxicity associated with organophosphate poisoning, therefore, is characterized by a disruption of nervous system function due to an accumulation of acetylcholine in the nerve synapses.

Another example of agents that affect a specific metabolic process are the inhibitors of mitochondrial energy production. Dinitrophenols and several halogenated phenols uncouple oxidative phosphorylation, possibly by perturbing the mitochondrial membrane (19). Other agents, such as cyanide or rotenone, combine with specific electron carriers of the electron transport system and thereby prevent the flow of electrons through the transport system.

CONCLUSION

An understanding of fundamental biochemical mechanisms of toxicity can in many instances serve as a foundation for predicting potential mechanisms and toxicities for a large variety of chemicals. Nonetheless, it must always be remembered that such speculation may be confounded by variables such as organ-specific distribution, and activation, detoxification, and repair capacities in the target tissue(s). However, a continued exploration of biochemical mechanisms of toxicity, along with the factors that influence the development of toxicity, is clearly needed in order to enable the toxicologist to better extrapolate from general mechanisms to defining the potential toxicity of specific chemicals.

REFERENCES

1 Malmfors, T. Toxicology as science. *Trends Pharmacol. Sci.* 2:2–4 (1981).

2 Heath, D., and P. Smith. The pathology of the lung in paraquat poisoning. In A. P. Autor (ed.), *Biochemical Mechanisms of Paraquat Toxicity*, pp. 39–51. New York: Academic Press (1977).

3 Rose, N. S., and L. L. Smith. The relevance of paraquat accumulation by tissues. In A. P. Autor (ed.), *Biochemical Mechanisms of Paraquat Toxicity*, pp. 71–91. New York: Academic Press (1977).

4 Manson, M. M. Epoxides—Is there a health hazard? *Br. J. Ind. Med.* 37:317–336 (1980).

5 Weisburger, E. K. Metabolism and activation of chemical carcinogens. *Mol. Cell. Biochem.* 32:95–104 (1980).

6 Potter, W. Z., S. S. Thorgeirsson, D. J. Jollow, and J. R. Mitchell. Acetaminophen-induced hepatic necrosis. V. Correlation of hepatic necrosis, covalent binding and glutathione depletion in hamsters. *Pharmacology* 12:129–143 (1974).

7 DeVries, J. Hepatotoxic metabolic activation of paracetamol and its derivatives phenacetin and benorilate: Oxygenation of electron transfer. *Biochem. Pharmacol.* 30:399–402 (1981).

8 Haber, F., and J. Weiss. The catalytic decomposition of hydrogen peroxide by iron salts. *Proc. R. Soc. Lond.* [A] 147:332–351 (1934).

9 Fong, K., P. B. McCay, J. L. Poyer, B. B. Keele, and H. Misra. Evidence that peroxidation of lysosomal membranes is initiated by hydroxyl free radicals produced during flavin enzyme activity. *J. Biol. Chem.* 248:7792–7797 (1972).

10 Farrington, J. A., M. Ebert, E. J. Land, and K. Fletcher. Bipyridylium quaternary salts and related compounds. V. Pulse radiolysis studies on the reaction of paraquat radical with oxygen. Implications for the mode of action of bipyridyl herbicides. *Biochim. Biophys. Acta* 314:372–381 (1973).

11 Heikkila, R. E., and G. Cohen. 6-Hydroxydopamine: Evidence for the superoxide radical as an oxidative intermediate. *Science* 181:456–457 (1973).

12 Heikkila, R. E., and G. Cohen. Cytotoxic aspects of the interaction of ascorbic acid with alloxan and 6-hydroxydopamine. *Ann. N. Y. Acad. Sci.* 258:221–230 (1975).

13 McCord, J. M., and I. Fridovich. Superoxide dismutase—an enzymic function for erythrocuprein (hemocuprein). *J. Biol. Chem.* 244:6049–6055 (1969).

14 Hassan, H. M., and I. Fridovich. Regulation of synthesis of superoxide dismutase in *E. Coli. J. Biol. Chem.* 252:7667–7672 (1977).

15 Hassan, H. M., and I. Fridovich. Superoxide radical and the enhancement of oxygen toxicity of paraquat in *E. coli. J. Biol. Chem.* 253:8143–8148 (1978).

16 Bus, J. S., and J. E. Gibson. Lipid peroxidation and its role in toxicology. *Rev. Biochem. Toxicol.* 1:125–149 (1979).

17 Bus, J. S., S. D. Aust, and J. E. Gibson. Lipid peroxidation: A possible mechanism for paraquat toxicity. *Res. Commun. Chem. Pathol. Pharmacol.* 11:31–38 (1975).

18 Main, A. R. Cholinesterase inhibitors. In E. Hodgson and F. E. Guthrie (eds.), *Introduction to Biochemical Toxicology*, pp. 193–223. New York: Elsevier (1980).

19 Moreland, D. E. Effect of toxicants on oxidative phosphorylation. In: E. Hodgson and F. E. Guthrie (eds.), *Introduction to Biochemical Toxicology*, pp. 245–260. New York: Elsevier (1980).

Chapter 5

Overview of Molecular Parameters that Relate to Biological Activity in Toxicology

Colin F. Chignell

All substances are poisons; there is none which is not a poison. Only the right dose differentiates between a poison and a remedy.
> Paracelsus (1493–1541)

EARLY CORRELATIONS

The idea that a relationship exists between the chemical structure of a compound and its pharmacological or toxicological properties is not new but stretches back more than a century. Blake suggested as early as 1848 that the biological activity of a salt is due to its basic or acidic component rather than the whole salt (1). He proposed, for example, that the poisonous properties of lead acetate or lead nitrate were due to the lead and not the acidic components of these salts. This revolutionary idea is all the more significant when one realizes that it was not until 1884 that Arrhenius introduced his theory of the electrolytic dissociation of salts.

In 1858 the Russian chemist and composer Borodin (2) wrote in his dissertation as follows: "By comparing poisonous substances with each other one came to realize that their toxicological properties and chemical makeup are closely related. The first thing to be noted was the fact that many substances consisting of the same element or taking part in similar reactions also exert similar actions in the organism."

Crum Brown and Fraser published a paper in 1869 in which they reported that when several alkaloids (e.g., atropine, strychnine) were quaternized with methyl iodide they lost their characteristic pharmacological properties and acquired instead the muscle-relaxant powers of tubocurarine, a drug known to act at the neuromuscular junction (3). These authors wrote: "There can be no reasonable doubt that a relation exists between the physiological action of a substance and its chemical composition and constitution" (3). Langley (4) was the first to propose that drugs act on specific components in the body. After studying the opposing actions of pilocarpine and atropine on the flow of saliva in the cat Langley wrote in 1878: "We may, I think, without much rashness assume that there is some substance or substances in the nerve endings or gland cells with which both atropine and pilocarpine are capable of forming compounds. On this assumption then, the atropine or pilocarpine compounds are formed according to some law of which their relative mass and chemical affinity for the substance are factors" (4).

The beginning of the twentieth century marked a dichotomy of approach to structure-activity relationships. One school of thought continued to pursue the idea that chemical constitution was the basis for understanding the biological activity of compounds. Ehrlich coined the word "receptor" for chemical groups in the body that elicit a given biological response by combining with complementary groups of drugs or chemical agents (5). He proposed, for example, that the mercapto group was the arsenic receptor in trypanosomes and that blockade of this receptor by arsenic results in the death of these organisms. The ideas of Ehrlich laid the foundation for many of the subsequent developments in pharmacology, immunochemistry, biochemistry, and toxicology. The structure-activity studies of Landsteiner on the serological specificity of stereoisomers of tartaric acid (6) and the work of Clark on pilocarpine and acetylcholinesterase (7) provide later examples of Ehrlich's original receptor concept.

At the same time that Ehrlich was developing his concept of the receptor, other workers began to focus attention on the importance of the physical properties of organic compounds in predicting their biological activities. In a treatise entitled "Lipid Theory of Cellular Depression," Meyer proposed that chemically inert substances of widely different molecular structures exert their depressant effect on those cells, e.g., those found in the central nervous system, that are rich in lipids (8). This idea was also suggested independently 2 years later in 1901 by Overton (9). In his studies, Meyer showed that a correlation existed between the olive oil/water partition coefficients of a group of diverse chemicals and the minimal concentration required to suppress the mobility of tadpoles. Thus, those chemicals that are highly lipophilic cause depression at much lower concentrations than those that are more soluble in the aqueous phase. In 1939 the relationship between lipophilicity and depressant action was restated in thermodynamic terms by Ferguson (10), who pointed out that the chemical potentials of isohypnotic solutions of various hypnotic substances must be the same.

In addition to lipophilicity, many other physicochemical properties may be used to predict the toxic effect of chemicals. More recently, Filov et al. have attempted to correlate 38 physicochemical properties of volatile organic compounds with four toxicity indexes (11). They found that the best correlations were obtained with properties determined at the molecular level, particularly those that related to the energy of interaction of molecules with one another.

The modern approach to quantitative structure-activity relationships, in which both physical and chemical properties of molecules are used to predict their biological activities, has its origin in the pioneering work of Hansch and his colleagues (12-14). For a more detailed discussion of the Hansch approach, see Dunn, Chapter 6, this volume.

MOLECULAR PARAMETERS IN QUANTITATIVE STRUCTURE-ACTIVITY RELATIONSHIPS

Hydrophobicity

Before discussing the importance of hydrophobicity (lipophilicity) in predicting biological activity it is essential to understand precisely what is meant by this term. The term "hydrophobic interaction" generally refers to the tendency of the nonpolar portions of molecules or ions to associate in aqueous solution (15). It is important to realize that the peculiar structural properties of water itself are responsible for this tendency. In ice, water usually takes the form of a hexagonal lattice. When solute molecules are introduced, the water molecules may take up a variety of other orientations, including the pentagonal dodecahedral arrangement in inert gas hydrates and the heptakaidecahedral configuration in the t-butylamine clathrate hydrate. While the structure of liquid water is still a matter of conjecture, it seems likely that it retains at least some "icelike" structure. Aqueous solutions of apolar molecules are characterized by a negative excess entropy ($T\Delta S$) of solution. Dissolution of an apolar molecule in water is thus accompanied by some process in which motional freedom is reduced and the degree of structure is increased. Spectroscopic studies confirm that hydrophobic solutes hinder the rotational motion of water and enhance the degree of hydrogen-bonding between water molecules. The association of two apolar solute molecules can be thought of as a partial reversal of the thermodynamically unfavorable process of solution. As a result of this interaction, some of the entropy loss is recovered, with the consequent partial release of structured hydration water. However, when the concentration dependence of many of the thermodynamic properties of apolar molecules dissolved in water is examined, this "classic" model is obviously inadequate. Franks (16) has recently suggested that the interaction between apolar molecules in aqueous solution may be stabilized by longer ranging interactions in which the water molecules act like a "cement." An excellent discussion of the role of water in the hydrophobic interaction has recently been provided by Suggett (17).

A large number of hydrophobicity parameters have been used as predictors of biological activity, including partition coefficients, chromatographic coefficients, molecular refractivity, and parachor. Since molar refractivity and parachor also contain steric components they will be discussed later.

In his work, Hansch has employed the octanol/water partition coefficient (P) as a hydrophobicity index. This parameter may be defined as

$$P = \frac{C_{octanol}}{C_{H_2O} (1 - \alpha)}$$

where $C_{octanol}$ and C_{H_2O} are the concentrations in the octanol and aqueous phases, respectively, and α equals the degree of ionization in the aqueous phase. Although many other organic solvents have been employed, octanol has several advantages (18), including the availability of data on a wide variety of compounds. In addition, octanol has a wide measurable range of partition coefficients. Since octanol has a hydroxyl group it will dissolve a small amount of water, which facilitates the dissolution of hydrogen-bonding compounds. From a practical point of view, the ready phase separation of octanol-water mixtures is also an advantage (18). Other solvents that have been employed include oleyl alcohol, *iso*butanol, chloroform, ether, benzene, and carbon tetrachloride. It is of interest to note that it is possible to predict the partition coefficient of a molecule in one solvent from a knowledge of its partition coefficient in another solvent (19).

One very important feature of the partition coefficient is its additive and constitutive nature. Thus the contribution of a single group to the overall hydrophobic character of a molecule can be determined from the partition coefficients of the parent molecule and the corresponding substituted analog. For example, the effect of introducing a methyl group into benzene (19) can be determined from the following relationship:

$$\Pi_{CH_3} = \log P_{toluene} - \log P_{benzene}$$
$$2.69 - 2.13 = 0.56$$

The additive character of log P and Π can be used to predict the partition coefficient a complex molecule, such as diethylstilbestrol (19), from a knowledge of the contributions made by each of the groups present in the molecule. This approach can be used for molecules that are either very lipophilic, e.g., tetrachlorodibenzodioxin or very hydrophilic, e.g., dimethyltubocurarine (18).

As might be expected, the hydrophobic parameters Π and log P are good predictors of simple *in vitro* interactions in which hydrophobic interactions are known to be important (19). Scholtan has studied the binding of a wide variety of drugs, e.g., sulfonamides, tetracyclines, penicillins, to plasma albumin and has found a good correlation between Π and the free energy of binding (20). However, when attempts are made to relate solvent partition coefficients to *in vivo* biological activity, nonlinear relationships are often found (18, 19). Thus, the activity of nitroimidazoles against *Trichomonas foetus* in mice is related to log P in a parabolic fashion (21). Hansch has pointed out that *in vivo* toxicity depends not only on simple interactions, such as protein binding and membrane penetration, but also on the rate of transport through successive compartments (21). Hansch has shown that if a model is considered in which a molecule moves through successive compartments alternating between water and a lipid substance, then a parabolic relationship exists between the amount of a substance arriving at its site of action and its partition coefficient. The two limbs of the parabola may have different slopes (bilinear relationship) due to diffusion-controlled rate of membrane penetration. One consequence of the parabolic relationship is that, in a given system, there exists an optimal partition coefficient that allows a molecule to reach its site of action and exert a biological effect. Molecules possessing lower partition coefficients are ineffective since they cannot penetrate membranes. Molecules with high partition coefficients never reach the target site because they are dissolved in the lipid portion of the membrane and never appear at the site of action in a high enough concentration.

Reactions involving enzyme inhibition can be studied in the absence of obscuring side reactions. Under these special conditions another type of nonlinearity may be observed called positional or direction hydrophobicity. Thus, Novinson et al. have found that the inhibition of cyclic adenosine monophosphate (cAMP) phosphodiesterase by 3-substituted-5,7-dilkyl[1,5-a] pyrimidines is dependent on the hydrophobicity of substituents at the 3- and 5- positions, while the 7- position contributes nothing to the interaction (22). Inhibition of bacterial dihydrofolate reductase by 2,4-diaminoquinazolines depends not on overall hydrophobicity but on the hydrophobicity of the 5-position substituents (23). Interestingly enough the antimalarial activity of these compounds *in vivo* obeys a parabolic relationship.

Polar or Electronic Parameters

The most popular electronic parameter for predicting the biological activity of molecules is the Hammett sigma (σ) value (24–26). Hammett measured the ionization constants for a series of *meta-* or *para*-subtituted benzoic acids and defined a constant (σ_x) for a given substituent as follows:

$$\sigma_x = \log \frac{K_x}{K_h}$$

where K_x and K_h are the ionization constants for the substituted and unsubstituted benzoic acid, respectively. The Hammett sigma values for *para*-substituents range from −0.20 for *tert*-butyl group (electron releasing) to +0.88 for the trimethylammonium moiety. In 1953 Taft determined a similar set of values for aliphatic systems based on acetic acid (27). Since that time a number of modified Hammett sigma values have been proposed to describe a variety of different chemical reactions (25, 26).

Ormerod was the first to use Hammett constants to explain substituent effects on the rate of hydrolysis of benzoylcholine esters by acetylcholinesterase (28). Hansen (29) showed that a relationship existed between the toxicities of substituted benzoic acids to mosquito larvae and the Hammett sigma values of the substituents. However, Hansch (14) has pointed out that an even better relationship is obtained by considering only the lipophilicity of these compounds. Metcalfe and Fukuto (30) found that the cholinesterase-inhibiting effects of phenyldiethylphosphates correlate well with the sigma values of the different substituents.

Steric Parameters

Steric parameters have been found to be extremely important in the prediction of biological activity. Taft (25, 26, 31, 32) studied the effect of different substituents on the acid hydrolysis of esters of aliphatic acids:

$$XCOOR' \xrightarrow[\text{H}^+]{\text{H}_2\text{O}} XCOOH + R'\,OH$$

He defined a steric parameter (E_s) using the following relationship:

$$\delta E_s = \log \frac{K_x}{K_o}$$

where K_x and K_o are the rate constants for hydrolysis of the substituted and unsubstituted ester, respectively, and δ is a constant for the given system under study. For the acid hydrolysis of esters $\delta = 1.00$ and methyl was chosen as the reference substituent, thus

$$E_s, CH_3 = 0.000$$

In formulating this approach Taft ignored the polar and resonance effects of the substituents since they are expected to be negligible based on a knowledge of the transition state

$$
\begin{array}{c}
\text{H} \\
| \\
\text{O } \delta^{+} \\
\| \\
\| \\
\| \\
\text{X--C--OR}' \\
| \\
| \\
\delta^{+} \text{ OH}_2
\end{array}
$$

Electron-donating groups assist initial protonation of the carbalkoxy group (*vide supra*) but they inhibit subsequent nucleophilic attack by water. Taft steric constants (E_s) range from $+1.25$ for H to -2.43 for $(C_2H_5)_3C$, with the more bulky groups having negative values.

In general the Taft steric parameter is used in conjunction with other parameters to predict biological activity. For example, Fukuto (33) studied the inhibition of fly brain cholinesterase by methyl-2,4,5-trichlorophenyl-*N*-alkyl-phosphoramidates and found that while the activity of analogs containing simple *N*-alkyl substituents, e.g., CH_3, C_2H_5, were predicted well by their Hammett sigma parameters, analogs containing bulky groups, e.g., *iso*propyl and *tert*-butyl, showed marked deviations. A much better correlation was obtained when Taft E_s parameters were also considered.

Verloop and co-workers have introduced "sterimol" constants in an attempt to quantitate the overall shapes of molecules and their substituents. This approach arose from a consideration of the fit of a molecule at its receptor site. The length (L) of the substrate along its longest axis will obviously affect binding depending on the shape of the receptor site. The width of a given substituent (perpendicular to the L-axis) may also be important if the receptor is considered as a three-dimensional structure. Verloop and co-workers (34) defined four parameters (B_1-B_4) to measure the thickness of a given substituent along its main axis. These substituent parameters have two main advantages, namely they describe more adequately nonsymmetrical substituents and emphasize the vectoral character of steric effects while at the same time offering additional information on the actual conformation of the receptor surface. Sterimol constants have now been determined for approximately 240 different substituents (34). The correlative power of the sterimol parameters may be illustrated by studies of the *in vitro* microsomal *para*-hydroxylation of substituted anilines of the type

$$
R_1 \text{—}\bigcirc\text{—NHR}_2
$$

Hansch, in his original analysis employing the Taft E_s parameter, excluded the *meta*-OCH_3 aniline because it caused a considerable deterioration in the correlation (35). However Motoc (36) has reanalyzed the data using the appropriate sterimol constants and found a good correlation for all of the analogs, including the *meta*-OCH₃ aniline.

In an attempt to provide a quantitative formulation for Ruzicka's (37) stereochemical theory of olfaction, Amoore introduced a steric parameter, $\overline{\Delta}$ (38). This parameter was calculated from the silhouettes (front, top, right) of a molecule by tracing out radii from the weight center. While the Amoore parameter has found application in olfaction structure-activity studies, it has not been used extensively in other biological situations.

Indicator variables were introduced into structure-activity studies by Bruice et al. (39), and their use was substantiated by Free and Wilson (40). This approach attempts to assign structural characteristics of the molecule under study to biological activity. The assumption is that each time a substituent group appears in the same position it makes a constant contribution to the biological activity of the molecule.

Molar refractivity (MR) can also be used as a steric parameter instead of or together with the Taft parameter, E_s. Molar refractivity is defined by the Lorentz-Lorentz equation:

$$MR = \frac{n^2 - 1}{n^2 + 2} \cdot \frac{MW}{d}$$

where n is the refractive index, MW is the molecular weight, and d is density. Like Π and log P, molar refractivity is an additive parameter. However, molar refractivity contains both a dielectric component, measured by London dispersion forces, as well as one of steric repulsion. Molar refractivity is linearly related to both Π and van der Waals volume (*vide infra*) and thus care must be taken when it is used in correlations containing other molecular parameters. Hansch and Moser have employed molar refractivity in conjunction with Π and σ to quantitate the binding of substituted phenylsuccinates to an antibody raised against 3-azopyridine (41).

The van der Waals volume of a substituent may be calculated by numerical integration (Monte Carlo technique) of its envelope (41). The van der Waals volume can also be obtained from the molar refractivity. Yamamoto (42) studied the effect of N-acylamido substituents on the hydrolysis of several p-nitrophenyl 2-acylamino-2-deoxy-β-D-glucopyranosides by Taka-N-acetyl-β-D-glucosaminidase. He found a good correlation between the relative rate of hydrolysis and the van der Waals volume of the substituents. The correlation was improved by including Π and σ constants.

Parachor (P) may be regarded as the molecular volume of a liquid of a surface tension equal to unity and is defined by

$$P = MW \cdot d^{-1} \cdot \gamma^{1/4}$$

where γ = surface tension, MW = molecular weight, and d = density. Like Π and molar refractivity, the parachor is a truly additive and constitutive property of a molecule and may be expressed as a sum of the atomic parachors. Ahmad et al. (43) have shown that there is a good correlation between parachor and biological activity for three classes of drugs: the thyromimetic activity of 3'-substituted thyroxine analogs, the blood clotting inhibitory activity of 5-substituted pentylamines, and the local anesthetic activity of the paracaines. Correlations comparable to Π were obtained for six more classes of drugs.

Reduction Potential

The reduction potential of a compound is a measure of the ease of addition of one or more electrons to form a reduced product or products. For example, aromatic nitro compounds undergo a series of reductions (44) that may eventually lead to the formation of the corresponding amine:

$$\text{R-NO}_2 \xrightarrow{e^-} \text{R}\overset{\centerdot}{\text{N}}\text{O}_2^- \xrightarrow[4\text{H}^+]{3e^-} \text{R-NHOH} \xrightarrow[2\text{H}^+]{2e^-} \text{R-NH}_2$$

The first step is a one-electron reduction to the corresponding nitro anion radical. Under aerobic conditions the radical may react with oxygen to yield superoxide $(\text{O}_2 \overset{\centerdot}{{}^-})$ and regenerate the parent nitrocompound:

$$\text{R}\overset{\centerdot}{\text{N}}\text{O}_2^- + \text{O}_2 \longrightarrow \text{RNO}_2 + \text{O}_2 \overset{\centerdot}{{}^-}$$

Thus it is not surprising that Adams and co-workers have found that the aerobic toxicity of a series of nitroaromatic compounds (phenyl, imidazole, furan) correlates well with their respective reduction potentials (45). The test system used by these workers was the Chinese hamster V79 cells grown in culture. Not only did they find that the more easily reduced nitro compounds are more toxic but also that unrelated quinones, which on reduction also form superoxide, showed an identical relationship.

Bond-Dissociation Energy

Carbon tetrachloride is a potent hepatotoxin. In 1961 Butler proposed (46) that the trichloromethyl radical, formed by homolytic cleavage, is the proximate toxic species:

$$\text{CCl}_4 \longrightarrow \text{Cl}^{\centerdot} + \text{CCl}_3^{\centerdot}$$

Although the radical does bind covalently to protein and lipid, it now seems probable that its toxic effect is due to the initiation of lipid peroxidation by abstraction of a methylene hydrogen atom from polyunsaturated fatty acids (47). The hepatotoxicities of four halogenated methanes and their corresponding bond-dissociation energies are shown in Table 1. It can be clearly seen that the easier it is to cause homolytic bond fission the more toxic the halogenated methane. More recent evidence suggests (44) that carbon tetrachloride does not undergo homolytic cleavage but rather is reductively cleaved:

$$CCl_4 \xrightarrow{\;e\;} Cl^- + \overset{\cdot}{C}Cl_3$$

If this is the case, then toxicity should be related to the reduction potential. The data in Table 1 (47–50) for carbon tetrachloride and chloroform suggest that such a relationship may indeed exist.

Other Molecular Parameters

In addition to those already discussed there are many other molecular parameters that have been used to correlate structure with biological activity. Hansch and co-workers have found (51) that hydrogen bonding is important in the anesthetic potency of gases. Hydrogen bonding is also a factor in the antiallergic activity of 2-phenyl-8-azapurin-6-ones (52). A relationship exists between odor and infrared frequencies for homologs of benzaldehyde and nitrobenzene (53). Hopfinger and Battershell (54) have demonstrated a correlation between the conformation of phenothrin analogs and their insecticidal activity. McKinney and co-workers (55, 56) have related the polarizability of chlorinated biphenyls to their toxicity. Cohen et al. have tentatively shown a dependence of toxicity on molecular symmetry for a

Table 1   Hepatotoxicity of Halogenated Methanes

Bond	Bond dissociation energy[*] (kcal mol^{-1})	Half peak potential[†] (volts)	Relative hepatotoxicity[§]
CCl$_3$-Br	49	NA[‡]	++++
CCl$_3$-Cl	68	−1.33	+++
CCl$_3$-H	90	NA[‡]	++
CHCl$_2$-Cl	NA	−1.90	++
CCl$_3$-F	102	NA[‡]	+

[*]Data from Slater (47).
[†]Data from Lambert et al. (50).
[‡]Data not available.
[§]Data from Slater (47), Kochi et al. (48), and Reynolds (49).

diverse group of chemicals (57). Molecular orbital calculations of electron densities for polycyclic aromatic hydrocarbons and their oxidative metabolites have provided additional insights in their mechanisms of toxicity (58).

In this chapter it has been possible to present only an overview of the molecular parameters that can be used to predict toxicity. More extensive discussions of this extremely important topic are available (59-64).

REFERENCES

1 Blake, J. *Am. J. Med. Sci.* 15:63 (1848).
2 Borodin, A. Concerning the analogy between arsenic and phosphoric acids in chemical and toxicological respects. Dissertation, St. Petersburg (1858).
3 Crum Brown, A., and T. Fraser. On the connection between chemical constitution and physiological action. *Trans. R. Soc. Edinburgh* 25:151-160 (1869).
4 Langley, J. N. On the physiology of the salivary secretion. *J. Physiol.* 1:339-369 (1878).
5 Ehrlich, P., and J. Morgenroth. In P. Ehrlich (ed.), *Studies in Immunity*, 2nd ed., pp. 23, 24, 47. New York: Wiley (1910).
6 Landsteiner, K., and J. van der Scheer. Serological differentiation of steric isomers (antigens containing tartaric acids). *J. Exp. Med.* 50:407-417 (1929).
7 Clark, A. J. In A. Heffler and W. Heubner (eds.), *Handbuch der experimentellen Pharmakologie*, Erganz 4, 63. Berlin: Springer (1937).
8 Meyer, H. Lipoidtheorie der Narkose. *Arch. Exp. Pathol. Pharmakol.* 42:109 (1899).
9 Overton, E. Studien über die Narkosen, Jena, Gustav Fischer, (1901).
10 Ferguson, J. Chemical potentials as indexes of toxicity. *Proc. R. Soc. B.* 127:387-397 (1939).
11 Filov, V. A., A. A. Golubev, E. I. Liublina, and N. A. Tolkontsev. *Quantitative Toxicology (Selective Topics)*, pp. 312-360, translated by V. E. Tatarchenko. New York: Wiley-Interscience (1973).
12 Hansch, C., and T. Fujita. Rho, sigma and pi analysis-correlations of biological activity and chemical structure. *J. Am. Chem. Soc.* 86:1616-1626 (1964).
13 Valkenburg, W. V. (ed.): Biological correlations- The Hansch Approach. *Adv. Chem.*, vol. 114 (1970).
14 Hansch, C. On the predictive value of QSAR. In J. A. Keverling Buisman (ed.), *Biological Activity and Chemical Structure*, vol. 2, pp. 47-61. Amsterdam: Elsevier (1977).
15 Tanford, C.A. *The Hydrophobic Effect*. New York: Wiley Interscience (1973).
16 Franks, F. *Water—A Comprehensive Treatise*, vol. 1, ch. 14. New York: Plenum Press (1975).
17 Suggett, A. Hydrophobic interactions and water structure. J. A. Keverling Buisman (ed.), *Biological Activity and Chemical Structure*, vol. 2, pp. 95-105. Amsterdam: Elsevier (1977).

18 Leo, A. J. Hansch analysis and the use of partition coefficients. In I. M. Asher and C. Zervox (eds.), *Structure Correlates of Carcinogenesis and Mutagenesis, Proceedings of the Second FDA Office of Science Summer Symposium*, pp. 55–62, (1977).

19 Hansch, C. Quantitative structure-activity relationships in drug design. In E. J. Ariens (ed.), *Drug Design*, vol. 1, pp. 271–342. New York: Academic Press (1971).

20 Scholtan, W. The hydrophobic binding of drugs to human albumin and ribonucleic acid. *Arzeim.-Forsch.* 18:505–517 (1968).

21 Wardman, P., E. D. Clarke, I. R. Flockhart, and R. G. Wallace. The rationale for the development of improved hypoxic cell radiosensitizers. *Br. J. Cancer* 37(suppl. III):2–5 (1978).

22 Novinson, T., J. P. Miller, M. Scholten, R. K. Robins, L. N. Simon, and D. E. O'Brien. Adenosine cyclic $3'$, $5'$-monophosphate phosphodiesterase inhibitors. 2. 3-Substituted-5, 7-dialkylpyrazolo[1,5-a] pyrimidines. *J. Med. Chem.* 18:460–464 (1975).

23 Hansch, C., J. Y. Fukunaga, and Y. C. Jow. Quantitative structure-activity relationships of antimalarial and dihydrofolate reductase inhibition by quinazolines and 5-substituted benzyl-2,4-aminopyrimidines. *J. Med. Chem.* 20:96-102 (1977).

24 Hammett, L. P. Effect of structure on the reactions of organic compounds. *Chem. Rev.* 17:125–139 (1935).

25 Charton, M. Linear free energy relationships. Part 1. An entry. *Chemtech.*, pp. 502–511, (Aug., 1974).

26 Charton, M. Linear free energy relationships. Part 2. Proximity effects. *Chemtech.*, pp. 246–255 (Apr, 1975).

27 Taft, R. W. Polar and steric constants for aliphatic and *o*-benzoate groups from rates of esterification and hydrolysis. *J. Am. Chem. Soc.* 75:4231 (1953).

28 Ormerod, W. E. Hydrolysis of benzoylcholine derivatives by cholinesterase in serum. *Biochem. J.* 54:701–709 (1953).

29 Hansen, O. R. Hammett series with biological activity. *Acta Chem. Scand.* 16:1593–1600 (1962).

30 Metcalf, R. L., and T. R. Fukuto. *m*-Sulfurpentafluorophenyl diethylphosphate and *m*-sulfurpentafluorophenyl *N*-methylcarbamate as insecticides and anticholinesterases. *J. Econ. Entomol.* 55:340–341 (1962).

31 Balaban, A. T., A. Chiriac, I. Motoc, and Z. Simon. *Steric Fit in Quantitative Structure-Activity Relations*. Berlin: Springer-Verlag (1980).

32 Taft, R. W. In M. S. Newnan (ed.), *Steric Effects in Organic Chemistry*, chap. 3. New York: Wiley (1956).

33 Fukuto, T. R. Physico-organic chemical approach to the mode of action of organophosphorus insectides. *Residue. Rev.* 25:327–332 (1969).

34 Verloop, A., W. Hoogenstraaten, and J. Tipker. Development and application of new steric parameters in drug design. In E. J. Ariëns (ed.), *Drug Design*, vol. II, pp. 165–207 (1976).

35 Hansch, C. Quantitative relationships between lipophilic character and drug metabolism. *Drug Metab. Rev.* 1:1–14 (1972).

36 Motoc, I. Steric and other structural parameters of QSAR. In A. T. Balaban, A. Chiriac, I. Motoc, and Z. Simon, *Steric Fit in Quantitative Structure-Activity Relations*, p. 16. Berlin: Springer-Verlag (1980).

37 Ruzicka, L. *Chem. Ztg.* 44:129 (1920).

38 Amoore, J. E. Stereochemical theory of olfaction. *Ann. N.Y. Acad. Sci.* 116:457–467 (1964).

39 Bruice, T. C., N. Kharasch, and R. J. Winzler. A correlation of thyroxine-like activity and chemical structure. *Arch. Biochem. Biophys.* 52:305–317 (1956).

40 Free, S. M., and J. W. Wilson. A mathematical contribution to structure-activity studies. *J. Med. Chem.* 1:395–399 (1964).

41 Motoc, I. Steric and other structural parameters for QSAR. In A. T. Balaban, A. Chiriac, I. Motoc, and Z. Simon, *Steric Fit in Quantitative Structure-Activity Relations*, p. 12. Berlin: Springer-Verlag (1980).

42 Yamamoto, K. A quantitative approach to the evaluation of 2-acetamide substituent effects on the hydrolysis by Taka-N-acetyl-β-D-glucosaminidase. *J. Biochem. (Tokyo)* 76:385–390 (1974).

43 Ahmad, P., C. A. Fyfe, and A. Mellors. Parachors in drug design. *Biochem. Pharmacol.* 24:1103–1109 (1975).

44 Mason, R. P. Free radical metabolites of foreign compounds and their toxicological significance. In E. Hodgson, J. R. Bend, and R. Philpot (eds.), *Reviews in Biochemical Toxicology*, pp. 151–200. Amsterdam: Elsevier North Holland (1979).

45 Adams, G. E., E. D. Clarke, R. S. Jacobs, I. J. Stratford, R. G. Wallace, P. Wardman, and M. E. Watts. Mammalian cell toxicity of nitrocompounds: Dependence upon reduction potential. *Biochem. Biophys. Res. Commun.* 72:824–829 (1976).

46 Butler, T. C. Reduction of carbon tetrachloride *in vivo* and carbon tetrachloride and chloroform *in vitro* by tissues and tissue constituents. *J. Pharmacol. Exp. Ther.* 134:311–319 (1961).

47 Slater, T. F. *Free Radical Mechanisms in Tissue Injury*, ch. 9. London: Pion (1972).

48 Kochi, R. R., E. A. Glende, and R. O. Recknagel. Hepatotoxicity of bromotrichloromethane-bond dissociation energy and lipoperoxidation. *Biochem. Pharmacol.* 23:2907–2915 (1974).

49 Reynolds, E. S. Comparison of early injury to liver endoplasmic reticulum by halomethanes, hexachloroethane, benzene, tolune, bromobenzene, ethionine, thioacetamide and dimethylnitrosamine. *Biochem. Pharmacol.* 21:2555–2561 (1972).

50 Lambert, F. L., B. L. Hasslinger, and R. N. Franz. The total reduction of CCl_4 at the glassy electrode. *J. Electrochem. Soc.* 122:737–739 (1975).

51 Hansch, C., C. Vittori, C. Silipo, and P. Y. C. Jow. Partition coefficient and the structure-activity relationship of the anesthetic gases. *J. Med. Chem.* 18:546–548 (1975).

52 Broughton, B. J., P. Chaplen, P. Knowles, E. Lunt, S. M. Marshall, D. L. Pain, and K. R. H. Wooldridge. Antiallergic activity of 2-phenyl-8-azapurin-6-ones. *J. Med. Chem.* 18:1117–1121 (1975).

53 Wright, R. H., and A. Robson. Basis of odour specificity: Homologues of benzaldehyde and nitrobenzene. *Nature* 222:290–291 (1969).

54 Hopfinger, A. J., and R. D. Battershell. Conformational studies of phenothrin analogs and implications on insecticidal activity. In H. Geissbuehler (ed.), *Adv. Pestic. Sci. Plenary Lect. Symp. Pop. Int. Congr. Pestic. Chem. 4th*, pp. 196–200. Oxford, England: Pergamon (1978).

55 McKinney, J. D., and P. Singh. Structure-activity relationships in halogenated biophenyls: Unifying hypothesis for structural specificity. *Chem.-Biol. Interact.* (in press).

56 Albro, P. W., and J. McKinney. The relationship between polarizability of polychlorinated biphenyls and their induction of mixed function oxidase activity. *Chem.-Biol. Interact* 34:373–378 (1981).

57 Cohen, J. L., W. Lee, and E. J. Lien. Dependence of toxicity on molecular structure group theory analysis. *J. Pharm. Sci.* 63:1068–1072 (1974).

58 Loew, G., J. Phillips, J. Wong, L. Hjelmeland, and G. Pack. Quantum chemical studies on the metabolism of polycyclic aromatic hydrocarbons: Bay region reactivity as a criterion for carcinogenic potency. *Cancer Biochem. Biophys.* 2:113–122 (1978).

59 Asher, I. M., and C. Zervos (eds.). Structure correlates of carcinogenesis and mutagenesis. In *Proceedings of the Second FDA Office of Science Summer Symposium* (1977).

60 McKinney, J. D. (ed.). *Environmental Health Chemistry. The Chemistry of Environmental Agents as Potential Human Hazards.* Ann Arbor, MI: Ann Arbor Science (1981).

61 Waters, D. B. (ed.). *Safe Handling of Chemical Carcinogens, Mutagens, Teratogens and Highly Toxic Substances*, vol. 2. Ann Arbor, MI: Ann Arbor Science (1980).

62 Buisman, J. A. K. (ed.): *Biological Activity and Chemical Structure.* Amsterdam: Elsevier (1977).

63 Albert, A. *Selective Toxicity. The Physicochemical Basis of Therapy.* London: Chapman and Hall (1979).

64 Cramer, R. D. Quantitative drug design. *Ann. Rep. Med. Chem.* 11:301–310 (1976).

Part Three

Correlative Methods

Studies of Relationships between Structural Properties and Biological Activity by Hansch Analysis

Yvonne C. Martin

The Hansch or linear free energy (LFER) method of investigating quantitative structure-activity relationships (QSAR) is widely used by many types of scientists. It is especially well liked by those who are not mathematically inclined because it is conceptually simple and easy to apply to one's data. The fundamental hypothesis behind the method is that there is some mathematical relationship between the physicochemical and biological properties of molecules. It quantitates and extends to several properties the practice of plotting one variable, such as log (LD_{50}) against another, such as pK_a. This quantitation and extension to several properties has proved to be worth the effort (1). Some examples of the application to toxic effects are found in the literature (2-5). A comment on the limitations of the predictability of toxicity has also been published (6).

This chapter will serve as a general introduction to the subject. It will be illustrated with the data presented in Table 1 on the hemolytic activity of N-alkyl piperidines (7). The reader is referred to more lengthy publications for details of how to actually perform such an analysis (8, 9), recent advances in

Table 1   Hemolytic Activity of *N*-Alkyl Piperidines

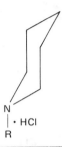

N
| · HCl
R

| R | log *P* | log (1/*C*) | |
		obs.	calc.
Heptyl	0.27	1.61	1.56
Octyl	0.77	1.97	2.04
Nonyl	1.27	2.55	2.53
Decyl	1.77	3.02	3.01
Undecyl	2.27	3.40	3.47
Dodecyl	2.77	3.92	3.87
Tridecyl	3.27	4.18	4.17
Tetradecyl	3.77	4.38	4.32
Pentadecyl	4.27	4.28	4.33
Hexadecyl	4.77	4.12	4.20
Heptadecyl	5.27	3.97	3.92

From Hansch and Glave (7).

the methodology and parameters (10–12), experiences with the method in industry (13), and other reviews (1, 14–20).

BASIS AND UNDERLYING ASSUMPTIONS
OF THE APPROACH

The method is based on three basic assumptions. The first is that one can quantitate the molecular properties that determine the biological activity of a molecule. These molecular properties are assumed to be physicochemical. They are typically a combination of measured and calculated values; for example, the octanol-water partition coefficient and the pK_a of the molecules might be used. Although the truth of this assumption and the choice of physicochemical properties seems unquestionable to many, it is contrary to the philosophy of those who consider small molecule-large molecule inter-actions, be they drug-receptor or substrate-enzyme interactions, to be governed solely by a lock-and-key type of spatial fit. In the latter terms, the

Hansch methodology may be thought to quantitate the effect of a variable substituent positioned at noncritical portions of the molecule on the reactivity of the critical or pharmacophore portion of the molecule.

The historical precedent for the assumption that one can accurately describe a molecule numerically is found in the Hammett equation. Fits to the Hammett equation showed that the relative effect of various remote substituents on the rate or equilibrium constant of an organic reaction is often a linear function of the effect of these substituents on the pK_a of benzoic acid. In other words, the substituent effect on pK_a is a model for the substituent effect on the other chemical reactions. It was a logical extension to assume that substituent effects in biological reactions might be parallel to those in chemical reactions.

The second assumption in the Hansch methodology is that one can measure the appropriate biological response in a quantitative fashion. Implicit in the method is the notion that all members of the series have the same mode of action, i.e., they interact with the same set of receptors.

The third assumption is that one can mathematically describe the relationship between the chemical and biological properties of the molecules. For a linear relationship the mathematics are straightforward (8); for nonlinear cases they can be complex and obscure (9). If one can mathematically investigate the proposed relationships, the outcome is that the method is quantitative and gives quantitative predictions. If one makes the usual statistical assumptions then the relationships and predictions have the usual statistical features as well. For example, this means that a predicted activity is a number with associated 95 percent confidence limits. The quantitative aspect of the predictions makes it possible to design compounds that will evaluate the relative predictive merits of several possible QSAR relationships of one data set.

From the assumptions it can be seen that the Hansch method is most suitable for a data set that has the following characteristics: (a) the compounds should be structural analogs that are identical in the structure of the pharmacophore, (b) all analogs should produce their biological effect by interacting with the same biological receptor(s), (c) it should be possible to derive reliable quantitative measures of the physical properties of the analogs, and (d) there should be enough compounds in the set that one can statistically examine a number of properties. It will be shown later that two additional characteristics of the data set are also important: (a) the variation in potency between different analogs should be substantially larger than the error in measuring potency, and (b) the relevant physicochemical properties should be varied properly within the series (21).

TYPE OF BIOLOGICAL DATA NECESSARY

It is understood that the biological data must be relevant. The predictions based on a QSAR will be only as relevant to the cure of a disease or prevention of toxic effects as are the data on which the predictions are based.

Since the LFER method is based on the assumption of parallelism between the substituent effect on rate or equilibrium constants, an attempt should be made to transform the biological response to a similar parameter (8). Consequently, the biological parameter is typically based on a dose-response curve, not just a single point determination. This also allows one a chance to detect differences in mechanism between analogs, to compare analogs of widely different potency, and to investigate structural effects on affinity and maximum effect separately. The second typical requirement for the LFER analysis is that the potency be converted into a molar value. Because of the assumption of parallelism of substituent effects on free energies, the logarithm of these concentrations is used. Accordingly, the Hansch equation is typically written with the biological data expressed as log $(1/C)$ values in which C is the molar concentration of the analog required to produce some specified level of biological response, such as 50 percent lethality.

The usual mathematical technique in Hansch analysis is regression analysis. This requires that the data be continuous, i.e., all-or-none, or incremental responses cannot be treated with this method. They will be discussed in chapter 7.

How precisely should the log $(1/C)$ value be measured? In essence, after a typical least squares fit, regression analysis portions the sum of squares of deviation of log $(1/C_i)$ from the mean log $(1/C)$ (SS_{mean}) into the sum of squares due to the model (SS_{reg}), i.e., that that can be attributed to differences in physicochemical properties, and that due to error (SS_{error}). The R^2 statistic is defined by Eq. 1:

$$R^2 = \frac{SS_{reg}}{SS_{mean}} = \frac{SS_{mean} - SS_{error}}{SS_{mean}} \tag{1}$$

The error term is fixed by the precision of the biological test; if all analogs are approximately equal in potency, then the SS_{mean} will be close in value to SS_{error} and the corresponding R^2 will be small. On the other hand, if there is a wide range in potency within the series, then the SS_{mean} will be large compared to SS_{error} and the R^2 will be large. Although the standard deviation from the fit may be the same in such different cases, that with a larger R^2 will describe more of the universe of compounds. Accordingly, for a QSAR to be of predictive value it is just as important to measure the relative potency of comparatively inactive analogs as it is to work on increasing the precision of estimate of the most potent analogs.

The SS_{mean} for the data in Table 1 is 9.57, whereas that from the fit to be reported later is 0.03. Hence:

$$R^2 = \frac{9.57 - 0.03}{9.57} = 0.997 \tag{2}$$

SELECTION AND CALCULATION
OF PHYSICOCHEMICAL PARAMETERS

The objective is to derive quantitative measures of the effects of substituents on the major types of noncovalent interactions; accordingly, log P parameterizes the substituent effect on hydrophobic interactions, pK_a parameterizes the substituent effect on some types of electronic interactions, the Taft E_s value and related quantities parameterize the substituent effect on steric hindrance, and molar refractivity parameterizes the substituent effect on dispersion or van der Waal's interactions. A whole book has been devoted to this topic (22). It includes a discussion of the various parameters and an extensive tabulation of them. The subject has been reviewed by others (11), and discussion and examples fill another book (10).

Hydrophobic Effect of Substituents

It has long been recognized that the tendency of compounds to partition into nonaqueous phases is a characteristic that is important to its biological activity. Both compounds that have too little a tendency to partition into nonaqueous phases and those that have too great a tendency to partition into nonaqueous phases are likely to have little biological activity. They simply deposit in only one phase of the biological system.

The partition coefficient is defined as the equilibrium ratio of the concentration of the compound in the nonaqueous phase to that in the aqueous phase. The usual partition coefficient for QSAR work is that between 1-octanol and water (22). In order to keep hydrophobic and ionization equilibria separate (23), the log P value is defined as the equilibrium constant for the neutral form in both phases:

$$P = \frac{C_{\text{octanol}}}{C_{H_2O} \, (1 - \alpha)} \tag{3}$$

in which P is the true partition coefficient, α is the degree of ionization, and C refers to the total concentration of the compound in the indicated phase. Provided one has an analytical method for the compound and its log P is neither extremely high nor low, it is relatively straightforward to measure the log P. Partition coefficients may also be established by chromatography, either reversed-phase thin layer or reversed-phase high-pressure liquid chromatography (HPLC) (12, 13). These methods are faster than shake flask methods and make fewer purity demands on the compounds.

One of the reasons QSAR has become possible is the demonstration that it is possible to calculate the partition coefficient of log P from values of related compounds. For example, a *meta*-Cl group adds 0.83 to the log P of benzoic acid, 0.86 to that of benzene, 0.76 to that of phenoxyacetic acid, 0.84 to that of benzyl alcohol, and 0.61 to that of nitrobenzene (24). As a result of such observations, the Hansch-Fujita π value was formulated:

$$\pi_X = \log P_{RX} - \log P_{RH} \qquad (4)$$

Although the rules become complex for structurally complex molecules (22, 25), several groups are writing computer programs to make this procedure automatic (26, 27).

Table 1 includes the calculated or measured log P values of the compounds in the example. Only that of the decyl analog was measured; in this case the log P value is of the hydrochloride, that is as measured in 0.01 M HCl. The other values were calculated using the old value of 0.50 per CH_2 group.

In recent years several groups have demonstrated that the *rate* of transfer of a compound from an aqueous to a nonaqueous phase may not be proportional to the ultimate *extent* of transfer or partition coefficient (28-30). That is, the kinetics (rate) and thermodynamics (extent) of partitioning are not linearly correlated. It is not clear how such *in vitro* model systems apply to *in vivo* systems, but at the moment these data cannot be ignored.

Electronic Effects of Substituents

In the introduction it was noted that the classic linear free energy relationships are used by physical organic chemists to correlate the substituent effect on chemical reactivity. The Hammett sigma constant describes the substituent effect on the electron density at a remote center. It is defined by Eq. 5:

$$\sigma_X = \log K_{a_{BX}} - \log K_{a_{BH}} \qquad (5)$$

in which log $K_{a_{BH}}$ is the logarithm of the acid dissociation constant of benzoic acid and log $K_{a_{BX}}$ is the corresponding value of the substituted benzoic acid. Hence σ values come from pK_a values. They have been shown to correlate with pK_a values in many systems, with redox potentials, as well as with rates of esterification of acids, solvolysis of many compounds, alkylation of amines, bromination of acetophenones, polymerization of styrenes, wavelength of ultraviolet (UV) absorption, and nuclear magnetic resonance (NMR) chemical shifts.

Other σ scales have been devised for substituents in an aliphatic system. Additionally, σ constants can be subdivided into the inductive-field and resonance effects of the substituents. The substituent effect on charge-transfer reactions (31, 32) or hydrogen bonding (33) may also be considered. The reader is referred to the book by Hansch and Leo for more information (22).

Another avenue to substituent electronic effects is from quantum chemical calculations on the molecules in question or on models of them (34). For example, the relative antibacterial potency of members of a series of tetracyclines appears to be correlated with the charge on the oxygen atoms (35). At the moment such calculations are time-consuming and expensive to do; however, it is likely that this situation will change in the near future. The problems with such calculations are that they are not necessarily a reliable predictor of measurable physical properties (36) and they yield such a vast array of numbers (37). Presumably, some pattern recognition technique will in the future aid in the reduction of these numbers to fewer meaningful ones. Another approach is to use biological mechanistic data to select a few properties to consider in regression analysis, as has been done with analogs of cephalosporins (38).

Investigation of the effects of substituent changes in electronic effects on changes in potency in a series is complicated by the fact that such changes are often accompanied by changes in pK_a of an ionizable group. As a result the ratio of various species present in the aqueous phases is different for the different compounds. The situation becomes even more complex when one remembers that different aqueous compartments of the body may have different pHs; for example, the gut, blood, and urine are not all the same pH. A further complication is that the drug-receptor interaction may involve the ion, the neutral compound, or both in the same or unequal proportions. The model-based approach to solving this problem has been recently reviewed (9); suffice it to say that the situation can be very complicated and unravelling it may require both good biological and chemical data.

Steric Effects of Substituents

In classic linear free energy analysis, the steric effects of substituents are considered to retard the reaction, i.e., larger substituents reduce the rate or equilibrium constant. For such effects the Taft E_s value has been experimentally determined from the substituent effect on the rate of ester hydrolysis. More recently, Verloop and co-workers have calculated five steric parameters of each substituent: L, the length in the direction of the bond to the parent molecule, and B_1–B_4, the breadth perpendicular to this axis. B_1 is the smallest breadth and B_2–B_4 are measured at $90°$ to $180°$ to it in increasing magnitude. These parameters have been reviewed (22).

Certain aspects of the shape of molecules may be derived from an analysis of the pattern or connections between molecules. Two approaches, connectivity (39) and steric difference (40), have been used with some success. This problem is also partially addressed by the consideration of position-dependent substituent effects discussed below.

It was noted in a previous chapter that the conformational properties of molecules may be important to the determination of activity. To date, only tentative attempts have been made to combine such considerations into QSAR (41). Further exploration of this topic is warranted.

Molar Refractivity (MR) of Substituents

This is an additive property of substituents that parameterizes their tendency to participate in dispersion or van der Waal's interactions. Since it increases in magnitude with increasing numbers of atoms in the group, it is sometimes collinear with steric parameters. Hence, in a regression equation a positive coefficient of MR suggests dispersion bonding, whereas a negative coefficient suggests steric hindrance and that another parameter should be chosen.

All-or-None Effects of Substituents:
Indicator Variables

This type of variable takes on only two values: it is used to indicate the presence or absence of a particular property in a series. For example, an indicator variable might be used to distinguish secondary from tertiary amines in a series or to distinguish an $-O-$ from an $-S-$ bridge between two aromatic rings. Such indicator variables for substructural features of molecules bridge the gap between LFER methods and the Free-Wilson and pattern recognition methods.

Global vs Local Properties of Compounds

An important difference between physical organic chemistry and QSAR is that in physical organic chemistry the reactions are studied in solution and there are very few steric restrictions except at the reaction site. In contrast, when studying molecules in biochemical or whole animal systems one may not know the atoms that interact, and there usually are more steric or spatial constraints on the interaction. Simply put, the active site of an enzyme is much more structurally complicated than is a hydroxide ion. As a consequence, it has become a practice to use position-dependent substituent effects. This means that for a series in which variable substituents are present at several positions, the π, σ, and MR value of the substituent at each position would be considered. In successful cases the regression equation describes a receptor map with, for example, hydrophobic binding at one position, dispersion binding at another, etc. For example, such a method was used to map the dihydrofolate reductase receptor site (42). This approach also allows one to treat stereoisomers in a sensible fashion; the substituents in one orientation with respect to the chiral center would form one set of properties and those in the other would form another (43).

Design of the Series of Analogs

As in any scientific study, in QSAR one will get more information from a study if it is properly planned. In the case of QSAR one is presumably interested in investigating the relationship between biological potency and the hydrophobicity, electronic effects, steric properties, and molar refractivity of the substituents. Clearly, one will get unambiguous answers only if one varies each of these properties widely enough that their effect on potency will be seen above the background variation, if one varies each property independently of all others. Additional increases in efficiency in answering the questions can be realized if there are no compounds with duplicate physical properties (21). Various strategies to accomplish these goals have been suggested (44-47).

CHARACTERISTICS OF REGRESSION ANALYSIS

It was mentioned above that the mainstay of the LFER methodology is the statistical technique of regression analysis to fit the Hansch equation:

$$\log\left(\frac{1}{C_i}\right) = a + b\,\pi_i + c\,\sigma_i + d\,E_{s_i} + e\,MR_i \qquad (6)$$

Details on the subject in this section are found elsewhere (8).

Linear vs Nonlinear Models
and Linear vs Nonlinear Regression

Early in the development of QSAR it was recognized that the relationship between log P and log $(1/C)$ is not linear but rather is nonlinear. The classic solution to this problem is to use a parabolic fit to log P in addition to the linear fits with σ, E_s, and MR:

$$\log\left(\frac{1}{C}\right) = a + b\,\pi_i - c\pi_i^2 + \ldots \qquad (7)$$

A parabola has a continuously changing slope symmetric around the optimum. As early as 1970 it was suggested that the relationship between log $(1/C)$ and log P may not be parabolic but rather that the slope at low log P may be different from that at high log P, and that indeed the slope at high log P may be zero (48). This subject has been reviewed recently (12). The consequence is that one may choose to fit a compartment model-based equation of the type:

$$\log\left(\frac{1}{C_i}\right) = X - \log\left(1 + cP_i^d + \frac{1}{aP_i^b}\right) + \ldots \tag{8}$$

or the bilinear equation (49):

$$\log\left(\frac{1}{C_i}\right) = a + b \log P_i - c \log (P_i^d + 1) + \ldots \tag{9}$$

Both equations 8 and 9 require the use of nonlinear regression analysis, which is considerably more difficult to use than linear regression (9).

Chosing the "Best" Equation

One advantage of the regression methodology compared to nonmathematical methods is that one tests the possibility that more than one property may work in concert to influence potency. How is such an analysis carried out in practice? The first step in the analysis is to prepare a matrix of all of the properties of the various analogs. This data matrix is then analyzed by a regression analysis program and plots of the log $(1/C)$ values versus each of the physicochemical properties are made. The steps are described in detail elsewhere (8). In essence one examines all possible regression equations and plots to choose those few relationships that are worthy of more study.

Four factors influence the choice of equations as those of interest. The first is the statistical significance of each term in the equation. Usually only equations in which all terms are significant at the 5 percent level are considered: one may choose to follow up equations with less significant terms with the synthesis of analogs that will allow a decision to be made on such parameters. The second criterion is the R^2: if the addition of another statistically significant term dramatically increases the R^2 then the more complex equation is probably of interest, if the increase in R^2 is small then the additional term may not be important. Again, testing of the proper additional analogs may answer this question. The third criterion is the magnitude of the standard deviation from the fit: this should be approximately the value of the standard deviation of a single determination. If it is smaller, then the data are overfit and error is being correlated. If it is substantially larger, then the physicochemical properties may not adequately describe the structural changes or there may be undetected nonlinearities in the data. In either case, the use of plots may help to decide this. The fourth point is that as a rule of thumb one usually likes to have three or four data points for each parameter estimated in the equation.

The data in Table 1 are *in vitro* data for which an equilibrium model may be considered. Accordingly, a fit to Eq. 8 was attempted. Although this was successful, the coefficients b and c were equal. Hence, they were fit as one. The result is:

$$\log\left(\frac{1}{C_i}\right) = 4.46 - \log\left[1 + dP_i^b + \left(\frac{1}{aP_i^b}\right)\right] \tag{10}$$

$\log a = -3.16 \pm 0.08$
$\log d = -4.76 \pm 0.31$
$b = 0.98 \pm 0.04$
$X = 4.46 \pm 0.08$

The statistics of fit are:

$R^2 = 0.997, s = 0.066, n = 11.$

The data and the calculated curve are shown in Fig. 1. The parabolic fit has an R^2 of 0.98 and an s of 0.141 (7).

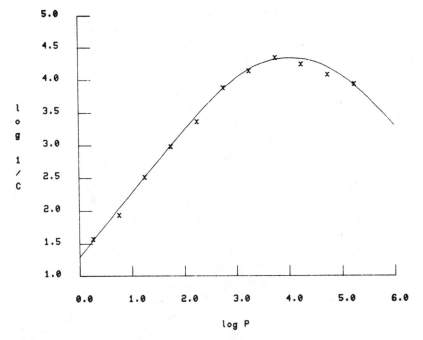

Figure 1 Plot of log (1/C) for hemolytic activity vs octanol-water log *P*. The curve is calculated from the reported fit to Eq. 10. The $R^2 = 0.997$ and $s = 0.066$. Data are from Hansch and Glave (7).

Availability of Computer Software

Computer programs for multiple linear and nonlinear regression analysis are very common. Those especially recommended by this author are the program HANSCH, available from the Pomona College Medicinal Chemistry Project, and those found in SAS (Statistical Analysis System) and BMDP (Biomedical Computer Programs). The desirable and essential characteristics of a multiple regression program have been discussed in detail (8).

INTERPRETATION OF RESULTS

Regression equations can be used as the basis for predictions of potency of untested analogs. Predictions are expected to be accurate within the bounds of the substituent space included in the data set examined. In other words, if the unknown compounds are similar to ones that have already been tested, then the predictions should be correct. For the example this would mean that accurate predictions could be made for straight chain N-alkyl piperidine hydrochlorides with a range of log P from 0.27 to 5.27. However, all such possible analogs are in the original data set, so no such forecasts are possible. On the other hand, extrapolations outside of the substituent space explored in the test set may lead to inaccurate predictions. In the example, the equation may be extrapolated to forecast the activity of other amines or piperidines with a branched or aryl R group. Such extrapolations may be considered hypotheses to be tested in further work, and indeed they frequently are correct (17). For example, if one were to examine the hemolytic activity of selected members of another series of amines, one may decide to test only that of log P closest to the optimum from the previous series or to test that analog plus the two 2.0 log units in the positive and negative direction from the optimum. Testing these three analogs would give one an idea if the new series follows the QSAR of the previous one.

Since in the example there was no variation in pK_a, one cannot use the resulting QSAR to decide if variations in pK_a affect hemolytic activity, nor can many conclusions be drawn with respect to steric effects. Rather, the only correct conclusion is that changes in hydrophobicity result in changes in hemolytic activity.

A second use of regression equations is to explore the physical properties associated with activity in an attempt to study the drug-receptor interaction at a molecular level. Only if the series is well designed, that is, only if the physical properties are varied widely and independently, can one draw valid conclusions about the forces involved in the drug-receptor interaction. Of course the caveat that the measured biological property must correspond to that being hypothesized goes without saying: one would be foolish to postulate drug-receptor properties based on whole animal potency data.

SUMMARY

The Hansch method has found wide application in the pharmaceutical and agricultural industry. The reasons for this are, first, the perceived reasonableness of using physicochemical properties to describe the difference between structurally related compounds; second, the ease with which the statistical analyses may be done; and third, the many published QSAR equations and correct predictions (1).

REFERENCES

1 Martin, Y. C. A practitioners' perspective of the role of quantitative structure activity analysis in medicinal chemistry. *J. Med. Chem.* 229–237 (1981).

2 Bass, G. E., W. H. Lawrence, W. P. Purcell, and U. Autrian. Further evaluation of a quantitative mathematical model for predicting acute toxicity of acrylates and methacrylates. *J. Dent. Res.* 53:756 (1974).

3 Buznikov, G. A., A. Kabankin, V. M. Kolbanov, M. A. Landau, A. A. Aroyan, T. R. Ovsepyan, and N. A. Teplits. Correlation of embryotoxicity and lipophilicity in alkoxybenzylalkylamines. *Khim. Farm. Zhur.* 10:23–27 (1976).

4 Freese, E., B. C. Levin, R. Pearce, T. Sreevals, J. J. Kaufman, W. S. Koski, and N. M. Semo. Correlation between the growth inhibitory effects, partition-coefficients and teratogenic effects of lipophilic acids. *Teratology* 20:413–439 (1979).

5 Enslein, K. LD50 toxicity estimation model—An update. *Genesee Statistics Newsletter* 6:3–4 (1978).

6 Rekker, R. F. LD50 values: Are they about to become predictable?. *Trends Pharmacol. Sci.,* pp. 383–384 (1980).

7 Hansch, C., and W. R. Glave. Structure-activity relationships in membrane-perturbing agents: Hemolytic, narcotic, and antibacterial compounds. *Mol. Pharmacol.* 7:337–354 (1971).

8 Martin, Y. C. *Quantitative Drug Design. A Critical Introduction.* New York: Dekker (1978).

9 Martin, Y. C. The quantitative relationships between pKa, ionization, and drug potency: Utility of model-based equations. In S. H. Yalkowsky, A. A. Sindula, and S. C. Valvani (eds.), *Physical Chemical Properties of Drugs,* pp. 49–110. New York: Dekker (1980).

10 Yalkowsky, S. H., A. A. Sinkula, and S. C. Valvani (eds.). *Physical Chemical Properties of Drugs.* New York: Dekker (1980).

11 Osman, R., H. Weinstein, and J. P. Green. Parameters and methods in quantitative structure-activity relationships. In E. C. Olson and R. E. Christoffersen (eds.), *Computer-Assisted Drug Design,* pp. 21–77. Washington, D.C.: American Chemical Society (1979).

12 Martin, Y. C. Advances in the methodology of quantitative drug design. In E. J. Ariëns (ed), *Drug Design,* 8:1–72. New York: Academic Press (1979).

13 Unger, S. H. Consequences of the Hansch paradigm for the pharmaceutical industry. In E. J. Ariëns (ed.), *Drug Design*, 9:47–119. New York: Academic Press (1980).

14 Charton, M. Linear free energy relationships. *Chemtech.*, pp. 502–511 (1974).

15 Charton, M. Linear free energy relationships. *Chemtech.*, pp. 245–255 (1975).

16 Grieco, C., C. Silipo, and A. Vittoria. Physiochemical parameters in biological correlation analysis—Meaning and limits. *Farmaco [Sci.]* 34: 433–464 (1979).

17 Hansch, C. On the predictive value of QSAR. In J. A. Keverling Buisman (ed.), *Biological Activity and Chemical Structure*, vol. 1, pp. 47–61. Amsterdam: Elsevier (1977).

18 Franke, R. Interpretability of quantitative structure-activity-relationships (QSAR). *Farmaco [Sci.]* 34:545–570 (1979).

19 Franke, R. *Optimierungsmethoden in der Wirkstofforschung*. Berlin: Akademie-Verlag (1980).

20 Seydel, J. K., and K. J. Schaper. *Chemische Struktur und biologische Aktivitat von Wirkstoffen*. Weinheim: Verlag Chemie (1980).

21 Martin, Y. C., and H. N. Panas. Mathematical considerations in series design. *J. Med. Chem.* 22:784–791 (1979).

22 Hansch, C., and A. J. Leo. *Substituents Constants for Correlation Analysis in Chemistry and Biology*. New York: Wiley (1979).

23 Martin, Y. C., and J. J. Hackbarth. Theoretical model-based equations for the linear free energy relationships of the biological activity of ionizable substances. 1. Equilibrium-controlled potency. *J. Med. Chem.* 19:1033–1039 (1976).

24 Fujita, T., J. Iwasa, and C. Hansch. A new substituent constant, pi, derived from partition coefficients. *J. Am. Chem. Soc.* 86:5175–5180 (1964).

25 Rekker, R. F., and H. M. de Kort. The hydrophobic fragmental constant: An extension to a 1000 data point set. *Eur. J. Med. Chem.* 14:479–488 (1979).

26 Chou, J. T., and P. C. Jurs. Computer-assisted computation of partition-coefficients from molecular-structures using fragment constants. *J. Chem. Inf.* 19:172–178 (1979).

27 Heller, S. R., and G. W. Milne. The NIH/EPA chemical information system. In W. J. Howe, M. M. Milne, and A. F. Pennell (eds.), *The Retrieval of Medicinal Chemical Information*, pp. 144–167. Washington, D.C.: American Chemical Society (1978).

28 Lippold, V. C., and G. F. Schneider. Zur Optimierung der Verfugbarkeit Homologer Quartarer Ammoniumverbindungen. *Arzneim.-Forsch.* 24:1952–1956 (1974).

29 Dearden, J. C., and J. Williams. The variation of forward and reverse partitioning rate constants with lipophilicity. *J. Pharm. Pharmacol.* 30:50P (1978).

30 VandeWaterbeemd, H., S. VanBoeckel, A. Jansen, and K. Gerritsma. Transport in QSAR. II. Rate-equilibrium relationships and the interfacial transfer of drugs. *Eur. J. Med. Chem.* 15:279–282 (1980).

31 Foster, R., R. M. Hyde, and D. J. Livingston. Substituent constant for drug design studies based on properties of organic electron donor-acceptor complexes. *J. Pharm. Sci.* 67:1310–1313 (1978).

32 Hetnarski, B. Application of the charge-transfer constant for correlation of acetylcholinesterase affinity reciprocals vs physicochemical properties of aromatic inhibitors. *Res. Commun. Chem. Pathol. Pharmacol.* 26:171–178 (1979).

33 Fujita, T., T. Nishioka, and M. Nakajima. Hydrogen bonding parameter and its significance in quantitative structure-activity studies. *J. Med. Chem.* 20:1071–1081 (1977).

34 Richards, W. G. *Quantum Pharmacology*, Boston: Butterworths (1977).

35 Peradejordi, F., A. N. Martin, and A. Cammarata. Quantum chemical approach to structure-activity relationships of tetracycline antibiotics. *J. Pharm. Sci.* 60:576–582 (1971).

36 Smith, R. L., D. W. Cochran, P. Gund, and E. J. Cragoe. Proton, carbon-13, and nitrogen-15 nuclear magnetic resonance and CNDO/2 studies on the tautomerism and conformation of amiloride, a novel acylguanidine. *J. Am. Chem. Soc.* 101:191–201 (1979).

37 Topliss, J. G., and R. P. Edwards. Chance factors in QSAR studies. In E. C. Olson and R. E. Christoffersen, (eds.), *Computer Assisted Drug Design*, pp. 131–145. Washington, D.C.: American Chemical Society (1979).

38 Boyd, D. B., D. K. Herron, W. W. Lunn, and A. Spitzer. Parabolic relationships between antibacterial activity of cephalosporins and beta-lactam reactivity predicted from molecular orbital calculations. *J. Am. Chem. Soc.* 102:1812–1814 (1980).

39 Kier, L. B. Molecular connectivity as a description of structure for SAR analyses. In S. H. Yalkowsky, A. S. Sinkula, and S. C. Valvani (eds.), *Physical Chemical Properties of Drugs*, pp. 277–319. New York: Dekker (1980).

40 Balaban, A. T., A. Chiriac, I. Motoc, and Z. Simon. *Steric Fit in Quantitative Structure-Activity Relations.* Berlin: Springer-Verlag (1980).

41 Hopfinger, A. J. A QSAR investigation of dihydrofolate reductase inhibition by Baker triazines based upon molecular shape analysis. *J. Am. Chem. Soc.* 102:7196–7206 (1980).

42 Dietrich, S. W., R. N. Smith, S. Brendler, and C. Hansch. The use of triazine inhibitors in mapping the active site region of *Lactobacillus casei* dihydrofolate reductase. *Arch. Biochem. Biophys.* 194:612–619 (1979).

43 Lien, E. J., J. F. Rodrigues de Miranda, and E. J. Ariëns. Quantitative structure-activity correlation of optical isomers. A molecular basis for Pfeiffer's rule. *Mol. Pharmacol.* 12:598–604 (1976).

44 Hansch, C., S. H. Unger, and A. B. Forsythe. Strategy in drug design. Cluster analysis as an aid in the selection of substituents. *J. Med. Chem.* 16:1217–1222 (1973).

45 Wootton, R., R. Cranfield, G. Sheppey, and P. J. Goodford. Physiochemical-activity relationships in practice. 2. Rational selection of benzenoid substituents. *J. Med. Chem.* 18:607–613 (1975).

46 Streich, W. J., S. Dove, and R. Franke. On the rational selection of test series. I. Principal component method combined with multidimensional mapping. *J. Med. Chem.* 23:1452–1456 (1980).

47 Dove, S., W. J. Streich, and R. Franke. On the rational selection of test series. 2. 2-Dimensional mapping of intra-class correlation matrices. *J. Med. Chem.* 23:1456–1459 (1980).

48 Higuchi, T., and S. S. Davis. Thermodynamic analysis of structure-activity relationships of drugs: Prediction of optimal structure. *J. Pharm. Sci.* 59:1376–1383 (1970).

49 Kubinyi, H. Quantitative structure-activity relationships. 7. Bilinear model. A new model for nonlinear dependence of biological activity on hydrophobic character. *J. Med. Chem.* 20:625–629 (1977).

Chapter 7

Studies of Relationships between Molecular Structure and Biological Activity by Pattern Recognition Methods

Peter C. Jurs

INTRODUCTION

The attempt to rationalize the connections between the molecular structures of organic compounds and their biological activities comprises the field of structure-activity relations (SAR) studies. Correlations between structure and activity are important for the understanding and the development of pharmaceutical agents, agricultural agents, and chemical communicants (olfactory and gustatory stimulants) and for the investigation of chemical and genetic toxicity (mutagenic and carcinogenic potential). Practical importance attaches to this type of study because the potential exists for prediction of the biological activity of untested or even hypothetical compounds. In addition the insights generated by SAR studies can guide a researcher's attention to molecular features that are correlated with the biological activity of interest, thus confirming or contradicting mechanisms of action or suggesting further experiments. The techniques of SAR have been applied in the pharmaceutical field (drug design) and, to some extent, in agricultural chemicals. The methods are beginning to be applied to problems in the areas of chemical and genetic toxicity.

The most desirable way to develop the capability to predict the activity of untested compounds is to exploit a molecular level theory of action or mechanism. Unfortunately, this knowledge is not yet available for most classes of biologically active compounds and this approach is ordinarily blocked in problems of immediate interest. Thus one must use correlative methods to look for relationships between the molecular structures of tested compounds and their experimentally observed biological activity. Generally, one has available a set of compounds that have been tested in a standard bioassay and the results of these experiments. One can then use the methods of SAR to search for relationships between the structures and activities. This approach attempts to simultaneously take into account the entire process of uptake, transport, distribution, metabolism, cell penetration, binding, and excretion by correlating the structure of the administered compound with the final observed activity.

Several different approaches to the study of SAR have been reported. The most widely employed is the semi-empirical linear free energy (LFER) or extrathermodynamic model proposed by Hansch and co-workers (1-3), which is described elsewhere in this volume. This chapter will focus on an approach to SAR that brings together techniques of chemical structure information handling and pattern recognition in an attempt to find relationships between molecular structure and biological activity.

The fundamental premises involved in applying pattern recognition methods to SAR studies of chemicals with genetic toxicity are as follows:

Molecular structure and biological activity (genetic toxicity) are related.

The structures of compounds having genetic toxicity and compounds of similar structural classes that are nontoxic can be adequately represented by a set of molecular structure descriptors.

A relation can be discovered between the structure and activity by applying statistical and pattern recognition methods to a set of tested compounds.

The relation can be extrapolated to untested compounds.

The heart of the approach is finding a set of adequate descriptors for a particular data set consideration, that is, a set of descriptors for which a discriminating relation can be found.

The fundamental steps involved in performing an SAR study are shown in Fig. 1. The individual steps are as follows:

1 Identify, assemble, input, store, and describe a data set of structures for chemicals that have been tested for biological activity.

2 Develop computer-generated molecular descriptors for each of the members of the data set. The descriptors may be derived directly from the

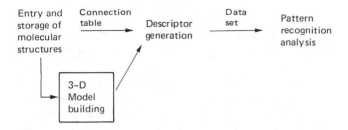

Figure 1 Flow chart of steps involved in structure-activity studies using chemical structure information handling and pattern recognition methods.

stored topological representations of the structures, or they may require the development of three-dimensional molecular models.

3 Using pattern recognition or statistical methods, develop classifiers to discriminate between active and inactive compounds based on the sets of molecular descriptors.

4 Test the predictive ability of these discriminants on compounds of unknown activity.

5 Systematically reduce the set of molecular structure descriptors employed to the minimum set sufficient to retain discrimination between the active and inactive compounds and to retain high predictive ability.

This approach to SAR studies has been implemented in a computer software system called ADAPT (*a*utomatic *d*ata *a*nalysis using *p*attern recognition *t*echniques) (4, 5). The ADAPT system currently consists of approximately 60 FORTRAN language routines that implement the steps necessary for an SAR study. It is designed to be run on a dedicated minicomputer or a time-sharing system, and it is highly interactive and must be guided by the user. The system is a set of tools that the user can apply to problems involving up to several hundred compounds at a time.

REPRESENTATION OF MOLECULAR STRUCTURE

The central problem of any correlative analysis is the choice of independent variables (here, molecular structure descriptors) that are used. The researcher's knowledge and intuition are brought to bear on the problem at hand through descriptor choice and refinement. Current hypotheses on mechanism of action, metabolism, transport, binding, etc., can be expressed through appropriately chosen descriptors. If a set of molecular structure descriptors that do contain the essential structural information relevant to the biological activity of interest is developed, then the analysis phase of the project will succeed. If an inadequate set of descriptors is analyzed, then no pattern recognition or statistical procedure will unearth relationships. The search for adequate or good sets of descriptors forms one of the most challenging aspects of SAR studies.

A number of different approaches to descriptor development coexist in the SAR field. Historically, substituent constants—coding for structural differences among compounds in a homologous series—have enjoyed the most use (6). These descriptors include Hammett sigma constants for electronic effects, Taft steric parameters, π lipophilicity parameters, Verloop steric constants, and many others. This type of structural descriptor is fully described elsewhere in this volume and will not be stressed here. Electronic parameters resulting from quantum mechanical calculations have also been used in SAR work, either alone or in conjunction with other parameters (7). These too are described elsewhere in this volume.

The approach to structural representation to be described here involves the entry of storage of molecular topologies graphically, the modeling of the structures, and the calculation of the descriptors from these internal representations. This approach permits the study of large sets of compounds, heterogeneous sets of compounds, and the prediction of activity of unknown from only a sketch of the structure. Of course, if experimental data are found to be critical to the development of a structure-activity relationship, then such data can easily be included in the analysis.

The following paragraphs describe one approach to the development of structural descriptors for SAR studies.

Entry of Molecular Structures

The ADAPT computer system has as one of its components all the modules necessary to enter, modify, retrieve, and draw molecular structures of organic molecules. The routines allow the convenient, interactive entry of structures by sketching them on the screen of a graphics display terminal. This can be done in 30 s to several minutes per compound, depending on structural complexity. No special techniques beyond those used in sketching molecular structures on a blackboard are needed. Thus, structure files on the order of hundreds of compounds can be entered in reasonable amounts of time. The structure files are stored permanently on disc files for further processing. Information saved for each compound includes a compressed connection table, ring information, a list of associated numerical information, and identification number, the chemical name of the compound, and the two-dimensional coordinates of the atoms as entered (for possible redrawing later or for starting coordinates for modeling).

Molecular Mechanics Model Builder

The three-dimensional molecular model builder routine is used to derive information on the spacial conformation of molecules. A molecule can be viewed as a collection of particles held together by simple harmonic or elastic forces. These forces can be defined by potential energy functions whose terms are the atom coordinates of the molecule. This function can then be minimized to obtain a strain-free three-dimensional model of the molecule. In the strain minimization section, the atom coordinates are systematically altered until a minimum is found in the strain or potential energy function. The strain function used is:

$$E_{strain} = E_{bond} + E_{angle} + E_{torsion} + E_{non-bond} + E_{stereo}$$

The first four terms of the function are commonly found in all molecular mechanics strain functions and are modified Hooke's law functions. The last term of the function has been added to assure the proper stereochemistry about an asymmetrical atom. An adaptive pattern search routine is used to minimize the strain energy because it does not require analytical derivatives. The amount of time necessary to obtain good molecular models depends on the number of atoms in the molecule, the initial strain of the molecule, and the degrees of freedom in the structure.

Descriptor Generation

The heart of SAR studies is the development of molecular structure descriptors. One of the major premises of the approach is that one can find an "adequate" set of descriptors to represent the compounds of interest. The existence of an adequate set of descriptors does not necessarily imply that they will be easily found. Thus descriptor development is the area in which chemists test their ingenuity most intensively, bringing to bear on the problem at hand all their insight and knowledge. It is in the area of descriptor development that the most difficult and most potentially rewarding parts of SAR research occur.

Fragment Descriptors These include counts of the number of atoms of each type, the number of bonds of each type, the number of basis rings, and the number of ring atoms.

Substructure Descriptors ADAPT has a substructure searching routine that can be used to develop descriptors. Each of the structures comprising a set of compounds under study is searched for the presence of the substructure of interest. If it is present, then the number of occurrences is computed. If not, then the descriptor is given the value of zero. The substructures to be used are problem dependent and must be found through the application of experience and outside knowledge by the researcher.

Environment Descriptors The information present in the fragment and substructure descriptors indicates the components of the molecular structure. However, the manner of interconnection is missing. Environment descriptors supply information about the connections by coding the immediate surroundings of substructures. To generate an environment descriptor, the molecule being coded is searched for the presence of the substructural fragment that forms the heart of the environment being sought. If no match is found, the descriptor is given the value of zero. If the substructure is found, then the descriptor is computed by performing a path one molecular connectivity calculation on the atoms comprising the substructure, as imbedded within the structure, and, in addition, the first nearest neighbor atoms. Thus, the value of the path one molecular connectivity represents the immediate surroundings of the substructure as imbedded within the molecule being coded.

Molecular Connectivity Descriptors The molecular connectivity (8) of a molecule is a measure of the branching of the structure. It is formed by summing contributions for each bond in the structure, where the contribution of each bond is determined by the connectivity of the atoms that are joined by that bond. This is the path one molecular connectivity. Higher order molecular connectivities can also be computed by considering all paths of length two, three, etc. These descriptors have been shown in several published reports to be correlated with a number of physicochemical parameters, such as partition coefficients and steric parameters.

Geometric Descriptors Once the molecules being studied have been modeled, then descriptors can be generated from these models. Geometrical descriptors that have been used in many SAR studies are the three principal moments of inertia of the molecules, the three ratios of these three principal moments, and the molecular volume. Many other geometrical descriptors can be envisioned, and the development of new descriptors is an active area of research.

Path and Path Environment Descriptors Molecular structures can be viewed in the abstract as graphs, in the mathematical sense. Graphs have a number of properties that can be readily computed, among them paths. A *path* is a sequence of connected atoms in which no atom appears more than once. The tracing of paths in highly connected graphs, e.g., polycyclic aromatic hydrocarbons, is tedious but can be done. A method for finding all the paths contained in a graph has been published, with a discussion of the chemical utility of this measure of bonding complexity (9). A descriptor generation routine has been implemented and interfaced to ADAPT using this concept. The routine calculates the total number of paths of all lengths contained within the structure being coded.

The path environment descriptor is similar to the molecular connectivity environment descriptor. A substructure is matched against the structure being coded. If it is present, then a pseudomolecule is formed from the substructure atoms and their first nearest neighbor atoms. Then the number of paths originating from the set of atoms forming the pseudomolecule is found. The maximum path length to be considered is input by the user. The descriptor for a particular structure consists of the number of paths originating from the substructure atoms and their first nearest neighbors. This environment can be made sensitive to the immediate surroundings of the substructure by making the maximum path length to be considered very small, e.g., two or three. Alternatively, it can be made sensitive to the overall structure of the molecule by making the maximum path length larger.

Partition Coefficient Estimation The log P, the logarithm of the partition coefficient of a compound between an aqueous phase and a model lipid phase, is highly correlated with various types of biological activities. Its inclusion as a descriptor allows the system to have access to information regarding transport and partioning that may not be as clearly represented in the other descriptors. The calculation of log P can be done using a "constructionist approach" (6). This formulation starts with a set of fundamental fragments the values of which are summed with appropriate weightings. Corrections are added to refine the calculation if necessary. The equation used is as follows:

$$\log P = \sum_{i=1}^{n} a_i f_i + \sum_{j=1}^{m} c_j$$

where f_i is the fragment constant for the ith fragment, a_i is the number of occurrences of the ith fragment, and c_j is the jth correction factor. The fundamental assumption of this approach is that hydrophobicity is an additive-constitutive property of molecules.

Recently, this fragment constant method has been implemented in a routine and interfaced to ADAPT (10). Thus, the estimated log P value for a molecule can be used as a descriptor along with all the other descriptor types.

Descriptor Manipulation Routines In addition to the individual descriptor generation routine, the ADAPT system contains several support routines. There is a general maintenance and interrogation routine for the descriptor files that allows the user to review descriptor values by listing them and to delete unwanted descriptors. Another routine allows the user to input from cards descriptors obtained from any source so that they can be studied along with the computer-generated descriptors. A manipulation routine allows the user to alter previously generated or stored descriptors to form new descriptors. Addition, subtraction, multiplication, division, exponentiation, logarithmic transformation, autoscaling, and inversion are allowed.

The development of adequate sets of descriptors for the compounds forming a data set comprises the most difficult part of SAR research. With an adequate set of descriptors, the analysis portion of the study is relatively straightforward. With a set of descriptors that is inadequate, one has no choice but to keep searching for better descriptors. Thus, descriptor development for a particular data set can consume quite a lot of time and can be a trial-and-error operation.

A key goal in descriptor development is to find descriptors that are related to the mode of action and the mechanism or metabolism responsible for the biological activity of interest. This will insure the most meaningful representation of the structures under investigation.

PATTERN RECOGNITION ANALYSIS

Once each compound in a data set under investigation has been represented by a set of descriptors, then the analysis phase of the structure-activity study begins. In this chapter, pattern recognition analysis methods will be discussed. Other alternative methods of data analysis are described elsewhere in this volume.

Pattern recognition is a subfield of artificial intelligence developed largely by electrical engineers and computer scientists. It comprises a set of parametric and nonparametric techniques used to study data sets that do not conform to well-characterized probability density functions. A voluminous literature describes the field (11-13).

Most of the pattern recognition methods share a set of common properties, including the method of representation of the data. Each compound is represented by a vector

$$\mathbf{X} = (x_1, x_2, \ldots, x_n)$$

wherein each individual component of the pattern vector, $\mathbf{x}_j$, is the value for the jth descriptor. To reference the ith compound in a data set, the notation $\mathbf{X}_i$ is used. An equivalent view of this representation is to consider each component to be represented by a point in n-dimensional space.

For a given compound, which is represented by a given point, the value of each coordinate is just the numerical value for one of the molecular structure descriptors comprising the representation. The expectation is that the points representing compounds of common biological activity (e.g., toxic compounds) will cluster in one limited region of the space separate from those compounds of another biological activity (e.g., nontoxic compounds), which will cluster elsewhere. The clusters are regions of high local density relatively far apart from each other. Pattern recognition consists of a set of methods for investigating data represented in this manner to assess the degree of clustering and general structure of the data space.

Preprocessing

Preprocessing operations alter the form of the representations of the compounds and include operations such as scaling, normalization, and other mathematical transformations designed to make the analysis easier at a later stage.

Scaling and normalization are required to convert the given units from different descriptors to a compatible form. For example, molecular weights ranging from 300–500 should not be studied simultaneously with log P values ranging from 3–5. In such cases the larger valued descriptors could dominate those of smaller value and lead to numerical instabilities in the pattern recognition programs. One preprocessing method that is quite useful in correcting this type of imbalance is autoscaling.

This method simultaneously scales and normalizes the data by translating it so that the mean is zero and normalizing it so that each descriptor has a standard deviation of S. The equations describing this process are given below.

$$x_{ij} = \frac{S(x_{ij} - x_j)}{\sigma_j}$$

$$x_j = \frac{1}{n} \sum_{i=1}^{n} x_{ij}$$

$$\sigma_j^2 = \frac{1}{n} \sum_{i=1}^{n} (x_{ij} - x_j)^2$$

The x_{ij} are the elements of the matrix representation of the data formed from the column vectors representing each data point, and the x'_{ij} are the elements of the data matrix resulting from the scaling operation. Autoscaling can be looked upon as "squaring up the space," since it places the data inside a hypercube. Although autoscaling alters the spread of the data, it does not alter the number of features or the basic geometry of the clustering.

Mapping and Display

One powerful method for analyzing the structure of a data set (here, a set of compounds) is to map the points from the high-dimensional space to a plane for direct viewing. It has long been recognized that people are adept at recognizing patterns in two-dimensional plots, and this has been exploited in many pattern recognition display methodologies. A number of useful and imaginative graphic techniques exist for directly displaying multivariate data in just one or two dimensions (14). Their use has been largely neglected in the physical sciences in favor of more common rectangular plots and histograms. However, techniques such as metroglyphs, linear and circular data profiles, Andrews plots, and Chernoff faces can be valuable tools for visualizing relationships between observations, for identifying outliers, and for classification purposes (15, 16).

A method that combines both mapping and display operations along with feature selection operations is principal components analysis, also known as the Karhunen-Loeve transformation (11). This involves taking the eigenvalues and eigenvectors of the variance-covariance matrix of a data set and then using the eigenvectors to perform a linear rotation. The multidimensional data set can be plotted in the two dimensions determined by the two principal eigenvectors and displayed for visual analysis. Alternatively, the data set can be rotated by multiplication with any desired number of elgenvectors to reduce the dimensionality of the data set. This operation commonly involves using just enough of the available eigenvectors to retain 95 to 99 percent of the total sum of the values. An advantage of this feature selection procedure is that the number of descriptors per compound is reduced, thus making further analysis more convenient in some ways. A disadvantage is that the individual descriptors resulting from this transformation are mixtures of the original descriptors, thus complicating analysis of later results.

Another mapping strategy is to attempt to find a two-dimensional display in which each point in the original data set is represented by a point in the two-dimensional array of points. Of course, a certain amount of error in the mapping is to be expected. The literature contains reports of many approaches to perform these nonlinear mapping operations (17–19). Iterative nonlinear mapping routines have been implemented using the following error function:

$$E = \frac{1}{\sum_{i<j} d_{ij}^{*}} \sum_{i<j} \frac{(d_{ij}^{*} - d_{ij})^2}{d_{ij}^{*}}$$

where d_{ij}^{*} is the euclidean distance between points i and j in the original n-dimensional space and d_{ij} is the two-dimensional interpoint distances. The method of steepest descent can be used to minimize E. The starting estimates may be chosen by the user; they could be the results of a previous principal components analysis, for example. Many other starting configuration options are also available. The results of the mapping routine could be presented graphically for visual analysis.

Classification by Discriminants

Commonly in SAR studies, the compounds available for study have been placed in a few discrete categories such as "active" versus "inactive." After the compounds have been represented by molecular structure descriptors and expressed as points in a high-dimensional space, then the question becomes, "Are the two sets of points representing compounds separable from one another?" That is, can a discriminant surface be placed between the point sets so that all points representing the active compounds fall on one side of the surface and all of the points representing inactive compounds fall on the other side of the surface? The search for such discriminants comprises the operation of classification and discriminant development.

Two different approaches to the development of discriminants are feasible: parametric and nonparametric methods. Parametric methods of pattern recognition attempt to find classification surfaces or clustering definitions based on statistical properties of the members of one or both classes of points. For example, bayesian classification surfaces are developed using the mean vectors for the members of the classes and the covariance matrices for the classes. If the statistical properties cannot be calculated or estimated, then nonparametric methods are used. Nonparametric methods attempt to find clustering definitions or classification surfaces by using the data themselves directly, without computing mean vectors, covariance matrices, etc. Examples of nonparametric methods would include error-correction feedback linear learning machines (threshold logic units or perceptrons) and simplex optimization methods of searching for separating classification surfaces.

Parametric Pattern Recognition Programs The parametric pattern recognition programs use the mean vectors and covariance matrices (or other statistical measures) of the two classes into which the patterns fall as their basis for development of discriminants (11).

One parametric approach implements a quadratic discriminant function using the Bayesian theorem. The equation for the discriminants is as follows:

$$d_k(X) = \ln p_k - \tfrac{1}{2} \ln |C_k| - \tfrac{1}{2} [(X - \mathbf{m}_k)^{\mathrm{T}} C_k^{-1} (X - \mathbf{m}_k)] \qquad k = 1,2$$

where p_k is the a priori probability for class k, C_k is the covariance matrix for class k, and $\mathbf{m}_k$ is the mean vector for class k. This discriminant assumes a multivariate normal distribution of the data. A pattern, $\mathbf{X}_i$, is put in the class for which $d_k(\mathbf{X}_i)$ is greatest.

If the assumption is made that the covariance matrices for the two classes are the same, then the discriminant function developed using the Bayes theorem and the multivariate normal assumption simplifies from that above to the following:

$$s = d_1(X) - d_2(X) = \ln p_1 - \ln p_2 + X'X^{-1}(m_1 - m_2)$$
$$- \tfrac{1}{2}m_1'C^{-1}m_1 + \tfrac{1}{2}m_2'C^{-1}m_2$$

where s is greater than zero for one class and less than zero for the other class.

Another parametric approach implements a discriminant function by the method commonly called linear discriminant function analysis (LDFA). It is nearly identical to the linear bayesian discriminant, except that instead of using the covariance matrix, the sum of cross-products matrix is used. Results obtained with LDFA are ordinarily very similar to those obtained using a Bayes routine.

Nonparametric Pattern Recognition Programs The nonparametric pattern recognition programs develop their discriminants using the training set of patterns to be classified rather than statistical measures of their distributions.

The k nearest neighbor method is conceptually the simplest. An unknown pattern is assigned to the class to which the majority of its nearest neighbors belong. The metric that is used to determine proximity is ordinarily the euclidean metric, but any metric can be used. Another widely used nonparametric method is the linear learning machine or perceptron (11). The algorithm is heuristic. A decision surface is initialized either arbitrarily or using the result from another linear discriminant development routine. Then the learning machine classifies one member of the training set at a time. When the current discriminant function correctly classifies a pattern, the discriminant is left unchanged. However, when an incorrect classification is made, then the discriminant is altered in such a way that the error just committed is eliminated. The learning machine continues to classify the members of the training set repeatedly until no errors are committed or until the user terminates the routine. This algorithm for development of linear discriminant functions has the desirable property that if a training set of patterns is separable into the two classes, i.e., if a solution exists, then this method will find a solution. This routine is the one ordinarily used to train a set of slightly different weight vectors to be used for the variance method of nonparametric feature selection method.

Another nonparametric method develops a linear discriminant function through an iterative least squares approach (12). The following function is minimized:

$$Q = \sum_{i=1}^{m} [Y_i - F(s_i)]^2$$

where m is the total number of patterns in the training set, Y_i equals +1 for one pattern class and -1 for the other class, s_i is the dot product of the weight vector with the ith pattern vector, and $F(s_i)$ is the hyperbolic tangent function of s_i. The hyperbolic tangent function has the values of positive one for all positive values of s_i and negative one for all negative values of s_i. Therefore, minimizing Q is equivalent to minimizing the number of incorrect classifications. The function is nonlinear in the independent variables and thus cannot be solved directly, so an iterative algorithm is employed. This routine has been found to be particularly useful for dealing with data that are not separable into the two classes.

Recently, Moriguchi and co-workers (20) have reported an adaptive least squares method for the development of a multiclass discriminant function, and they have applied the method to a structure-activity problem.

The search for a good discriminant that separates two clusters of points in an n-dimensional space from one another can be formulated as a linear programming problem (21). The objective function whose value is to be minimized can be defined as the fraction of the training set of patterns that are incorrectly classified. Because two different discriminants can easily have the same classification power, it has been suggested that a secondary objective function be defined as the sum of the distances from the discriminant plane to the misclassified points. The secondary objective function is invoked only if the primary function is equal for two different discriminants being compared. The simplex optimization procedure described above has been applied to a number of chemical problems.

Once discriminants have been found that do separate the data set into the appropriate subsets, then these discriminants can be used to assess validity. This is usually done by a round-robin procedure involving leaving out a small number of data set members to act as "unknown" compounds. When available, true unknowns can also be input into the system for prediction of activity.

Clustering Methods

A subset of pattern recognition methods consists of clustering methods that attempt to determine structural characteristics of a set of data by organizing the data into subgroups or clusters. These methods are known as "unsupervised" because they attempt to define clusters solely on the basis of criteria derived from the data themselves (as opposed to finding clusters after knowing which data points belong to which categories). The most widely used clustering method is hierarchical clustering. This method works by measuring the distances between all pairs of points, identifying the closest pair, combining them into a single point at the midpoint, recalculating the distances from this new point to every other point in the data set, finding the nearest pair, combining them, etc. The process is repeated until all the points have been combined. The resulting structure can be displayed as a dendogram, which shows at what degree of similarity each pair of points was combined. The overall purpose is usually to simplify a data matrix that is too extensive for direct analysis. The product of hierarchical clustering analysis is a dendogram or treelike structure that shows visually the hierarchy of similarity relationships inherent in the original data. The techniques are independent of the nature of the material to be classified, and they have been applied to a wide variety of problems drawn from engineering, the social sciences, the physical sciences, medicine, and biology (19, 22-24). Clustering routines must be considered to be an exploratory tool (25), and the absolute validity of dendograms generated may be less important than the insights and suggestions generated regarding the data structure.

Simca Pattern Recognition

A pattern recognition method has been developed by Wold and co-workers called SIMCA (26-28). SIMCA is a set of procedures with which each class of pattern recognition problems is separately modeled with a principal components model. Unknowns to be classified are fitted to the class models, and the classifications are made according to the statistics of the fits. An unknown pattern is assigned a probability for each class; if all probabilities are low, then the pattern may be an outlier belonging to none of the original classes.

PATTERN RECOGNITION IN STRUCTURE-ACTIVITY RELATIONSHIP STUDIES

The methods of pattern recognition have been applied to the problem of searching for correlations between molecular structure and biological activity. The types of biological activity studied include pharmaceutical activity (drug design), agricultural chemicals, chemical communicants (olfactory stimulants), and toxicity (chemical, mutagenic, and carcinogenic activity). Applications of pattern recognition to drug design have been reviewed by Kirschner and Kowalski (29) and briefly discussed by Varmuza (13). A book describing research on pattern recognition in SAR has appeared (5).

A few papers have appeared in the past several years dealing with specific structure-toxicity studies. Each of these will be described briefly in the following paragraphs.

A paper by Norden et al. (30) reported a study of 32 PAH using the SIMCA pattern recognition methodology. Each PAH was characterized by 23 variables. These included 15 theoretical variables (electronic descriptors, molecular orbital energies, charges of radical cations, symmetry descriptors, etc.) and eight measured variables (six spectroscopic values extracted from absorption spectra and two other spectroscopic variables). A procedure was developed to classify the 32 PAH as carcinogenic or noncarcinogenic and to provide a quantitative prediction about the level of activity of the active compounds. Validation studies showed the classification rate to be significantly better than chance. The correlation coefficient between predicted and observed activity during the validation test was 0.793.

A paper by Dunn and Wold (31) reported a study of 33 4-nitroquinoline-1-oxides using the SIMCA pattern recognition methodology. Each compound was characterized by 43 variables: six positions of possible substitution with six physicochemical substituent constants each (π, MR, σ_m, σ_p, L, and B_4), two positions with three additional substituent constants used (B_1, B_2, and B_3), and log P. A four-component principal components model was derived for the carcinogens, which was 82 percent successful in predicting the carcinogenic potential of the compounds. Validation of the classification procedure developed showed a highly statistically significant relationship to exist.

A paper by Jurs and co-workers (32) reported a study of 209 heterogeneous compounds drawn from more than 12 structural classes. Twenty-six calculated molecular structure descriptors were used; these supported a linear discriminant function capable of separating 192 compounds into the carcinogen and noncarcinogen classes. Validation of the linear discriminant achieved a classification success rate of 90 percent for carcinogens and 78 percent for noncarcinogens.

A paper by Chou and Jurs (33) described studies of 153 N-nitrosamines and N-nitrosamides. A set of 15 calculated molecular structure descriptors was found that supported a linear discriminant function capable of separating 116 carcinogens from 28 noncarcinogens. Randomized validation testing produced a classification ability of 93 percent for carcinogens and 85 percent for noncarcinogens. The inclusion of two electronic descriptors representing the electronic properties of the N–NO group and the α-carbon atom implicitly supports the α-hydroxylation hypothesis of action of N-nitroso compounds.

A paper by Yuan and Jurs (34) reported the application of pattern recognition to the study of carcinogenic potential of PAH compounds drawn from 16 structural subclasses. Each PAH was represented by 28 calculated molecular structure descriptors. Linear discriminants were found that could classify 191 of the 200 PAH as carcinogens versus noncarcinogens. Validation testing produced 91 percent correct classifications.

Dunn and Wold (35) have reported a study of N-nitroso compounds, including nitrosamines, N-nitrosoureas, and N-nitrosourethans. Each compound was represented by six substituent constants for two sites (Rekker lipophilicity constant, Taft's σ^* and E_s, MR, Verloop's steric constants L and B_4). The active compounds were subdivided into three classes and models were developed for each of the three: a two-component model correctly classified 23 of 27 in class 1; a one-component model correctly classified 7 of 9 in class

2; a three-component model correctly classified all 14 compounds in class 3. Thus 44 of 50 or 88 percent of the active compounds were classified correctly overall. All of the inactive compounds, except one, were classified as members of none of the three classes.

A paper by Yuta and Jurs (36) describes studies of aromatic amines using pattern recognition methods. The 157 aromatic amine compounds were divided into subsets according to active site (breast, ear duct, liver, other, all sites), route of administration (oral or other), and activity (carcinogen or noncarcinogen). Sets of calculated molecular structure descriptors were generated that could support linear discriminant functions able to separate sets of active carcinogens from inactive compounds. Prominent among the important structural descriptors were those coding sizes and shapes of the amines. The pattern recognition results were not strongly affected by differences in active site, and the study showed that mixed data could be used in computer-assisted structure-carcinogenicity studies.

A study by Whalen-Pedersen and Jurs (37) describes the results of a study of relationships between molecular structures of polycyclic aromatic compounds (PAC) and capillary column gas chromatographic retention indexes. Experimentally measured retention indexes, on a linear scale that involves interpolation between PAH standards, for 207 PAC were found to be well explained by a four-variable linear regression model. The four calculated structural descriptors were molecular volume, number of basis rings, path one molecular connectivity, and the number of nitrogen plus oxygen atoms. For 207 compounds the correlation coefficient obtained was 0.988 and standard error was 12.4 compared to the range of the dependent variable, which was 197 to 504.

REFERENCES

1 Hansch, C. Recent advances in biochemical QSAR. In N. R. Chapman and J. Shorter (eds.), *Advances in Linear Free Energy Relationships.* New York: Plenum Press (1979).
2 Martin, Y. C. *Quantitative Drug Design.* New York: Dekker (1978).
3 Unger, S. H. Consequences of the Hansch paradigm for the pharmaceutical industry. In E. J. Ariëns (ed.), *Drug Design*, vol. IX, pp. 48–119. New York: Academic Press (1980).
4 Stuper, A. J., W. E. Brugger, and P. C. Jurs. A computer system for structure-activity studies using chemical structure information handling and pattern recognition techniques. *A.C.S. Symp. Ser.* 52:165–191 (1977).
5 Stuper, A. J., W. E. Brugger, and P. C. Jurs. *Computer Assisted Studies of Chemical Structure and Biological Function.* New York: Wiley-Interscience (1979).
6 Hansch, C., and A. Leo. *Substitutent Constants for Correlation Analysis in Chemistry and Biology.* New York: Wiley-Interscience (1979).

7   Christoffersen, R. E. Quantum pharmacology: Recent progress and current status. In E. C. Olsen and R. E. Christoffersen (eds.), *Computer Assisted Drug Design*. Washington, D.C.: American Chemical Society (1979).

8   Kier, L. B., and L. H. Hall. *Molecular Connectivity in Chemistry and Drug Research*. New York: Academic Press (1976).

9   Randic, M., G. M. Brissey, R. B. Spencer, and C. L. Wilkins. Search for all self-avoiding paths for molecular graphs. *Comput. Chem.* 3:5–13 (1979).

10 Chou, J. T., and P. C. Jurs. Computation of partition coefficients from molecular structures by a fragment addition method. In S. H. Yalkowsky, A. A. Sinkula, and S. C. Valvani (eds.), *Physical Chemical Properties of Drugs*, pp. 163–199. New York: Dekker (1980).

11 Tou, J. T., and R. C. Gonzalez. *Pattern Recognition Principles*. Reading, Mass.: Addison-Wesley (1974).

12 Jurs, P. C., and T. L. Isenhour. *Chemical Applications of Pattern Recognition*. New York: Wiley-Interscience (1975).

13 Varmuza, K. *Pattern Recognition in Chemistry*. Berlin: Springer-Verlag (1980).

14 Gnanadesikan, R. *Methods for Statistical Data Analysis of Multivariate Observations*. New York: Wiley, (1977).

15 Mezzich, J. E. *Graphical Representation of Multivariate Data*. New York: Academic Press (1978).

16 Chernoff, H. *The Use of Faces to Represent Points in n-Dimensional Space Graphically*. Technical Rep. No. 71, Department of Statistics, Stanford University, Stanford, CA (1971).

17 Duda, R. O., and P. E. Hart. *Pattern Classification and Scene Analysis*. New York: Wiley (1973).

18 Sammon, J. W. A nonlinear mapping for data structure analysis. *IEEE Trans. Comput.* C-18:401 (1979).

19 Fukunaga, K. *Introduction to Statistical Pattern Recognition*. New York: Academic Press (1972).

20 Moriguchi, I., K. Komatsu, and Y. Matsushita. Adaptive least-squares method applied to structure-activity correlation of hypotensive N-alkyl-N''-cyano-N'-pyridylguanidines. *J. Med. Chem.* 23:20–26 (1980).

21 Ritter, G. L., S. R. Lowry, C. L. Wilkins, and T. L. Isenhour. Simplex pattern recognition. *Anal. Chem.* 47:1951 (1975).

22 Everitt, B. *Cluster Analysis*. New York: Wiley (1974).

23 Sokal, R. R., and P. H. A. Sneath. *Principles of Numerical Taxonomy*. San Francisco: Freeman (1963).

24 Hartigan, J. A. *Clustering Algorithms*. New York: Wiley (1975).

25 Dubes, R., and A. K. Jain. Validity studies in clustering methodologies. *Pattern Recog.* 11:235 (1979).

26 Wold, S. Pattern recognition by means of disjoint principal components models. *Pattern Recog.* 8:127–139 (1976).

27 Wold, S., and M. Sjostrom. SIMCA: A method for analyzing chemical data in terms of similarity and analogy. *A.C.S. Symp. Ser.* 52:243–282 (1977).

28 Dunn, W. J., III, and S. Wold. Relationships between chemical structure
    and biological activity modeled by SIMCA pattern recognition. *Bioorganic
    Chem.* 9:505–523 (1980).
29 Kirschner, G. L., and B. R. Kowalski. The application of pattern
    recognition to drug design. In E. J. Ariëns (ed.), *Drug Design*, vol. 8, pp.
    73–131. New York: Academic Press (1979).
30 Norden, B., U. Edlund, and S. Wold. Carcinogenicity of polycyclic
    aromatic hydrocarbons studied by SIMCA pattern recognition. *Acta
    Chem. Scand.* [B] 32:602–608 (1978).
31 Dunn, W. J., and S. Wold. A structure-carcinogenicity study of 4-nitro-
    quinoline 1-oxides using the SIMCA method of pattern recognition.
    J. Med. Chem. 21:1001–1007 (1978).
32 Jurs, P. C., J. T. Chou, and M. Yuan. Computer assisted structure-activity
    studies of chemical carcinogens. A heterogeneous data set. *J. Med. Chem.*
    22:476–483 (1979).
33 Chou, J. T., and P. C. Jurs. Computer assisted structure-activity studies of
    chemical carcinogens. N-nitroso compounds. *J. Med. Chem.* 22:792–797
    (1979).
34 Yuan, M., and P. C. Jurs. Computer assisted structure-activity studies of
    chemical carcinogens. Polycyclic aromatic hydrocarbons. *Toxicol. Appl.
    Pharmacol.* 52:294–312 (1980).
35 Dunn, W. J., III. and S. Wold. The carcinogenicity of N-nitroso
    compounds: A SIMCA pattern recognition study. *Bioorganic Chem.* (in
    press).
36 Yuta, K., and P. C. Jurs. Computer assisted structure-activity studies of
    chemical carcinogens. Aromatic amines. *J. Med. Chem.* (in press).
37 Whalen-Pedersen, E. K., and P. C. Jurs. Computer assisted structure-
    activity studies of polycyclic aromatic hydrocarbons. In *Fifth Inter-
    national Symposium on Polynuclear Aromatic Hydrocarbons.* Columbus,
    Ohio: Battelle Press (in press).

Chapter 8

Mechanistic Structure-Activity Studies Using Quantum Chemical Methods: Application to Polycyclic Aromatic Hydrocarbon Carcinogens

Gilda H. Loew, James Ferrell,
and Michael Poulsen

OVERVIEW

The evaluation of large numbers of diverse chemicals for a spectrum of potential toxic effects is an enormous task if the chemicals are to include not only those meant to be used as drugs for specific purposes but also those that could be industrial and environmental hazards.

In drug evaluation if a compound is found to be toxic, a reasonable goal is to find a close analog with similar beneficial pharmacological activity but reduced toxicity. Such studies benefit from their focused nature, dealing as they usually do with similar compounds with known pharmacological activity, which can often provide a clue to possible toxicity.

For example, in one such study (1) we have used the techniques of theoretical chemistry to investigate the toxicity of closely related haloester inhalation anaesthetics. One of these, the widely used methoxyflurane, was removed from clinical use because of renal and hepatic toxicity found to be associated with its metabolic products. In our study we were able to formulate plausible mechanisms for such metabolism, select molecular properties that were indicators of the extent of metabolism, and predict that a closely related analog would be less extensively metabolized and hence potentially less toxic. Such predictions have since been verified by experimental and clinical studies.

In the evaluation of toxicities of industrial and environmental chemicals, the complexities are increased by the more diverse class of chemicals involved and the frequent absence of prior knowledge of any of their pharmacological effects.

Computational structure-activity studies can be very useful in such evaluations. However, independent of the computational methods or molecular descriptors used, they require an initial data set to test the reliability of selected molecular descriptors prior to their use in predictive screening. The question then arises as to how to design an iterative process that makes optimum use of combined experimental testing and computational screening methods.

A five-step process is suggested (Fig. 1). The first step is to divide the chemicals into subgroups according to structure and functional groups by any one of a number of procedures, the simplest being a "chemical reactivity" group categorization.

The next suggested step is selection of compounds from each class for a series of assays for adverse effects such as acute toxicity, mutagenicity, and carcinogenicity, thus providing an experimentally determined structure-activity data set, i.e., a "data base." The more specific the biological activity tested, the more useful the tests will be in relating structure to activity. For example, if a given toxicity can be related to inhibition or activation of a specific enzyme or chemical modification of a nucleic acid or protein component, then molecular properties related to the toxicity will be more apparent.

As a third step, mechanistic studies are suggested for limited number of representative compounds of different classes of chemicals that have been tested and found to be positive in any risk of interest. Any information coming from such studies that gives an indication of the origin of the adverse effect can be very useful in selecting mechanistically relevant molecular descriptors. While such in depth studies might appear to be relatively time-consuming, they should ultimately lead to more effective and rapidly converging schemes for obtaining reliable molecular descriptors, which also give insights into mechanisms of action since they will provide direct criteria for selection of relevant molecular indicators.

Once chosen, each set of candidate molecular descriptors must be calculated by some method, ranging from direct experimental determination through semiempirical evaluation to purely theoretical methods (step 4).

The reliability of the calculated molecular descriptors to account for known activity would them be tested (step 5). If successful, their use for large-scale screening is indicated. If not, they should be reexamined for their

1. CLASSIFICATION OF COMPOUNDS

Organize compounds into classes of chemicals according to structure and function; i.e. aromatic amines, halogenated hydrocarbons, etc.

2. PRELIMINARY DATA BASE

Select a limited number of compounds from each class for extensive series of tests; e.g., acute toxicities, mutagenicity/carcinogenicity, resistance to chemical and biological degradation.

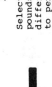

3. MECHANISTIC STUDIES

Select a limited number of compounds which have been screened for different types of adverse effects to perform in-depth mechanistic studies relevant to each risk; e.g. by mechanisms of degradation, specific toxicities

4. SELECTION OF MOLECULAR DESCRIPTORS

Use the insights obtained from in-depth studies of limited numbers of compounds to identify and select a set of appropriate "molecular descriptors" with mechanistic relevance to each risk.

No

Yes

Reexamine mechanistic basis for selection of parameters (more experiments/calculations)

Go to Step #3 and try again

Use as screening procedure for large numbers of compounds.

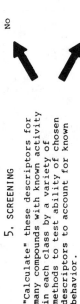

5. SCREENING

"Calculate" these descriptors for many compounds with known activity in each class by a variety of methods to test ability of chosen descriptors to account for known behavior.

Figure 1 Suggested scheme for optimal collaboration between experimental testing and computational screening methods for toxicities of diverse chemicals.

113

mechanistic relevance and for the procedures by which they were obtained. Thus a number of sets of putative descriptors, each corresponding to a possible mechanism, would be calculated and used to correlate to known adverse activity in a series of related compounds. The set that gives best correlation would also allow insight into the most probable mechanisms.

The techniques of theoretical chemistry can be particularly useful in three different steps of the process outlined in Fig. 1: (*a*) *elucidation* of mechanisms (step 3), (*b*) *selection* of molecular descriptors mechanistically relevant to a specific risk (step 4), and (*c*) *calculation* of selected molecular descriptors of potential use in screening large numbers of molecules (step 5).

The inherent capabilities of theoretical chemistry relevant to the selection of molecular descriptors are (*a*) the ability to model chemical and biochemical reactions, and (*b*) the ability to model complex formation with environmental components and tissue macromolecules. Table 1 summarizes the information that can be obtained from such calculations and how it can be translated to

Table 1   Capabilities of Theoretical Chemistry Relevant to the Selection of Molecular Descriptors (Steps 3 and 4)

A. Characterization of chemical/biochemical reactions	
What can we calculate?	**How can it be useful?**
1. Mechanisms: identification of reacting groups and the properties determining their reactivity	1. Allows identification of chemical reactivity parameters of compounds
2. Activation energies	2. Estimates of relative rates of reaction
3. Heats of reaction	3. Estimate of energy requirements for reaction
4. Identification and characterization of transition states and intermediates	4. Identification and characterization of intermediates too unstable to be examined experimentally but which could be implicated in toxicity, persistency, or other adverse environmental effects

B. Characterization of nonbonding interactions (complex formation)	
What can we calculate?	**How can it be useful?**
1. Complex geometry	1. Identify *conformational* requirement for complex formation
2. Complex stability	2. Select electronic properties contributing to stability
3. Kinetics of complex formation	3. Estimate the importance of complex formation in the time scale of interest

Table 2 Capabilities of Theoretical Chemistry Relevant to Calculation of Molecular Descriptors: Screening (Step 5)

What can be calculated?	How can it be useful?
Electronic properties Net atomic charges Dipole and higher moments Ionization potentials Electron affinities Electrostatic potential	As a measure of the extent of complex formation with polar or nonpolar solvents and a variety of tissue macromolecules—DNA, proteins, and membranes
Conformational energies A set of low-energy conformers	As a measure of the nature and stability of complex formation with macromolecules
Chemical reactivity properties Group or atomic electrophilicities and/ or nucleophilicities	Estimate of the relative ease and selectivity in transformation to specific intermediates Estimate of the extent and specificity of covalent adduct formation with tissue macromolecules

identification of specific molecular properties that could be relevant to a given risk.

For example, modeling of a chemical reaction (Table 1, A) allows the identification of groups in the interacting systems most intimately involved in the reaction and the properties of these groups, such as electrophilicity and nucleophilicity, which are important in the reaction. From such information, chemical reactivity parameters for isolated reactants can be extracted and calculated for a large number of compounds. In addition, intermediates can be identified and characterized that might be too transient to be examined experimentally but which could be implicated in toxicity or other adverse environmental effects.

The techniques of theoretical chemistry also allow the characterization of nonbonding interactions (Table 1, B), i.e., complex formation such as H-bonding and van der Waals complexes, which are typified by inhibitor-enzyme and drug-receptor molecular complexes. This characterization also leads to selection of extractable molecular descriptors, which can be readily calculated for each component of the molecular complex. Thus conformational and electronic properties related to requirements for complex formation can be selected that should be relevant to the ability of chemicals to bind to solvents, to solid state organic and inorganic materials, and to tissue macromolecules.

In addition to help in identification and selection of molecular descriptors, the techniques of theoretical chemistry can also be useful in calculating these descriptors. Examples of the types of properties that can be calculated and how they can be useful are given in Table 2. A number of electronic and chemical reactivity properties related to complex formation or chemical transformations are indicated. Energy conformation studies can also be made yielding a set of low energy conformers and isomers and their relative energies, which are indications of the flexibility of a given compound and how its conformation, volume, and shape can play a role in determining observed adverse effect.

Most of the techniques of theoretical chemistry are embodied in large-scale computer programs, rendering computers the "laboratory" where chemical reactions, complex formation, and properties of individual molecular systems can be modeled and calculated. These techniques are not limited to one particular method. In fact, an extensive library of diverse methods is currently available, with programs of varying degrees of sophistication. The types of specific methods in our library and their usefulness are summarized in Table 3. Diverse empirical energy methods, known also as molecular mechanics and empirical potential procedures, are now available. These methods utilize multiterm energy expressions with empirical parameters and are best suited for intermolecular and intramolecular energy conformational calculations. Electronic properties are best calculated using semiempirical and *ab initio* quantum chemical procedures, for which many different methods and programs are also available. The particular theoretical method used should depend on the property to be calculated and the degree of accuracy needed to use it as a reliable molecular indicator.

In this section we have outlined a general approach to a collaborative experimental and theoretical effort in risk assessment and indicated how the techniques of theoretical chemistry can be useful in this approach.

In the remaining section an application of this approach is given: the identification, selection, and calculation of molecular descriptors relevant to carcinogenic activity in a series of polycyclic aromatic hydrocarbons and their methyl derivatives.

Table 3   Classes of Specific Methods of Theoretical Chemistry

---

I. Empirical energy methods
   A. Rapid calculation of three-dimensional structures with or without geometry optimization
   B. Rapid characterization of energies and geometries of intermolecular complexes
II. Semiempirical quantum chemical methods
   A. Calculate energy conformation profile to obtain a set of low-energy conformers
   B. Calculate all relevant electronic properties
   C. Calculate chemical/biochemical reactivity parameters
   D. Model chemical/biochemical reactions
   E. Model complex formation
III. Ab initio quantum chemical methods
   Same capabilities as semiempirical methods, with greater accuracy but with much greater time constraints

---

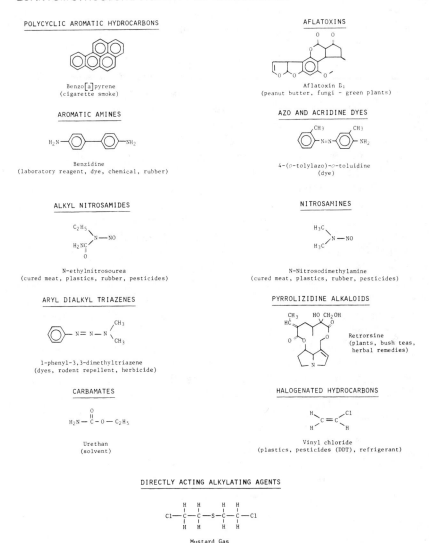

Figure 2 Classes of chemical carcinogens.

MECHANISTIC STRUCTURE–ACTIVITY STUDIES OF POLYCYCLIC AROMATIC HYDROCARBON CARCINOGENS

Background and Methods

A wide variety of chemicals (Fig. 2) have been shown to exhibit mutagenic and carcinogenic activity by a number of assays including *in vivo* animal testing, bacterial mutagenicity, cell culture transformations, and sedimentation analysis of DNA.

Polycyclic aromatic hydrocarbons (PAH) were selected for initial studies since they have long been implicated as mutagens and carcinogens (2). They are widely distributed throughout the environment, being found in urban air (3), cigarette smoke (4), and foodstuffs (5), and pose an important health threat. As a result, much experimental and theoretical effort has been aimed at understanding the mechanisms by which PAH initiate carcinogenesis.

Early work established that reactive intermediates capable of binding to DNA and other tissue nucleophiles are formed in PAH metabolism (6). Indirect evidence accumulated that PAH require metabolic activation to become active carcinogens (7), but it was not until recently that the complete sequence of intermediates between a parent PAH and DNA adduct was demonstrated (8). Based on this work and subsequent studies of benzo-[a]pyrene (9), benz[a]anthracene (10), 7-methylbenz[a]anthracene (11), chrysene (12), dibenz[a,h]anthracene (13), and 3-methylcholanthrene (14, 15), the concept of bay region diol epoxides as proximate carcinogens was advanced. As shown in Fig. 3, activation of a parent PAH to a bay region diol epoxide involves three enzymatic reactions. The first is a cytochrome P-450-mediated epoxidation at the bond adjacent to the bay region (e.g., bond 3, 4 in benz[a]anthracene), which can be called a distal bay region bond. The second is an epoxide hydrase-catalyzed hydrolysis of the distal bay region epoxide to a *trans*-dihydrodiol. The third is another cytochrome P-450-mediated epoxidation yielding the bay region tetrahydrodiol epoxide.

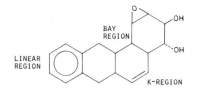

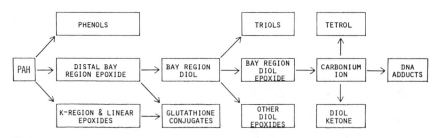

Figure 3 Detoxification and activation pathways for polycyclic aromatic hydrocarbons.

For the parent hydrocarbon, as well as the intermediate species, there are detoxification pathways competing with this activation pathway. For example, the parent compound can be oxidized to epoxides other than the distal bay region epoxide or to phenols. The distal bay region epoxide can rearrange to a phenol or a ketone or undergo competitive enzymatic reactions such as glutathione conjugation. The distal bay region diol can be oxidized to a diol-phenol or a nonvicinal diol epoxide. Finally, the bay region diol epoxide itself can be hydrolyzed to a tetrol or rearrange to a ketone. The algebraic sum of all these detoxification and activation processes determines the net amount of available diol epoxide. These species are thought to attack critical nucleophilic sites in DNA, either directly in an S_N^2 reaction (16) or after forming a carbocation in an S_N^1 (17) reaction.

If such nucleophilic attack is the critical event in tumor initiation, then the carcinogenic potency of a given PAH presumably is determined by the relative amounts of metabolic activation and detoxification and by the reactivity of the resulting ultimate carcinogen. Thus a thorough understanding of the metabolism of a series of PAH and the characterization of the ultimate carcinogens could be important in explaining their relative carcinogenicities and in predicting the carcinogenicity of untested molecules.

While every step involved in PAH activation and detoxification has not yet been totally elucidated, the significant progress outlined above makes it possible to use a mechanistic approach to structure-activity correlations for this class of carcinogens. Thus we report the results of quantum mechanical calculation of molecular properties for a series of (*a*) 17 aromatic hydrocarbons (Fig. 4) (18), (*b*) 14 methyl derivatives of benz[a]anthracene (Fig. 5) (19, 20), and (*c*) 13 methyl and fluoro derivatives of chrysene (Fig. 6) (21–24), which, in light of the bay region hypothesis, might correlate to their mutagenic or carcinogenic potencies.

In addition to the widely accepted bay region diol epoxide (BRDE) hypothesis, two other hypotheses were considered. One is the hypothesis that differential rates of transformation of the PAH to K-region oxides might relate to carcinogenic potencies. It was once thought that K-region oxides might be important ultimate carcinogens (25). In fact, it is still possible that some K-region oxides under *in vivo* conditions are not effectively detoxified by enzymes like epoxide hydrase and glutathione transferase and that K-region epoxidation could activate PAH and their methyl derivatives. The third hypothesis investigated is based on an alternative activation scheme suggested by Cavalieri and co-workers (26, 27). They envision PAH as undergoing one electron oxidation, yielding a reactive radical cation intermediate that acts as an ultimate carcinogen.

Many explanations for the effect of methyl groups on carcinogenic activity have been offered. These are summarized in Fig. 7. In the context of the BRDE hypotheses, enhanced metabolism to this species as well as

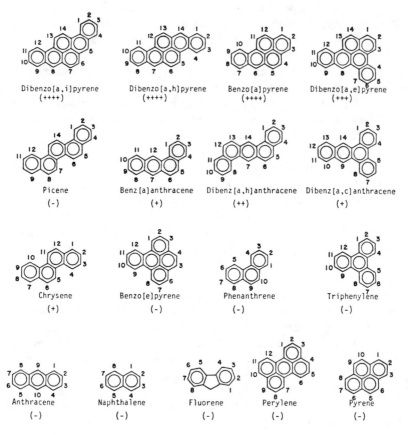

Figure 4 Structures of 17 percent polycyclic aromatic hydrocarbons studied. Qualitative carcinogenicities shown in parentheses are taken from Arcos and Argus (18).

enhanced ease of carbocation formation could be responsible. The earlier ideas of the nature of the ultimate carcinogens also have their implications for the origin of methyl group-enhanced activity. If K-region epoxide is the ultimate carcinogen, the effect of methyl groups on the extent of cytochrome P-450-mediated oxidation to this species should be relevant. If parent PAH radical cations are the active forms, then the effectiveness of methyl groups in decreasing ionization potentials and enhancing maximum ring carbon electron density should be important.

Finally, by any one of these mechanisms, if addition of methyl groups blocks phenol formation or formation of other detoxification products, then it could also enhance carcinogenic activity.

In the studies reported here, all three hypotheses were considered, and three types of properties were calculated: ability of parent compounds to

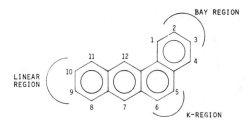

Figure 5 Structure of benz[a]anthracene (BA) and the methyl derivatives included in this study. Carcinogenicities taken from Dunning and Curtis (19) and Stevenson and Von Haam (20).

MBAs	CARCINOGENICITY	DMBAs	CARCINOGENICITY
1,2,3,4	−	9,10	++
5	−	6, 8	++++
6	++	5,12	−
7	+++	6,12	++++
8	++	7,12	++++
9	+	8,12	++++
10	±		
11	−		
12	++		

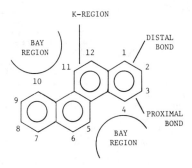

MC	CARCINOGENICITY	DMC	CARCINOGENICITY	n–F–5MC	CARCINOGENICITY
1	−	2,3	−	1	−
2	−	5,6	++ (?)	3	−
3	−	5,12	−	6	++++
4	−			7	++++
5	++++			9	++++
6	−			12	+

Figure 6 Structure of chrysene and the methyl and fluoro derivatives included in this study. Carcinogenicities taken from literature (21–24).

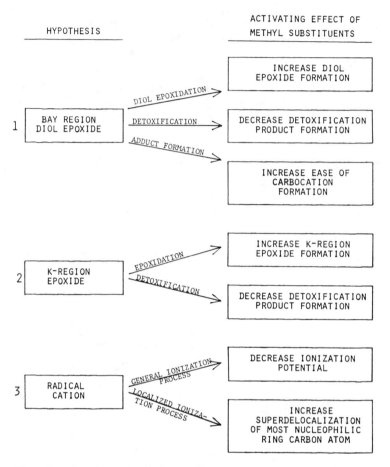

Figure 7 Three alternative hypotheses for origin of carcinogenic activity in polycyclic aromatic hydrocarbons and their consequences for the effect of methyl substituents on this activity.

form radical cations, ideal reactivities of parent compounds and dihydrodiols as substrates of cytochrome P-450, and energies of the diol epoxide carbocations relative to the diol epoxides. The ideal reactivities are electronic factors that in part determine the relative extents of activating and detoxifying metabolism for each PAH.

To predict the reactivity of the compounds toward radical cation formation, two calculated parameters were considered: the energy of the highest occupied molecular orbital from which the electron would be removed (a measure of the ionization potential) and the nucleophilic superdelocalizability of the most reactive ring carbon atom considered as a specific site of ionization of an electron.

Parameters relevant to epoxidation and hydroxylation by cytochrome by P-450 were chosen by consideration of probable mechanisms of cytochrome P-450 oxidations. All forms of cytochrome P-450 are thought to effect the transfer of an electrophilic oxygen to specific electron-rich sites in the substrate. Thus, insofar as the extent and specificity of metabolism is controlled by electronic properties of the substrate, the relative propensities of a PAH to undergo activation versus detoxification can be predicted from such calculations.

If epoxidation proceeds by electrophilic oxygen atom insertion across the double bond, then π-bond nucleophilic reactivity should be a reasonable property to monitor the relative extent of transformation of each double bond in a given PAH and within a series of PAH. If direct phenol formation proceeds by addition of an electrophilic oxygen to a ring carbon atom and rearrangement of a hydrogen atom to the phenol, then ring carbon atom nucleophilicity should be a measure of relative extent of phenol formation at different ring positions in a given compound and within a series of PAH. These nucleophilic parameters are defined below. They are the energy-weighted averages of π-bond densities (ρ_{AB}) and net atomic charges (q_A), respectively.

The atomic superdelocalizability is defined by

$$ S_A(\pi) = \sum_{k \text{ filled}}^{\text{MOs}} \frac{q_A^\pi(k)}{\epsilon(k)} $$

where $q_A^\pi(k) = \pi$-electron density on atom A in molecular orbital (MO) k
$\quad \epsilon(k) =$ energy of molecular orbital k in electron-volts.
The greater the absolute value of $S_A(\pi)$, the more likely direct phenol formation will occur at carbon atom A.

In similar fashion, the π bond reactivity to epoxidation was defined as:

$$ R_{AB} = \sum_{k \text{ filled}}^{\text{MOs}} \frac{\rho_{AB}^\pi(k)}{\epsilon(k)} $$

where $\rho_{AB}^\pi(k) = \pi$-bond density between atom A and B in molecular orbital k
$\quad \epsilon(k) =$ energy of molecular orbital k in electron-volts.
The greater the absolute value of π-bond reactivity, the more likely epoxidation by an electrophilic oxygen will occur at a given bond.

As a measure of ease of rearrangement of epoxide to phenols we have used differences in the nucleophilicity ($S_A - S_B$) at the two carbon atoms C_A and C_B forming the epoxide bond. The rationale for this choice of parameter is that large differences in the electron density at the two carbon atoms are assumed to facilitate the epoxide bond-breaking step. We further assume that C—O bond cleavage occurs at the carbon atom with the lesser electron density. All of these reactivity parameters were calculated using a semiempirical, all-valence electron molecular orbital method called iterative extended huckel theory (IEHT) (28).

To calculate the relative energies of each diol epoxide and its carbocation, the semiempirical molecular orbital method called INDO (intermediate neglect of differential overlap) (29) was used. The calculated energy difference, $^\Delta E = E$ (diol epoxide) $- E$ (carbocation), was used as a measure of the ease of formation of the benzylic carbocation from the bay region diol epoxide for each of the 44 analogs studied. This energy difference is presumed to be proportional to the transition state energy in the rate-determining step of carcinogens macromolecule adduct formation by an S_N^1 mechanism.

Both of the methods used require molecular geometries as input, and these were obtained from tables of standard bond lengths and angles, and x-ray crystal structures together with geometry optimization procedures.

Standard bond lengths and angles (29) were used to construct molecular geometries for all planar PAH and their methyl derivatives. In 12-methyl benzanthracene (MBA) and its n,12-DMBA derivatives, steric repulsion between the 1-hydrogen and 12-methyl groups forces the molecule into a gradually bent conformation, interfering with total electron delocalization. The geometries for these nonplanar molecules were based on a crystal structure of 7,12-DMBA (30). For the nonplanar 5,12-dimethylchrysene (5,12-DMC), the hydrocarbon geometry was also taken from its x-ray crystal structure (31). The structure of 5-MC was then created by removing the 12-methyl group.

For the bay region diol epoxides and carbocations, standard bond lengths and angles were again used for the intact aromatic rings of the planar compounds and the crystal structure of 7,12-DMBA and 5,12-DMC for the nonplanar derivatives. The diol epoxide ring geometry was obtained by total geometry optimization of 1β,2β-epoxy-3β,4α-dihydroxybenzene (benzene *anti*-diol epoxide) using the MINDO/3 method (32). This geometry has been described more completely elsewhere (16, 33) and, in the absence of a crystal structure, provides a self-consistent geometry for this series of calculations.

In addition, steric effects required that the structures of the 12-BA derivatives be more completely optimized. Important bond angles as well as torsion angles were chosen in these special cases for optimization using the perturbative configuration interaction using localized orbitals PCILO) program (34). The geometries for 6,12-DMBA and 3,12-DMBA were based on this more completely optimized structure for 12-DMBA, while the 5,12-DMBA required further local geometry relaxation and optimization because of the proximity of the 5-methyl group to the bay region diol epoxide. These changes primarily involved rotations of the 5-methyl group and the 4-hydroxyl group, with the overall ring conformation remaining largely the same.

Similarly, the geometries of the diol epoxide and triol carbocations of 5-MC and 5,12-DMC were optimized using a local optimization procedure of the PCILO program (34) to adjust the geometry of atoms that were most affected by the crowding of the methyl groups.

Results and Discussion

Metabolism Calculation of the π-bond and ring carbon nucleophilicities and the "skewing" of π-bond density at each epoxide bond site for all compounds has allowed predictions to be made of the major diol and phenol metabolites of each PAH and methyl benz[a] anthracene (BA) and methyl chrysene derivative studied. Unfortunately, except for a few well-characterized compounds such as benz[a] pyrene, BA, 1,12-diCH$_3$BA chrysene, and 5-CH$_3$ chrysene, only a limited amount of data of variable quality are available for these compounds. Nevertheless, the well-studied cases offered a good test of our reactivity parameters, and, in general, the calculated reactivity parameters are in fairly good agreement with what data are available. These results are discussed in detail elsewhere (35–39). A few salient features will be mentioned here.

On the basis of these results, some general conclusions can be drawn concerning the reactivities of aromatic bonds and atomic centers to cytochrome P-450–mediated hydroxylation and epoxidation and, more generally, to electrophilic substitution. It was found that saturating one bond in a benzo ring (4) makes the adjacent bond more reactive to epoxidation than any arene bonds. Next most reactive are K-region bonds (5). Of the remaining types, the anthracene-type (linear, non-bay region) bonds (6) are more reactive than distal bay region bonds (7A) while proximal bay region bonds (7B) are still less reactive. Bonds to atoms with three-ring junctions (8) are least reactive. For atomic centers, it was found that L-region positions (9) are most reactive to one-centered oxidation followed by K-region positions (10), α-carbons (11), and finally β-carbons (12). Proximal bay region α- and β-carbons were less reactive than distal-bay or non-bay α- and β-carbons, respectively.

A very interesting specific effect of addition of a 5-CH$_3$ group on chrysene metabolism is also obtained. Chrysene has two equivalent bay regions but has little or no carcinogenic potency. Addition of a 5-CH$_3$ group creates a potent carcinogen, makes the entire ring system nonplanar, and also renders the two bay regions inequivalent.

Comparing the calculated π-bond reactivities for chrysene and 5-MC (Table 4), two striking effects of the 5-methyl group are observed. First, there is a dramatic increase in reactivity of all π-bonds relative to chrysene. Second, and perhaps more importantly, the magnitude and order of bond reactivities in the two distinct bay regions is different. Our results show that while the 7,8,9,10 bay is activated relative to the 1,2,3,4 bay, the proximal (9,10) bond of the 7,8,9,10 bay is much more reactive than the distal (7,8) bond. The preferential epoxidation at the 9,10 bond, which this result suggests, would lead to the "wrong" bay region diol epoxide, i.e., the 7,8-oxide-9-10-diol, which is presumed to form a carbocation less readily than the reverse 9,10-oxide-7,8-diol. Thus the reactivity pattern of this bay region suggests that it would not contribute significantly to the greatly increased carcinogenic activity observed for 5-MC.

For the other (1,2,3,4) bay region, the calculated results are very different. Not only are the 1,2 and 3,4 bonds both activated relative to the chrysene, but the 1,2 bond is predicted to be epoxidated preferentially, leading to the "correct" diol epoxide, i.e., the one that more readily forms a carbocation.

A study of the metabolic products of 5-MC shows that diols are present in the order 1,2 $\geqslant$ 9,10 $\geqslant$ 7,8 (40). This result reinforces our conclusion that in one bay region, the 9,10-diol will be more abundant than the 7,8-diol; and for the other bay region, the 1,2-diol will form more than the 3,4-diol, which was not definitively identified but could possibly be the source of one of the undetermined high-pressure liquid chromatography (HPLC) peaks.

Table 4   Calculated π-Bond Nucleophilic Superdelocalizabilities for Chrysene Derivatives Using IEHT Method

Bond[*]	Chrysene	5-MC	5-MC (ΔS_{AB})[†]	C_A—OH[‡]
1–2	−22.35	−24.60	4.02	1—OH
3–4	−22.27	−23.73	2.57	3—OH
5–6	−24.73	−26.55	4.81	6—OH
7–8	−22.35	−23.52	2.00	7—OH
9–10	−22.27	−25.95	1.96	9—OH
11–12	−24.73	−25.56	2.67	12—OH

[*]See Fig. 6 for numbering scheme.

[†]ΔS_{AB} = Superdelocalizability and difference between the two carbon atoms, C_A and C_B of a given epoxide.

[‡]Predicted phenol product from rearrangement of epoxide.

Table 5   Radical Mechanism: Correlation between Reactivity toward One-Centered Oxidation and Carcinogenicity

Compound	Position	Reactivity[*]	Carcinogenicity
Dibenzo [a, h] pyrene	7	−65.0	++++
Dibenzo [a, i] pyrene	7	−64.7	++++
Benz [a] pyrene	6	−64.5	++++
Dibenzo [a, e] pyrene	8	−63.5	+++
Benz [a] anthracene	7	−63.5	+
Anthracene	9	−63.5	−
Dibenz [a, c] anthracene	9	−62.7	+
Dibenz [a, h] anthracene	7	−62.6	++
Perylene	3	−62.2	−
Pyrene	3	−61.5	−
Benzo [e] pyrene	7	−61.3	+
Picene	4	−60.8	−
Phenanthrene	1	−60.2	−
Napthalene	1	−60.0	−
Triphenylene	1	−59.8	−

[*]Maximum carbon atom π electron density.

The addition of a fluorine atom to either bay of 5-MC, presumably forcing metabolism at the other bay, does not produce a major electronic effect.

Correlation with Carcinogenicity 1. *Differences in reactive toward one-electron oxidation do not explain relative carcinogenicities of PAH and MBA.* As shown in Table 5, using carbon atom nucleophilicity as a criterion for one-electron oxidation for PAH, there appear to be some correlation to carcinogenic activity. However, this criterion fails (Table 6) for BA and MBA and does not hold if both tables are interdigitated. As shown in Table 6, the ionization potential, as measured by the energy of the highest occupied molecular orbital, is insensitive to methyl group substitution, and even the small variations do not correlate to relative carcinogenicities. Thus one-electron oxidation of parent compounds does not appear to lead to their active carcinogenic form.

2. *Differences in K-region bond reactivities do not correlate with carcinogenic activities of PAH and MBA.* While there is some trend toward decreased carcinogenic activity with decreased K-region π-bond reactivity in MBA and DMBA (Table 7), there is absolutely no such correlation for diverse PAH in general (Table 8), and combining the two sets of data further reduces the correlations. Thus K-region epoxidation appears to be neither activating nor detoxifying.

Table 6 Calculated Reactivity toward One-Electron Oxidation in Methylbenz[a] anthracenes

	Using ionization potential			Using maximum electron density in ring carbon atom (n)	
Compound	HOMO energy (eV)	Carcinogenicity	Compound	Reactivity	Carcinogenicity
7-MBA	10.95	+++	5,12-DMBA	−66.1 (7)	−
6,8-DMBA	10.96	++++	8,12-DMBA	−65.9 (9)	++++
5-MBA	10.97	−	7-MBA	−65.5 (12)	+++
9,10-MBA	10.98	++	5-MBA	−64.9 (7)	−
7,12-DMBA	10.98	++++	12-MBA	−64.9 (7)	++
4-MBA	11.02	−	6,12-DMBA	−64.9 (7)	++++
8-MBA	11.02	++	6-MBA	−64.8 (5)	++
6-MBA	11.03	++	9,10-DMBA	−64.8 (8)	++
9-MBA	11.04	+	9-MBA	−64.6 (7)	+
11-MBA	11.04	−	10-MBA	−64.3 (11)	±
10-MBA	11.06	±	11-MBA	−64.1 (7)	−
6,12-DMBA	11.06	++++	2-MBA	−63.9 (7)	−
5,12-DMBA	11.08	−	4-MBA	−63.8 (7)	−
3-MBA	11.08	−	3-MBA	−63.7 (7)	−
8,12-DMBA	11.09	++++	BA	−63.5 (7)	±
2-MBA	11.09	−	6,8-DMBA	−63.4 (11)	++++
BA	11.10	±	8-MBA	−63.3 (11)	++
12-MBA	11.14	++	7,12-DMBA	−62.3 (9)	++++

Table 7   K-Region Epoxide as Ultimate Carcinogen: Parent PAH K-Region Reactivity and Carcinogenicity

Compound	Reactivity[*]	Carcinogenicity
Benz[a] anthracene	−26.1	+
Dibenzo[a,i] pyrene	−25.7	++++
Benzo[e] pyrene	−25.6	+
Phenanthrene	−25.5	−
Benzo[a] pyrene	−25.4	++++
Dibenz[a,h] anthracene	−25.2	++
Pyrene	−24.9	−
Chrysene	−24.7	+
Dibenzo[a,h] pyrene	−24.6	++++
Picene	−24.3	−
Dibenzo[a,e] pyrene	−24.1	+++
Dibenz[a,c] anthracene	No K-region	+
Triphenylene	No K-region	−
Anthracene	No K-region	−
Naphthalene	No K-region	−
Perylene	No K-region	−
Fluorene	No K-region	−

[*]Reactivity expressed in units of thousandths of an electron charge per electron-volt (eV).

Table 8   Calculated K-Region π-Bond Reactivity to Epoxidation: Benz[a] anthracene and Its Methyl Derivatives

Compound	Reactivity	Carcinogenicity
5,12-DMBA	−28.43	−
6,12-DMBA	−28.42	++++
7,12-DMBA	−27.98	++++
8,12-DMBA	−27.87	++++
12-MBA	−27.86	++
6,8-DMBA	−26.66	++++
6-MBA	−26.64	++
5-MBA	−26.54	−
7-MBA	−26.32	+++
4-MBA	−26.23	−
9-MBA	−26.21	+
8-MBA	−26.18	++
9,10-DMBA	−26.16	++
2-MBA	−26.12	−
11-MBA	−26.12	−
10-MBA	−26.11	±
3-MBA	−26.10	−
BA	−26.09	±

3. Differences in detoxification reactivities might explain the relative carcinogenicities of benz[a]anthracene and its methyl derivatives. Since phenols are not by themselves carcinogenic and, in fact, appear to inhibit PAH metabolism (41), phenol formation could be a detoxification pathway for PAH.

In Table 9 is given the reactivity of ring carbon positions in BA to direct phenyl formation. The data for BA in Table 9 appear to support the suggestion that methyl groups added to BA could enhance carcinogenic activity by blocking detoxification by phenol formation. Thus, 7,12-DMBA, with the two most reactive sites blocked to phenol formation, is the most carcinogenic of these compounds, while 7- and 12-MBA, each with one reactive site blocked, are highly and moderately carcinogenic, respectively. The 6- and 8-MBA, with moderately reactive sites blocked and the reactive 7-position sterically hindered, are the only other moderately carcinogenic compounds.

However, the inviting explanation that the enhanced activity of some MBA is due to blocking of phenol formation is mitigated by the result that while the 7- and 12-MBA each have one reactive site blocked, the reactivity of the other site to phenol formation is enhanced, as shown in parentheses in this table; and yet, both compounds are highly active carcinogens. Taken together there is not enough evidence to implicate methyl groups clearly as blockers of detoxification pathways in PAH.

4. In the context of the bay region diol epoxide carbocation as the ultimate carcinogen, (a) differences in the first enzymatic transformation of the parent compounds to "distal" bay region epoxides correlate to some extent with relative carcinogenicity of PAH and MBA. This result is seen in

Table 9 Correlation Between Carcinogenicity of N-CH$_3$ Benz[a] anthracene and Reactivity of Blocked Sites

Site	C atom reactivity by π criterion in BA	Carcinogenicity
7	−63.5 (65.6)	+++
12	−62.1 (64.9)	++
8	−60.5	++
6	−60.4	++
5	−60.4	−
11	−60.4	−
4	−60.2	−
1	−59.1	−
2	−58.7	−
10	−58.6	± (?)
9	−58.5	± (?)
3	−58.3	−

Table 10   Correlation between Reactivity of Distal Bay Region Bond Parent Compound Reactivity and Carcinogenicity

Compound	Reactivity[*]	Carcinogenicity
Dibenzo[a,h]pyrene	−22.6	++++
Benzo[a]pyrene	−22.4	++++
Chrysene	−22.4	+
Dibenzo[a,e]pyrene	−22.3	+++
Dibenzo[a,i]pyrene	−22.1	++++
Phenanthrene	−22.0	−
Picene	−21.7	−
Benz[a]anthracene	−21.6	+
Benzo[e]pyrene	−21.4	+
Dibenz[a,h]anthracene	−21.3	++
Triphenylene	−21.0	−
Dibenz[a,c]anthracene	−20.7	+
Anthracene[†]	−23.9	−
Naphthalene[†]	−23.0	−
Fluorene[†]	−20.4	−
Perylene	No bay region	−
Pyrene	No bay region	−

[*]Reactivity expressed in units of thousandths of an electron charge per electron-volt (eV). Large negative reactivities denote reactive bonds.
[†]These compounds can form proximal diol epoxides but have no true bay region.

Tables 10 and 11. However, the reactivity of the distal bay region bond is not very sensitive either to fused ring structure or to methyl substitution, and this reaction does not appear to be a primary molecular determinant for activity.

  (b) Distal bay region diol reactivity to proximal bay region epoxidation (the third activating step) does not correlate to relative carcinogenic activity in PAH. As shown in Table 12, the reactivity of this isolated double bond is high and relatively constant in all PAH. Thus, once the distal bay region diol is formed, epoxidation should be enhanced and proceed to the same extent for all PAH with bay regions, making this a nondiscriminating activating step.

  (c) Differences in bay region diol epoxide carbocation stability correlate well to carcinogenicity in the 44 PAH and methyl derivatives studied. For the 44 PAH studied, Table 13 shows the calculated energy difference between their bay region diol epoxides and carbocations, with the most easily formed carbocation that of 6,12-DMBA, arbitrarily taken to have a $\Delta E = 0$. The calculated value of ΔE is an estimate of the energy of activation for the formation of the carbocation. As shown in Table 13, a striking correlation is obtained between ease of formation of carbocation and carcinogenic potencies. Among the methyl derivatives, the eight most stable carbocations have the nonplanar geometry of 12-MBA or 5-MC.

Table 11 Calculated Reactivity of the Distal Bay Region (3–4) Bond in Benz[a] anthracene and Its Methyl Derivatives

Compound	Reactivity	Carcinogenicity
7,12-DMBA	−22.212	++++
12-MBA	−22.198	++
5,12-DMBA	−22.164	−
6,12-DMBA	−22.149	++++
8,12-DMBA	−22.115	++++
6,8-DMBA	−21.689	++++
7-MBA	−21.684	+++
5-MBA	−21.667	−
6-MBA	−21.665	++
9-MBA	−21.664	+
8-MBA	−21.651	++
9,10-DMBA	−21.639	++
11-MBA	−21.619	−
10-MBA	−21.601	±
BA	−21.596	±

Table 12 Dihydrodiol Reactivity: Lack of Correlation between Intrinsic Reactivity to Second Epoxidation and Carcinogenicity

Compound	Reactivity[*]	Carcinogenicity
Dibenzo[a,e] pyrene	−32.2	+++
Picene	−32.2	−
Dibenz[a,c] anthracene	−32.2	+
Phenanthrene	−32.2	−
Triphenylene	−32.2	−
Dibenzo[a,i] pyrene	−32.1	++++
Dibenzo[a,h] pyrene	−32.1	++++
Benzo[e] pyrene	−32.1	+
Naphthalene	−32.1	−
Benz[a] anthracene	−32.0	+
Anthracene	−32.0	−
Benzo[a] pyrene	−31.9	++++
Dibenz[a,h] anthracene	−31.9	++
Chrysene	−31.9	+
Perylene	Cannot form proximal diol epoxide	−
Pyrene	Cannot form proximal diol epoxide	−

[*]Reactivity expressed in units of thousandths of an electron charge per eV. Large negative reactivities denote reactive bonds.

Table 13   Calculated Energy of Carbocation Formation and Observed
Carcinogenic Potency for 44 PAH and Their Methyl Derivatives

Compound	ΔE (kcal/mol)[*]	Carcinogenicity[†]
6,12-DMBA	0	++++
Dibenzo[a,i]pyrene	1.9	++++
Dibenzo[a,h]pyrene	3.2	++++
7,12-DMBA	3.8	++++
8,12-DMBA	5.1	++++
12-MBA	5.3	++
5,12-DMBA	6.8	–
Benzo[a]pyrene	7.2	++++
5,6-DMC	7.3	++ (?)
5,12-DMC	7.4	–
Dibenzo[a,e]pyrene	8.1	+++
5-MC	9.2	++++
6,8-DMBA	9.2	++++
6-F-5-MC	9.7	++++
6-MBA	9.7	++
9-F-5-MC	11.3	++++
7-F-5-MC	11.3	++++
9,10-DMBA	13.2	++
7-MBA	13.3	+++
10-MBA	13.7	–
Dibenz[a,h]anthracene	14.4	++
8-MBA	14.4	++
9-MBA	14.5	+
11-MBA	15.0	–
Benz[a]anthracene	15.0	–
5-MBA	15.2	–
Dibenz[a,c]anthracene	15.8	+
12-F-5-MC	17.4	+
Benzo[e]pyrene	18.0	+
6-MC	18.2	–
Picene	18.3	–
7,12-Dimethylbenzo[b]chrysene	18.3	–
2,3-DMC	19.0	–
Benzo[b]chrysene	19.1	–
3-MC	19.5	–
4-MC	19.8	–
1-MC	19.9	–
Triphenylene	20.0	–
2-MC	20.0	–
Chrysene	20.6	+

(See footnote on page 134.)

Table 13   Calculated Energy of Carbocation Formation and Observed
Carcinogenic Potency for 44 PAH and Their Methyl Derivatives (*Continued*)

Compound	ΔE (kcal/mol)[*]	Carcinogenicity[†]
Phenanthrene	22.2	−
5,10-Dimethylanthracene	24.6	+
Anthracene	27.7	−
Naphthalene	35.1	−

[*]Energies relative to 6,12-DMBA.
[†]Data from Dunning and Curtis (19), Hecht et al. (22, 24, 40), Hewlett (1940), Shear (1938), and Stevenson and Von Haam (20).

The major exceptions to the excellent correlations obtained can be explained in terms of the steric effect of a methyl group adjacent to the bay region, the 5-position in BA and the 12-position in chrysene. Called the *peri* effect (27, 35, 42), it has been proposed to inactivate PAH by blocking distal bay region diol formation, the second activating step which we have not modeled. However, the results of our studies offer an alternative explanation of the peri effect.

Energy conformation calculations performed on the *trans*-3,4-diol of 5,12-DMBA to determine its minimum energy conformation indicate that the diol substituents have a different conformation from that in any other MBA. Although it appears minor, this change in conformation could prevent the diol from being further epoxidized at the 1-2 position; or if the diol epoxide is formed, the altered conformation could sterically inhibit interaction of its carbocation with tissue nucleophiles.

CONCLUSIONS

Of all the hypotheses and molecular properties examined in this study, one specific molecular descriptor, the ease of bay region diol epoxide carbocation formation, yields excellent correlation with observed carcinogenic activity for 17 PAH. Moreover, this property can also account for the relative carcinogenicities of a series of methyl derivatives of benz[a]anthracene and chrysene. These results lend support to the bay region hypothesis for PAH activity and identify useful parameters for mass screening for PAH and related compounds for carcinogenic activity, calculated values of ΔE greater than 15 kcal/mol, indicating little or no activity. Similar mechanistic structure-activity studies have been made for aromatic amine carcinogens (43, 44), and work is in progress on structure-activity studies of the toxicity and carcinogenicity of halohydrocarbons.

REFERENCES

1 Loew, G., H. Motulsky, J. Trudell, E. Cohen, and L. Hjelmeland. Quantum chemical studies of the metabolism of the inhalation anesthetics methoxyflurane, enflurane and isoflurane. *Mol. Pharmacol.* 100:406–418 (1974).

2 Pott, P. Cancer scroti in chirurgical observations relative to the cataract, the polypus of the nose, the cancer of the scrotum, the different kinds of ruptures and the modification of the toes and feet, p. 63. London: Howes, Clarke and Collins (1775); reprinted in *Natl. Cancer Inst. Monogr.* 10:7 (1963).

3 National Academy of Sciences. *Particulate Polycyclic Organic Matter: Biological Effects of Atmospheric Pollutants.* Washington, D.C.: National Resource Council (1972).

4 Hoffman, D., and E. L. Wynder. The chemistry of tobacco smoke. In: I. Schmeltz (ed.), p. 123. New York: Plenum (1972).

5 Lijinsky, W., and A. E. Ross. Production of carcinogenic polynuclear hydrocarbons in the cooking of food. *Food Cosmet. Toxicol.* 5:343 (1967).

6 Boyland, E. The biological significance of metabolism of polycyclic compounds. *Biochem. Soc. Symp.* 5:40 (1950).

7 Dipple, A. Polynuclear aromatic carcinogens. In C. E. Searle (ed.), *Chemical Carcinogens*, pp. 245–307, Washington, D.C.: American Chemical Society (1976).

8 Borgen, A., H. Darvey, N. Castagnoli, J. T. Crocker, R. E. Rasmussen, hamster liver microsomes and binding of metabolites to DNA. *J. Med. Chem.* 16:502 (1973).

9 Sims, P., and P. L. Grover. Epoxides in polycyclic aromatic hydrocarbon metabolism and carcinogenesis. *Adv. Cancer Res.* 20:165 (1974).

10 Wood, W. A., R. L. Chang, W. Levin, R. E. Lehr, M. Schaefer-Ridder, J. M. Karle, D. M. Jerina, and A. H. Conney. Mutagenicity and cytotoxicity of benz[a]anthracene diol epoxides and tetrahydro epoxides: Exceptional activity of the bay region 1,2-epoxide. *Proc. Natl. Acad. Sci. (U.S.A.)* 74:2746 (1977).

11 Tierney, B., A. Hewer, C. Walsh, P. L. Grover, and P. Sims. The metabolic activation of 7-methylbenz(a)anthracene in mouse skin. *Chem.-Biol. Interact.* 18:179 (1977).

12 Wood, A. W., W. Levin, A. Y. H. Lu, D. Ryan, S. B. West, H. Yagi, H. D. Mah, D. M. Jerina, and A. H. Conney. High mutagenicity of metabolically activated chrysene 1,2-dihydrodiol: Evidence for bay region activation in chrysene. *Biochem. Biophys. Res. Commun.* 78:487 (1977).

13 Wood, A. W., W. Levin, R. L. Chang, J. M. Karbe, H. D. Mah, H. Yagi, D. M. Jerina, and A. H. Conney. Evidence that bay region diol epoxide of chrysene and dibenz[a,h]anthracene (DBA) are ultimate carcinogens. *A.A.C.R. Abstracts*, p. 109 (March 1975).

14   Thakker, D. R., W. Levin, A. W. Wood, A. H. Conney, T. A. Stoming, and D. M. Jerina. Metabolic formation of 1,9,10-trihydroxy-9,10, dihydro-3-methylcolthrene: A potential proximate carcinogen from 3-methylcholanthrene. *J. Am. Chem. Soc.* 100:645 (1978).

15   Thakker, D. R., W. Levin, A. W. Wood, A. H. Conney, T. A. Stoming, and D. M. Jerina. 9,10-Dihydrodiols of 1-hydroxy-t-methylcholanthrene: Potential proximate carcinogen derived from 3-methylcholanthrene. *A.A.C.R. Abstracts*, p. 204 (March 1978).

16   Ferrell, J. E., Jr., and G. H. Loew. Mechanistic studies of arene oxide and diol epoxide rearrangement and hydrolysis reactions. *J. Am Chem. Soc.* 101:1385 (1979).

17   Yang, S. K., D. W. McCourt, and H. V. Gelboin. The mechanism of hydrolysis of the non-K-region benzo[a]pyrene diol epoxide r-7, t-8-dihydroxy-t-9.10-oxy-7,8,9,10-tetrahydrobenzo[a]pyrene. *J. Am. Chem. Soc.* 99:5130 (1977).

18   Arcos, J. C., and M. F. Argus. Molecular geometry and carcinogenic activity of aromatic compounds. New perspectives. *Adv. Cancer Res.* 11:305 (1968).

19   Dunning, W. F., and M. R. Curtis. Relative carcinogenic activity of monomethyl derivatives of benz[a]anthracene in Fischer line 344 rats. *J. Natl. Cancer Inst.* 25:387 (1960).

20   Stevenson, J. L., and E. Von Haam. Carcinogenicity of benzo-[a]anthracene and benzo[c]phenanthrene. *J. Am. Ind. Hyg. Assoc.* 26:475 (1965).

21   Hoffman, D., W. E. Bondinell, and E. L. Wynder. Carcinogenicity of methylchrysenes. *Science* 18:215 (1974).

22   Hecht, S. S., W. E. Bondinell, and D. Hoffman. Chrysene and methyl-chrysenes: Presence in tobacco smoke and carcinogenicity. *J. Natl. Cancer Inst.* 53:1121 (1974).

23   Hecht, S. S., M. Loy, R. R. Maronpot, and D. Hoffman. A study of chemical carcinogenesis: Comparative carcinogenicity of 5-methylchrysene, benzo[a]pyrene, and modified chrysenes. *Cancer Lett.* 1:147 (1976).

24   Hecht, S. S., E. LaVoie, R. Mazzarese, N. Hirota, T. Ohmori, and D. Hoffmann. Comparative mutagenicity, tumor-initiating activity, carcino-genicity, and *in vitro* metabolism of fluorinated 5-methylchrysenes. *J. Natl. Cancer Inst.* 63:855 (1979).

25   Sims, P., and P. L. Grover. Epoxides in polycyclic aromatic hydrocarbon metabolism and carcinogenesis. *Adv. Cancer Res.* 20:165 (1974).

26   Cavalieri, E., and R. Auerbach. Reactions between activated benzo-[a]pyrene and nucleophilic compounds, with possible implications on the mechanism of tumor initiation. *J. Natl. Cancer Inst.* 53:2649 (1974).

27   Rogan, E., R. Ruth, P. Katomski, J. Benderson, and E. Cavalieri. Binding of benzo[a]pyrene at the 1,2,6 positions to nucleic acids in vivo on mouse skin and in vitro with rat liver microsomes and nuclei. *Chem.-Biol. Interact.* 22:35 (1978).

28   Zerner, M., M. Gouterman, and H. Kobayashi. Porphyrins. VIII. Extended

Huckel calculations on iron complexes. *Theor. Chim. Acta (Berl.)* 6:363 (1966).

29 Pople, J. A., and D. L. Beveridge. *Approximate Molecular Orbital Theory.* New York: McGraw-Hill (1970).

30 Iball, J. A refinement of the structure of 9,10-dimethyl-1:2-benzanthracene. *Nature* 201:916 (1964).

31 Glusker, J. Personal communication (1979).

32 Bingham, R. C., M. J. S. Dewar, and D. H. Lo. Ground state of molecules. XXV. MINDO/3. An improved version of the MINDO semiempirical SCFMO method. *J. Am. Chem. Soc.* 97:1285 (1975).

33 Loew, G. H., A. T. Pudzianowski, A. Czerwinski, and J. E. Ferrell. Mechanistic studies of addition of nucleophiles to arene oxides and diol epoxides: Candidate ultimate carcinogens. *Int. J. Quant. Chem. (QBS)* 7(1980).

34 Diner, S., J. P. Malrieu, F. Jordan, and M. Gilbert. Localized bond orbitals and the correlation problem. III. Energy up to third-order in the zero-differential overlap approximation. Application to σ-electron systems. *Theor. Chim. Acta (Berl.)* 15:100 (1979).

35 Loew, G. H., J. Wong, J. Phillips, L. Hjelmeland, and G. Pack. Quantum chemical studies of the metabolism of benzo[a]pyrene. *Cancer Biochem. Biophys* 2:123 (1978).

36 Loew, G. H., J. Phillips, J. Wong, L. Hjelmeland, and G. Pack. Quantum chemical studies of the metabolism of polycyclic aromatic hydrocarbons: Bay region reactivity as a criterion for carcinogenic potency. *Cancer Biochem. Biophys.* 2:113 (1978).

37 Loew, G. H., B. S. Sudhindra, J. E. Ferrell, Jr. Quantum chemical studies of polycyclic aromatic hydrocarbons and their metabolites: Correlations to carcinogenicity. *Chem.-Biol. Interact* 26:75 (1979).

38 Loew, G. H., M. Poulsen, J. Ferrell, and D. Cheat. Quantum chemical studies of methylbenz[a]anthracenes: Metabolism and correlations with carcinogenicity. *Chem.-Biol. Interact.* 31:319 (1980).

39 Poulsen, M. T., and G. H. Loew. Quantum chemical studies of methyl and fluoro analogs of chrysene: Metabolic activation and correlation with carcinogenic activity. *Cancer Biochem. Biophys.* (in press).

40 Hecht, S. S., E. LaVoie, R. Mazzarese, S. Aming, V. Bedenko, and D. Hoffman. 1,2-Dihydro-1,2-dihydroxy-5-methylchrysene, a major activated metabolite of the environmental carcinogen 5-methylchrysene. *Cancer Res.* 38:4191 (1978).

41 Thakker, D. R., W. Levin, H. Yagi, D. Ryan, P. E. Thomas, J. M. Karle, R. E. Lehr, D. M. Jerina, and A. H. Conney. Metabolism of benzo[a]anthracene to its tumorigenic 3,4 dihydrodiol. *Mol. Pharmacol.* 15:138 (1979).

42 Jerina, D. M., H. Yagi, R. E. Lehr, D. R. Thakker, M. Schaefer-Ridder, J. M. Karle, W. Levin, A. W. Wood, R. L. Chang, and A. H. Conney. The bay-region theory of carcinogenesis by polycyclic aromatic hydrocarbons. In: *Polycyclic Aromatic Hydrocarbons and Cancer*, vol. 1. New York: Academic Press (1978).

43 Loew, G. H., B. S. Sudhindra, J. M. Walker, C. C. Sigman, and H. L. Johnson. Correlation of calculated electronic parameters of fifteen aniline derivatives with their mutagenic potencies. *J. Environ. Pathol. Toxicol.* 2:1069 (1979).

44 Loew, G., B. S. Sudhindra, S. Burt, G. R. Pack, and R. MacElroy. Aromatic amine carcinogenesis: Activation and interaction with nucleic acid bases. *Int. J. Quant. Chem. (QBS)* 6:259 (1979).

Part Four

Applications of SAR in Toxicology

The Use of SIMCA Pattern Recognition in Predicting the Carcinogenicity of Potential Environmental Pollutants

William J. Dunn III
and Svante Wold

Estimating the potential for unknown or untested compounds to induce toxic or other harmful effects in a population is an exercise in learning from experience. As presently done, this estimate is obtained by simply comparing the structures of the unknown or untested compounds with those whose potential for inducing the toxic response has been quantitated in some way. Depending on the prior experience of the structure examiner, a qualitative estimate of the unknown's harmful effect can be obtained. While an experienced pharmacologist may be able to obtain estimates in this way, the qualitative nature of the estimate is a disadvantage to the approach, especially if something other than mere classification is desired.

For example, it may be estimated in this way that five or six compounds may be harmful and some decision must be made as to which two of the compounds should be submitted for further evaluation and testing. This requires that some ranking of the compounds be done, adding a nontrivial dimension to the problem. A number of methods of statistical data analysis, so called methods of classification, can be used in such classification problems. As formulated, this is not just a classification problem that can be approached by most readily available methods. The level of information required from the analysis may preclude their use.

A recently described method of pattern recognition, the SIMCA method (1) can be used when results beyond classification are required from the analysis. For example, it may be of interest to predict the relative level of carcinogenicity of a particular compound, to predict its location of tumor induction, or to determine which combination of physical properties of a class of compounds is common to those that induce tumors in a specific organ. A number of examples of such applications of SIMCA pattern recognition have been published (2–5) and these will be reviewed.

The objective of applying pattern recognition to a particular problem is to derive mathematical rules that can be used to estimate the probability that a particular object (in this case chemical compound) belongs to a defined class (in this case carcinogen). It should be noted at this point that, generally, noncarcinogens will not be considered as a definable class. This important point will be discussed later.

Since the type of response a chemical agent can effect is determined by its structure, it is necessary to convert the structure into a number or vector. This is done by describing each molecule in the analysis by physicochemical variables that are known to reflect their structure. Such descriptors as log P, molar refractivity, and Hammett-like constants are used. They have the advantage of being derived from systems that measure the analogous effects the agents may be expected to have in chemical and biological systems. In addition, they are continuous in the mathematical sense. This property of continuity satisfies one of the most important assumptions underlying the application of the various methods of classification to structure-activity data.

The description of classes of compounds in this way leads to a matrix, as is shown in Fig. 1. Here there are N compounds described by M variables. The compounds are divided into classes. Compounds of known classification are called the training sets, while those compounds of unknown class assignment are called the test set. It is the objective of the analysis to estimate their probability of being a member of any one of the known classes. The possibility also exists that they may be members of none of the classes and this must be considered a possible outcome of the classification.

A geometrical representation of the classification problem is given in Fig. 2. Here the problem is illustrated by two classes in three dimensions rather than in the M-dimensionality of the variables. The data for each compound are graphed in the descriptor coordinate system. The ideal and hoped-for result is that two well-defined clusters will result. In such cases, classification of the test compounds can be carried out by determining in which of the well-defined clusters, if any, the unknowns belong.

There are, methodologically, two general approaches to determining this: (a) inserting a plane between the classes and (b) describing the volume in

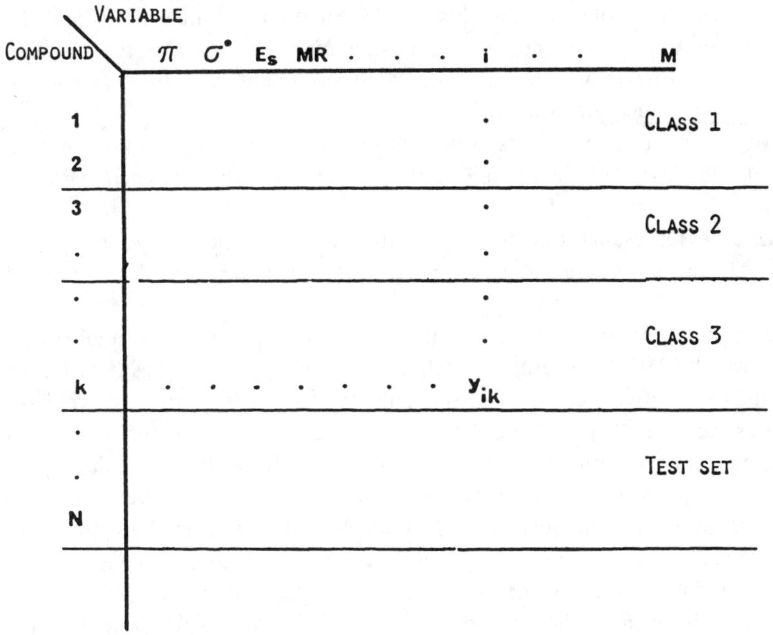

VARIABLE
COMPOUND
π σ* Es MR . . . i . . M
1
2
3
k
N
yik
CLASS 1
CLASS 2
CLASS 3
TEST SET

Figure 1 $N \times M$ chemical descriptor matrix for a three-class classification problem.

u1
2 RSDs
u2
u2
u1
Variable 3
Variable 2
Variable 1

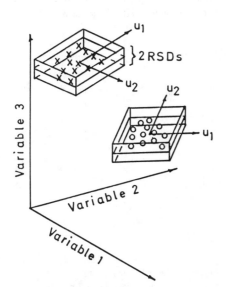

Figure 2 Symmetrical structure. Two well-structured classes projected into descriptor space.

space in which a particular class clusters. Linear discriminant analysis and the linear learning machine operate in the former manner. These are the so-called hyperplane methods, which calculate a discriminant function (plane or hyperplane) that separates the two classes.

SIMCA operates by the second method by obtaining a mathematical model of the class. This leads to a mathematical description of each class and the volume it occupies.

Figure 2 represents the problem with the classes clustering in separate regions of the coordinate space. Such data structure we have termed symmetric (6).

Figure 3 represents the data structure that has been observed in all of the cases in which SIMCA pattern recognition has been applied to classification of compounds as active versus inactive. This type of data structure we have termed asymmetric (6) and results from the active compounds forming a well-defined cluster while the inactives are randomly scattered in descriptor space around the active class. Asymmetric data structure, if observed, can have a profound effect on the analysis and should be anticipated in the application of pattern recognition to the classification of compounds as carcinogens.

The origin of this phenomenon and its effect on structure-biological activity classification studies has been discussed (7). An explanation for this type of data structure can be given if we consider some of the assumptions that lead to the establishment of the training sets. It is assumed in the construction of the training sets that each class represents a chemically and pharmacologically homogeneous class of carcinogens. This is to say that the

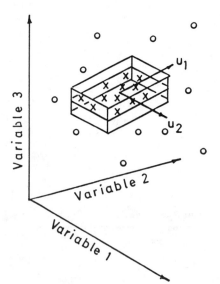

Figure 3 Asymmetrical data structure. One well-defined class (x) with a non-definable class (o) randomly distributed in descriptor space.

members of each respective training set exert their effect by a common mechanism of action and within this class there will be predictable changes in levels of activity, with small and regular changes in chemical structure. If a drastic structural alteration occurs, the regularity in the structure-activity relationship will be disrupted. This is equivalent to moving away from the active class in any one of the directions in Fig. 3. One result is inactivity and that the inactive compounds will be randomly scattered around the active class. The inactive class, noncarcinogens in this case, will not generally be mathematically definable.

The classification result of a compound outside of an active class means that it may be either a noncarcinogen or it may be a member of an as yet described (discovered class of carcinogens. Therefore, it is not possible to classify a compound with certainty as a noncarcinogen.

Asymmetric data structure can have another effect on the analysis in that if it is present in a problem, linear discriminant analysis and the linear learning machine cannot be applied to the data. With these methods, distinction of the carcinogen class from the other class(es) cannot be accomplished, as calculation of a discriminant plane or hyperplane separating them will not be possible.

SIMCA PATTERN RECOGNITION

The strategy of **SIMCA** pattern recognition is to search classes of compounds for similarities. With reference to Fig. 2, the strategy is to search for mathematical regularity within the data for each class. Provided that some assumptions can be justified (1), it is possible to approximate the data for a class by

$$y_{ik} = m_i + \sum_{a=1}^{A} b_{ia} u_{ak} + \epsilon_{ik}$$

This is a principal components model where y is the value of variable i for compound k, m_i is the mean value of variable i, A is the number of product terms in the model, b_{ia} is the loading or variable specific term and u_{ak} is the compound specific term with ϵ_{ik} being the residual for the respective variable. For $A = 1$ the result is that the data are approximated by a line while $A \geqslant 2$ approximates the data by a plane or hyperplane.

If Q classes are present it may be possible to derive Q disjoint similarity models. Using the residuals of the data for each object in each class, standard deviations for each object and for each class can be calculated. Standard deviations above and below the plane or hyperplane for each class then define a volume in descriptor space with a high probability for finding members of that class. Classification of unknown compounds then is based on determining which class they belong to. This results in a quantitative, probabilistic assessment of class assignment.

APPLICATIONS

A number of classes of organic compounds have been shown to have the potential for inducing cancer in experimental animals. Among these are the polycyclic aromatic hydrocarbons, N-nitroso compounds, and 4-nitroquinoline-1-oxides. For these substances, considerable, reliable carcinogenicity testing data have accumulated in the literature to justify the application of SIMCA pattern recognition in a classification study.

Polycyclic Aromatic Hydrocarbons

The most studied potential carcinogens are the polycyclic aromatic hydrocarbons (4). Most attempts to study their structure-activity relationships have given poor results. Such attempts have relied on univariate approaches to the analysis when clearly their carcinogenicity is a multivariable function of structure. A recent application of SIMCA to such multivariable data gave encouraging classification results (3).

Using 15 theoretical variables derived from molecular orbital calculations and 8 experimentally measured variables, it was possible to derive a similarity model for the 13 carcinogens in the training set. The 19 noncarcinogens were found not to be members of this class, giving a correct classification result. In addition, the relative carcinogenic potency of the carcinogens was correctly estimated by the models.

4-Nitroquinoline-1-oxides

SIMCA was applied to data on 33, 4-nitroquinoline-1-oxides (structure I), of which 10 were noncarcinogenic and 18 were carcinogens (2). Five analogs were 3-substituted compounds, which were apparently mechanistically heterogeneous from the active training set and could not be treated in the analysis. Such compounds are a natural result of SIMCA analyses, and this behavior of such compounds should be expected.

(I)

Of the 28 analogs treated, 89 percent of the active compounds were correctly predicted to be active while 70 percent of the inactive compounds were found to be outside of this described class.

N-Nitroso Compounds

In attempts to assess the carcinogenic potential of N-nitroso compounds, a number of laboratories have synthesized and tested a large number of N-nitroso compounds for their carcinogenic properties in test systems (7-10). From these sources, a set containing 61 nitrosamines, N-nitrosoureas, N-nitrosoamides, etc., resulted. Of the 61 compounds, 50 were carcinogenic in rats, 8 were noncarcinogens, and 3 had not been tested at the time the analysis was carried out. The inactive and untested compounds were considered test cases.

In the initial stages of the analysis it became obvious that the active compounds could not be treated as a chemically homogeneous class. This implied pharmacological heterogenicity in the class and the training set was divided into three groups of compounds. The basis for the subdivision was the expected fate of the respective chemical agents when they interact with biological systems.

This subdivision led to the derivation of three disjoint similarity models, which classified correctly 88 percent of the carcinogens. Most important was the classification of the untested compounds. After the analysis was completed, data became available on their carcinogenicity and two thirds were correctly classified.

SIMCA classified N-nitrosodiphenylamine as a member of none of the three classes of active compounds. It was initially found to be inactive (7), but in subsequent testing at higher doses it was shown to be carcinogenic (11). The results of the SIMCA analysis may appear to be inconsistent with these test results. They are not, however, as classification into none of the defined classes does not imply a noncarcinogen classification result. The possibility exists that the compound may be a member of a class of mechanistically different carcinogens from the three training sets. This is apparently the case with N-nitrosodiphenylamine (11).

In the use of pattern recognition techniques in the prediction of the harmful effects of chemical agents, various levels of information may be desired from the analysis. One aspect of the carcinogenicity of the N-nitroso compounds that is quite interesting is their tissue specificity. This property is a multivariable one, in that pharmacologically it could result from competing routes of distribution, metabolism, etc., within a class of N-nitroso compounds. Therefore, attempts to explain it considering a small structural change within the series as leading to a single change in physicochemical properties

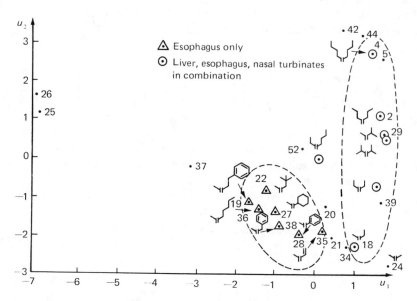

Figure 4 Eigenvector plot of alkylnitrosamines shows specificity in site of tumor induction as a function of eigenvectors u_1 and u_2.

will, and does, lead to a failure in explaining the organ specificity of these compounds.

By plotting the first two eigenvectors from the similarity model for the dialkylnitrosamines, Fig. 4 results. Each of the eigenvectors is a linear combination of 12 physicochemical variables, and it can be seen that the clustering due to organ specificity is a complex function of these physicochemical properties. This specificity can be sorted out and interpreted, and the reader is referred to the original discussion (4) for an explanation.

This example also illustrates a unique property of **SIMCA** pattern recognition—its two-way predictability: not only is it possible to predict from structural data an expected pharmacological response, it is also possible using **SIMCA** to construct a molecule that will have a particular defined response. This is not true of the other methods of pattern recognition being used in structure-biological activity analyses.

It is hoped that the examples of the use of **SIMCA** discussed here show the usefulness of the method in problems in which the objective is to predict toxicity. Further applications, to be published soon, will extend the method's usefulness.

REFERENCES

1 Wold, S. Pattern recognition by disjoint principal component models. *Pattern Recognition* 8:127–133 (1976).

2 Dunn, W. J., S. Wold. A strucutre-carcinogenicity of study of 4-nitro-quinoline-1-oxides using the SIMCA method of pattern recognition. *J. Med. Chem.* 21:1001–1007 (1978).

3 Norden, B., U. Edlung, and S. Wold. Carcinogenicity of polycyclic aromatic hydrocarbons studied by SIMCA pattern recognition. *Acta Chem. Scand. [B]* 32:602–606 (1978).

4 Dunn, W. J., and S. Wold. The carcinogenicity of N-nitroso compounds: A SIMCA pattern recognition study. *Bioorg. Chem.* 9:474–491 (1981).

5 Dunn, W. J., and S. Wold. Relationship between chemical structure and biological activity modeled by SIMCA pattern recognition. *Bioorg. Chem.* 9:505–523 (1980).

6 Albano, C., W. J. Dunn, U. Edlund, E. Johansson, B. Norden, M. Sjostrom, and S. Wold. Four levels of pattern recognition. *Anal. Chem. Acta* 103:429–435 (1978).

7 Dunn, W. J., and S. Wold. Structure-activity analyzed by pattern recognition: The asymmetric case. *J. Med. Chem.* 23:595–597 (1980).

8 Druckrey, H., R. Preussman, S. Ivankovic, and D. Schmall. Organotrope carcinogene wirkungen bei 65 verschiedenen N-nitroso-verbindngen an BD-ratten. *Z. Krebsforsch.* 69:103–201 (1967).

9 Kaneswar Rao, T., J. A. Young, W. Lijinsky, and J. L. Epler. Mutagenicity of nitrosamines in salmonella typhimurium. *Mut. Res.* 66:1–7 (1979).

10 Andrews, A. W., L. H. Libault, and W. Lijinsky. The relationship between mutagenicity and carcinogenicity of some nitrosamines. *Mut. Res.* 51:319–326 (1978).

11 Cardy, R. H., W. Lijinsky, and R. K. Hildebrandt. Neoplastic and nonneoplastic urinary bladder lesions induced in Fischer 344 rats and B6C3F₁ hybrid mice by N-nitroso diphenylamine. *Ecotoxicol. Environ. Safety* 3:29–35 (1979).

Chapter 10

Computer-Assisted Prediction of Metabolism

**W. Todd Wipke, Glenn I. Ouchi,
and J. T. Chou**

INTRODUCTION

The relationship between pharmacological activity and drug metabolism has
been a center of interest for a considerable period and has led to numerous
advances in the pharmaceutical sciences. Other papers in this symposium have
addressed the problem of relating the structure of a xenobiotic compound (a
compound foreign to the living system) to its observed toxicological activity.
However, in many cases the observed activity is not due directly to the
xenobiotic compound but instead is due to one or more metabolites of the
xenobiotic compound: that is, the parent compound may be a protoxicant
that is metabolically activated to become the biologically active agent, such as
a reactive electrophile, that then may lead to the observed activity. The

This work was supported by the National Cancer Institute Contract No.
N01-CP-75816. Computer support was provided by the Stanford SUMEX–AIM research
resource. We wish to acknowledge In Suk Kim for the work on structure-activity
prediction and Dave Rogers for assistance in converting XENO to F10 FORTRAN and
for helpful discussions.

purpose of this paper is to describe how computer methodology can be used to predict plausible metabolites of a xenobiotic compound.

The general scheme of xenobiotic metabolism is shown in Fig. 1. After the living system is exposed to a drug or chemical, either by skin contact, inhalation, or oral administration, several processes take place. The xenobiotic compound is first absorbed and is then distributed or transported to various organs or tissues in the body. The compound may then be biotransformed to a metabolite structurally different from the parent compound. The metabolite may be excreted from the living system (detoxification) or may interact with a receptor, either covalently or by complexation (potential biological activity expression), or the metabolite may be redistributed or transported to yet other organs or tissues, where it may interact with a receptor or again be biotransformed.

TYPES OF METABOLIC REACTION

Metabolism of xenobiotic compounds involves biotransformation by enzyme systems, although some transformations may not require enzymes. One of the major metabolizing enzyme systems is referred to as mixed function oxidase (MFO) or monooxygenases. It is highly concentrated in the liver, the principal organ responsible for metabolism of xenobiotics (1). The mammalian MFO system is capable of metabolizing vast, structurally diverse classes of substrates by various reactions. It is well established that MFO actually consists of a family of enzymes each having somewhat different specificities toward substrate and different sensitivities to induction or inhibition by chemicals (1).

In general, the metabolites derived from a xenobiotic are more hydrophilic, so that they are eliminated more readily from the body. For this reason, metabolism is sometimes referred to as a detoxifying mechanism for a living system. Basically, there are two types of metabolic reactions: phase I and phase II (2, 3).

Phase I reactions include those reactions that convert one functional group into another functional group (oxidations, reductions, hydrolyses) and those that alter the skeleton of the compound (condensations, fragmentations, rearrangements). The chemical groups or functionalities of a xenobiotic are

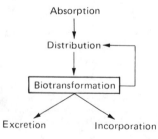

Figure 1 General scheme of xenobiotic metabolism.

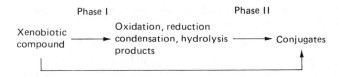

Figure 2 Types of metabolic reaction.

changed to more hydrosoluble moieties that facilitate the excretion of the foreign compound.

Phase II, sometimes called conjugation or synthesis reactions, involves a transfer of a chemical moiety (e.g., glucuronyl group) from a coenzyme to the xenobiotic itself or its phase I metabolites. These conjugating moieties are common metabolic intermediates that display strong hydrophilic properties due to ionic (e.g., sulfate) or other highly polar functional groups (e.g., polyhydroxy functionality in glucuronide). Conjugation changes the metabolite's physicochemical as well as biochemical properties from those of the unconjugated compound (2). These second phase reactions include the reactions that conjugate with glucuronate, sulfate, glutathione (mercapturic acid formation), methyl group, glycine, and other amino acids.

Very commonly, metabolic reactions proceed sequentially: that is, phase I reactions occur before phase II reactions, as shown in Fig. 2. For instance, oxidation of C–H to C–OH must proceed first before conjugation could occur at the hydroxyl group. The reverse sequence, although much less common, has been observed (4). Very often a xenobiotic is subjected to several pathways competitively. The extent of formation of various metabolites depends on the relative rates of these competitive reactions and various interactions.

RATIONALE

The complexity of metabolic processes precludes thorough systematic prediction of metabolites by manual methods. Yet to anticipate the potential toxicological effects of a xenobiotic compound, a thorough consideration of metabolism is required. Manual metabolism analysis is subject to inherent limitations: (*a*) people tend to be biased by their past experience, (*b*) they fail to utilize all available information (*c*) they introduce unnecessary constraints that the chemistry does not mandate, and (*d*) they tend toward selective rather than comprehensive analysis. The computer, in contrast, when properly programmed is not subject to these limitations. Thus, given the set of metabolic reactions applicable to xenobiotic compounds, together with appropriate logical algorithms for applying these reactions and generating the resulting metabolites, the computer could provide rapid, comprehensive, and unbiased analysis of a compound. The result would be a tree of metabolites derived from the substrate xenobiotic, including not only the structure of each metabolite but also all potential paths leading to that structure.

The program could thus be used for identifying unknown metabolites, for finding possible mechanisms of formation of a metabolite, for testing models of metabolism, and for aiding the scientist in planning an experiment as well as suggesting areas for further experiments. Direct SAR studies on the metabolites can then be performed using SAR techniques to assess or predict their potential biological activity.

IN CALCULO MODEL

In order to reduce the size and complexity of our metabolism model, we restrict our attention to the biotransformation block of Fig. 1. At this point we feel there is insufficient knowledge available to allow simulating transport in the general case. We thus have created a computer metabolic model (*in calculo* model) in which all metabolizing enzymes are present in "one reaction vessel," as shown in Fig. 3. The xenobiotic substrate is added to the vessel. Because there is no transport out of the vessel, the substrate and metabolites are retained in the presence of the biotransforming agents. Assuming that the *in calculo* model contains all the biotransforms that the *in vivo* system does, then in the *in calculo* model the xenobiotic is "exposed to" every biotransformation that exists in the *in vivo* system. Some of the reactions observed in the *in calculo* model are not observed *in vivo* because *in vivo* transport removes compounds before certain transformations may occur or because the compound may never reach the site of the transforming agent. We can conclude that the *in vivo* metabolites are a subset of the *in calculo* metabolites, which is exactly the relationship desired for toxicological assessment.

Our model does not attempt to predict the quantitative amount of metabolites per se. The quantitative aspects are dependent on many factors, including biological conditions, chemical induction or inhibition, and, of course, transport. However, the model does provide the general relative importance of each biotransformation performed, which for positional competition does reflect relative likelihood.

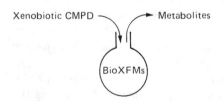

In vivo ⊂ in calculo   Figure 3   *In calculo* model.

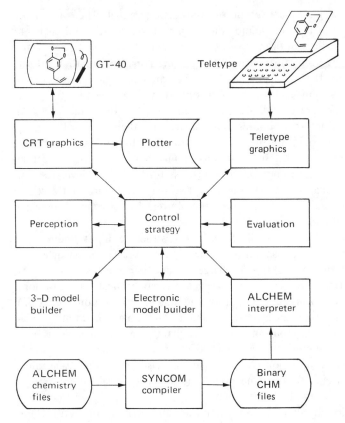

Figure 4 Block diagram of XENO.

DESIGN OF XENO

This computer metabolism program, called XENO, is an interactive domain-specific knowledge-based program. The knowledge, i.e., metabolic biotransformations, is extracted from experts and represented in the ALCHEM language (discussed later).

XENO is a modular FORTRAN program with a few assembly language functions for handling sets, list processing, and dynamic arrays. It is designed to be relatively machine-independent and is currently running on a Digital Equipment Corporation PDP-10 computer at the SUMEX–AIM (Stanford University Medical Experiment-Artificial Intelligence in Medicine) facility. A block diagram of XENO is shown in Fig. 4.

First, the investigator must transmit the parent molecule to the program by either drawing it in, using a GT40 graphics terminal and light pen, or typing it in, using a simple teletype or equivalent terminal. Then, when the user starts to process the compound, the program takes control and begins to perceive all chemically significant features of the parent compound, e.g., rings. Based on this perceived information, three-dimensional information (if the molecule is modelled) and calculated electronic parameters along with control and strategic constraints, chemical transformations are selected from the metabolic reaction library and are performed to generate metabolites. All these machine-generated metabolites are evaluated for their chemical stability. Then control is returned to the user, who also evaluates the metabolites generated. The user may delete or modify a metabolite and may select an interesting metabolite as a compound to process further. If the investigator is satisfied with the analysis, he or she may terminate the work and save the entire tree, which can then be output to the plotter. The program stops when the user is satisfied and tells it to stop.

The program utilizes the SECS chemical structure input and output modules (5). The structure diagram notations used by XENO consist of atoms, C, H, N, O, S, P, and X (halogens); charges, + and −; radical, $\sqrt{}$; and bonds, single, double, triple, and dotted or wedged (stereochemical configuration). Internally, the structure is represented as a redundant connection table (CT), which actually consists of an atom table and a bond table (5). An atom table contains the information about an atom type, charge type, number of valences explicitly used, the number of the attached explicit atoms, number of bonds, and stereochemical information. A bond table consists of a bond type, atom numbers of the atoms forming the bond, and stereochemical information of the bond with respect to the bond atoms.

The perception module derives from the fundamental connection table the high level perceptions about a structure that are required for functioning of control and biochemical manipulation modules. It perceives different functional groups, number of different atom types, bond types, basis rings, and redundancy or symmetry in molecular skeleton or network (5).

The model-building module utilizes heuristic classical-mechanical energy minimization algorithm to construct a three-dimensional model directly from a two-dimensional diagram or connection table without coordinates (5). The molecule is viewed as a collection of particles held together simply by harmonic or elastic forces. The minimization algorithm optimizes the bond lengths, bond angles, torsional, and nonbonded interaction plus stereochemical terms to minimize the strain energy of the molecule.

From the three-dimensional model XENO extracts new information such as the euclidean distances between atoms or dihedral angles, which enables XENO to evaluate the conformation-dependent proximity effect on metabolic reactions (6), and by using the SECS steric congestion function, XENO can evaluate steric congestion at a particular reactive site (7).

The control module of XENO examines each biochemical transform to see if it applies to the current substrate by mapping the required transform substructure onto the substructure in all possible ways. Each mapping is examined for the other ALCHEM scope and limitation statements. If the priority of the biotransform is above the cutoff priority (user selectable), then the manipulation statements are examined.

Basically, the manipulation module performs the chemical transformations symbolically to create the desired metabolite structures from the substrate structure based on the reaction manipulation instructions that are generated from the ALCHEM transforms. Routines in the module operate on the connection table to perform the symbolic metabolic conversion. The execution of these routines results in the making and breaking of bonds, addition or deletion of atoms, addition or loss of charges, and creation, deletion, retention, or inversion of stereocenters.

It is the role of the transform to *propose* potential metabolites. It is the role of the evaluation module to *dispose* of the metabolites if the structures are not chemically stable.

The factors for the chemical stability of a structure considered by the program are valence of atoms (violation of valence), electronic stability (unlikely charge distribution, e.g., dication, dianion), and implausible topological bonding (highly strained ring, etc., e.g., Bredt's rule). The ones that fail to survive these evaluations are deleted from the tree.

REPRESENTATION OF METABOLIC SCHEME

The *in vivo* metabolic fate of a xenobiotic compound is governed by many factors: the biochemical and physiological conditions of a living system, the structural influence of the substrate or xenobiotic compound, route of administration, dose, etc. (1, 8). The biological factors, such as species, sex, age, and hormonal disturbance, are very complicated and not well understood. The route of administration and dosing is more related to absorption, distribution, and transport phenomena in the body. The influence on metabolism of a substrate molecule depends on its molecular structure, connectivity of atoms, bond types, atom types, the positions and number of different functional groups, spatial arrangement, and physicochemical properties.

It is predominantly the latter structural dependencies that we are representing in our *in calculo* model because more is known about these effects, although we have included some other variables such as species.

ALCHEM

Each biotransformation is represented as a self-contained packet of knowledge described in ALCHEM, *a* language for *chem*istry (8). ALCHEM is an

English-like language with particular grammar and chemical vocabulary readable to the chemist.

An ALCHEM-described reaction consists of the following basic elements:

Reference: The literature reference substantiates the validity of the transform described below.

Name: This is a text string for identification of the transform.

Substructure: A linear notation for a pattern string of atoms and bonds required to be present in the substrate molecule.

Priority: This value is empirically assigned to establish the initial relative importance or plausibility of the transform. The value may be subject to adjustment on the influence of secondary structural features or other physicochemical properties.

Species: Specifies to what species the reaction being considered is applicable.

Qualifiers and Manipulations: This segment comprises the bulk of ALCHEM transforms. Qualifiers check for certain conditions in the structure being considered using conditional "IF .... THEN" situation-action rule. The action part may adjust the transform priorities, may terminate the transform, may be further structural queries, or may be a structure manipulation statement.

End: Signals the end of this reaction.

The biotransforms are interpreted from top to bottom, without any possibility of accidental loops. The reader is directed to reference 9 and later figures for examples of ALCHEM transforms.

Biotransformation Library

The ALCHEM transforms are gathered together in a sequential source file, i.e., the library. This source file is compiled by a compiler, called SYNCOM, into a binary direct access CHM file. The CHM file is then later interpreted by the XENO program to perform the metabolic transformations or the actions, as shown in Fig. 4. Each transform in the library is independent of the others. Consequently, a new transform can be added without interference with any other transform, although it might result in a duplication of an existing transform.

Since the library is not stored in the main memory, the number and length of transforms in the library is practically unlimited. The fact that the library is separate from the XENO program means that addition, modification, or deletion of transforms can be performed without changing the program and that the program may be changed without affecting the library.

We have chosen to represent biotransforms by a semimechanistic approach so fewer transforms are needed to cover the whole of xenobiotic metabolism and so XENO will have predictive power even in cases that have not been studied. The NIH shift shown in Fig. 5, for example, requires four steps (I-V) in XENO. All three intermediates are actually generated and remain in the metabolism tree. By representing the reactive intermediates explicitly, XENO is able to also consider alternative competing pathways, for example, reaction V in Fig. 5, which competes for the carbocation intermediate from step II. The balance between the competition is controlled in XENO by the scope and limitations of the biotransforms that describe structural influences on each path.

The current biotransform library was created by extracting information from books (1, 4) and the current metabolism literature.

Stereoselectivity

One of the important characteristics of drug metabolism is stereoselectivity. Many drug substrates are quite selectively metabolized (4, 10). One stereoisomer may be preferentially metabolized over the others, with retention or loss of the existing elements of stereoisomerism but without creation of new subsequent chiral centers (substrate stereoselectivity). Or, the generation of a chiral center at a prochiral center leads to the formation of one isomer predominantly over the other (product stereoselectivity). The reaction may also display both substrate and product stereoselectivity.

This requires that for the *in calculo* model to mimic this stereocontrol, ALCHEM must permit precise, unambiguous stereochemical descriptions. Since normal chemical nomenclature is inadequate, we developed an approach based on an imaginary graph theoretical plane. The plane is described by a sequence of atom numbers (at least three atoms). For example, in Fig. 6 the "plane" is defined by the path $<1,2,4,5>$. The "right hand rule" defines "up" as the direction of the thumb of the right hand when the fingers of that hand are curved along the path from atom 1 to atom 2 then to atom 4. Thus the NH_2

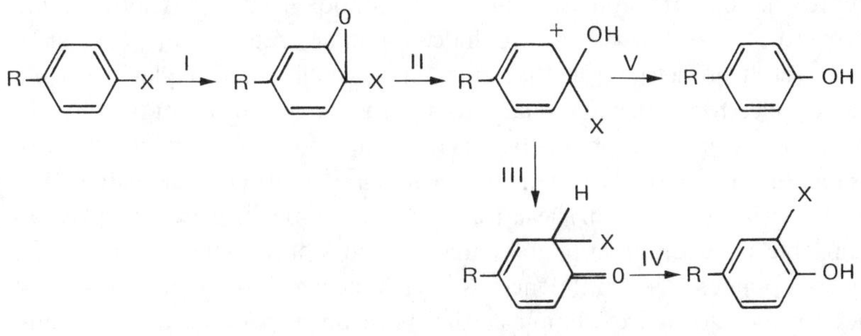

Figure 5 XENO representation of NIH shift. X = Cl, Br, F, CH_3, D, T.

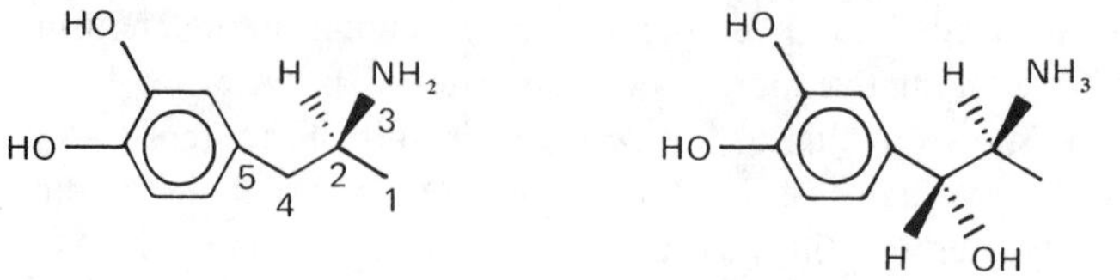

2S—(+)—α—methyldopamine   1R:2S—α—methylnorepinephrine

;Ref.: B. Waldeck, *Eur. J. Pharmacol.* 5: 114 (1968).
;
STEREOSPF
C—C(—N)—CC/
PRIORITY 10
SPECIES ALL
        DEFINE PLANE 1 USING ATOM 1 ATOM 2 ATOM 4 ATOM 5
        IF ATOM 3 IS UP WITH RESPECT TO PLANE 1 THEN ADD 30

;stereospecifically add up

        ADD 0 TO ATOM 4
        STEREOSPECIFICALLY UP AT ATOM 4 WITH RESPECT TO PLANE 1
END

Figure 6   ALCHEM-represented stereospecific reaction.

group is up with respect to plane 1, and the OH group in the metabolite is created "up" with respect to the same plane, but because the path curves in the opposite direction the right hand must flip to follow the curve 2,4,5. The priority of this transform is higher if the substrate has the right absolute stereochemistry and the hydroxyl group is introducted stereospecifically. This allows one to describe the complete stereospecificity of any metabolic process. Note that this particular stereochemical aspect is *independent* of conformation. If the stereospecificity is unknown, XENO generates the possible stereoisomers, assuming no stereoselectivity.

Electronic Effect

The hydroxylation of aromatic rings by monooxygenases usually occurs according to the rules of electrophilic aromatic substitution (11, 12). Activated (electron-rich) aromatic rings are readily hydroxylated, while deactivated (electron-deficient) ones are hydroxylated slowly or not at all. Hydroxylation occurs predominantly at the same position at which electrophilic substitution takes place, i.e., the *ortho-para* position in activated rings and in the *meta* position in deactivated rings. Steric effects also play an important role in determining metabolites formed from aromatic compounds. The most notable steric influence is the tendency for monosubstituted benzenes to undergo hydroxylation at the more open, *para*-position, as many examples have shown (13, 14).

The relative reactivities of the various positions on an aromatic ring toward electrophilic, nucleophilic, and radical attack have been approached by molecular orbital (MO) calculations (15). Using the Hückel LCAO method, the effects of a variety of groups on the π-electron energies of the pentadienate intermediates for electrophilic, nucleophilic, and free radical reagents have been calculated by Wheland (15). The aromatic module in XENO, HAREHM, is based on this computational method. The localization procedure is used to calculate the energy of an intermediate along the reaction path and to compare its energy to energy of the starting substrate. One of the π-electron centers of the aromatic ring, i.e., the point of potential substitution, is converted to a saturated atom, modelling the formation of the π-localized intermediate. The π-energy of the intermediate is calculated and compared to the π-energy of the initial state. The magnitude of this energy difference can be used as a measure of reactivity to predict the general pattern of aromatic substitution. XENO computes and stores these energy differences for each position on each aromatic ring system. Within an ALCHEM transform this information is accessed by a statement of the form:

IF ELENERGY ON ATOM 1 IS BETTER THAN AROMATIC ATOM

& THEN ADD 10 FOR EACH

XENO then automatically compares attack at atom 1 to all other aromatic atoms and the priority is raised by 10 for each noncompeting position. Thus the highest priority will arise by attack at the most favored position, but attack at other positions is not precluded.

ELENERGY stands for the calculated energy for electrophilic substitution at an atom. Nucleophilic and radical attack are also calculated but not currently used within XENO. Figure 7 shows how steric factors can also be included within an aromatic hydroxylation transform. The transform writer has wide latitude in how he or she relates priority to electronic and steric effects. For the priorities to have a consistent meaning, the transform writer must also be consistent in the way these effects are handled.

Table 1 shows the results of applying this biotransformation to many different classes of aromatic compounds and comparison of these results to some of the experimental data. These predictions were made by XENO using the electrophilic substitution mechanism with steric effects. On the compounds studied, which include substituted benzene, bicyclic, tricyclic, and polycyclic compounds, XENO's predictions are in excellent agreement with experimental results. In each case tested, the predicted metabolites with highest priority are also the major metabolites found experimentally and the priorities of predicted metabolites are in the same order as the relative amounts of isolated metabolites.

```
INSERTION
C/
PRIORITY 0
SPECIES ALL
        IF ATOM 1 IS NOT AROMATIC ATOM THEN KILL
        IF ATOM 1 IS ATTACHED TO 0 HYDROGEN THEN KILL
        IF ATOM 1 AND EPOXIDE ARE IN THE SAME RING THEN KILL
        IF EPOXIDE IS ONRING OF SIZE 6 THEN KILL
; Catechols are formed from arene oxide not from phenolic
; intermediates [Jerina, et al. JACS 89, 5488–5489 (1967)]
        IF ATOM ALPHA TO ATOM 1 IS AROMATIC ATOM (1) THEN
            BEGIN IF PRIMARY OXYGEN IS ALPHA TO (1) THEN KILL
            DONE
; Electronic factor is considered for aromatic oxygen insertion:
        IF ELENERGY ON ATOM 1 IS BETTER THAN AROMATIC ATOM THEN ADD 5
&           FOR EACH
; Steric influence on ortho : para ratio is considered :
        IF ATOM BETA TO ATOM 1 IS NOT AROMATIC THEN SUBT 15 FOR EACH
        IF ELENERGY ON ATOM 1 IS BETTER THAN (1) THEN ADD 10 FOR EACH
; Xform :
        ADD 0 TO ATOM 1
END
```

Figure 7   ALCHEM transform. Electronic effect on aromatic oxygen insertion.

Species Variations

One of the most important biological factors affecting the metabolism of a xenobiotic is the species variation (8, 25, 26). Species variations have been shown to occur both in phase I and in phase II metabolic reactions.

Species variations may appear as (a) qualitative differences in the actual pathways of metabolism, and/or (b) quantitative differences in the pathways of metabolism that are common to several species. The qualitative difference may result from the lack of a certain enzyme in a species which is generally present in other species or the presence of an enzyme in a particular species which is absent in the others. An example is that a cat lacks phenol glucuronyl transferase necessary for the formation of phenolic glucuronides; therefore most of the phenols are not excreted as glucuronide conjugates.

Quantitative differences could be due to variations in the relative amount and activity of an enzyme or its natural inhibitor, or to the occurrence of an enzyme reversing reaction, or to the presence of an enzyme competing for the same substrate.

Species metabolic variations might impose quantitatively or qualitatively different susceptibilities of the species to the biological activity of a compound (27). For instance, it has been shown that N–OH–2–AAF (acetylaminofluorene) is responsible for 2–AAF's carcinogenic activity (28). A guinea pig produces a negligible amount of N–OH metabolite of 2–AAF and is not susceptible to 2–AAF's carcinogenic effect, while other species are (29). Species variation is essential in the field of comparative drug metabolism, in which investigators want to find the best animal model for a drug. It is also important in the new field of comparative toxicology, wherein the focus is to find the most sensitive animal model for a specific toxic effect (30), since most of the toxic effects are due to metabolism.

In order to represent the quantitative and qualitative species variations in a transform, two types of ALCHEM statements have been developed. The first is a qualitative header statement, e.g.,

SPECIES RAT

Table 1 Comparison of XENO Predictions and Experimental Results for Aromatic Hydroxylation

No.	Compound	XENO predicted metabolite (priority)	Experimental results metabolite (% dose)	Reference
1	Acetanilide	4–OH (35)	4–OH (94)[*]	16
		2–OH (20)	2–OH (5)[*]	
			3–OH (1)[*]	
2	Aniline	4–OH (35)	4–OH (50)	17
		2–OH (20)	2–OH (9)	
		3–OH (10)	3–OH (0.1)	
3	Benzoic acid	3–OH (45)	3–OH (130)[*]	
		4–OH (5)	4–OH (100)[*]	
		2–OH (0)	2–OH (4)[*]	
4	Nitrobenzene	3–OH (45)	3–OH (9)	19
		4–OH (5)	4–OH (9)	
		2–OH (0)	2–OH (0.1)	
5	Imipramine	2–OH (50)	2–OH (25)	20
		4–OH (35)		
		3–OH (20)		
		1–OH (−5)		
6	Lidocaine	3–OH (10)	3–OH (31)	21
		4–OH (5)	4–OH (0)	
7	Xylidine	4–OH (35)	4–OH (73)[†]	
		3–OH (−5)	3–OH (0)	
8	Azapropazone	6–OH (10)	6–OH (5)	22
		5–OH (5)		
		8–OH (−5)		
9	Naphthalene	1–OH (50)	1–OH > 2–OH	23
		2–OH (30)		
10	Pyrene	1–OH (60)	1–OH (major)	24
		4–OH (40)		
		2–OH (10)		

[*]Ratio of the isomers.
[†]Percentage of lidocaine in humans.

meaning that the reaction is only applicable to the rat and not to other species. The other one is a query statement that reflects the quantitative variation by adjusting the priority as shown below:

IF SPECIES IS RAT THEN ADD 10

This means if the transform is applied to the rat, then the priority will be raised by 10. If the other species is used, the priority will not be increased. This can reflect the relative quantitative species difference.

EXAMPLE ANALYSIS

We test XENO by analyzing compounds whose metabolism has been thoroughly studied and see if XENO can generate all the metabolites that were found experimentally. We also look at metabolites generated *in calculo* but not observed *in vivo* to see if they are reasonable predictions or if they result from an improperly coded biotransform.

An example path generated for cyclophosphamide is shown in Fig. 8. In addition, of course, many other paths were found, some of which have been reported in the literature.

We are also currently collaborating with experimental research groups to try XENO on some ongoing research problems before the answers are known. Results of those studies will be reported in a later paper.

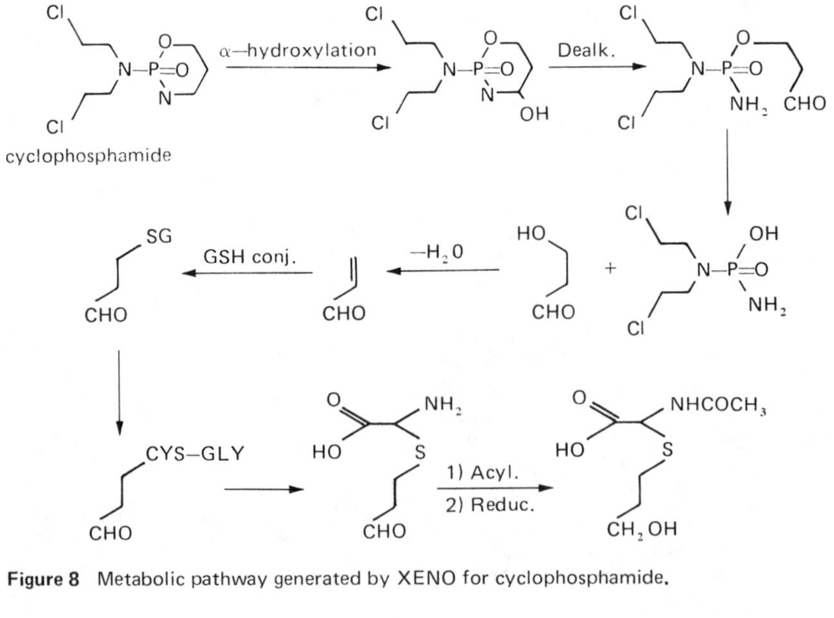

Figure 8   Metabolic pathway generated by XENO for cyclophosphamide.

EVALUATION OF BIOLOGICAL ACTIVITY

We now turn to a second part of our research—evaluating the plausible biological activity of each metabolite after it is generated. Our purpose is to draw the attention of the user to those metabolites that are potentially active so the structures are not overlooked in a large metabolism tree.

Many rational methods in structure-activity relations (SAR) have been developed: semiempirical linear free energy (LFER) model using multivariate statistical analysis method by Hansch and co-workers (30), de novo additivity Free-Wilson model (31), quantum mechanically based approaches (32, 33), and pattern recognition techniques (34, 35). However, these methods have been applied to the SAR studies of biological activity and parent compounds rather than metabolites. The relationship between parent xenobiotic chemical structures and rates of some metabolic reactions has been studied using the Hansch approach (36, 37). Quantum mechanical methods have also been used in SAR studies of metabolic activation and chemical carcinogenesis (38, 39), but structure-activity studies on metabolites themselves have not been reported.

In evaluating approaches to this problem it is obvious that simple, exact match library look-up using a library of known metabolites with known activity would be of limited utility since most metabolites would not be in the library. An alternative is to try to find the "nearest" match with a structure in the library using a function to compute structural similarity. Unfortunately, this can take a long time if the library is large.

Along these lines, a computerized decision tree for chemical carcinogenesis has been developed (40). It extracts the structural features from a molecule under study. The probability for carcinogenic risk of these structural features has been assessed by experts. By doing the substructure search, the activity tree is formed and carcinogenic risk is assessed statistically. One advantage of this approach is speed of operation.

We are exploring a new unique approach to this problem. Briefly, our objective is to be able to evaluate biological activity as well as be an expert in the field. We have developed a rule-based method for representing this expert knowledge. First, we extract from examples the structural requirement (pharmacophore) for the specific biological activities of interest. Next, we encode the rules in the ALCHEM language. All the power of ALCHEM known previously is available for examining the environment of the pharmacophore or toxicophore, including physicochemical properties of the molecule, species, and electronic, geometric, and steric factors.

The advantages of our approach is that it is easy to add new information as it becomes available, the method is computationally fast, and chemists can read the rules and understand precisely how the system works. It is also easy to represent exceptions by this method by simply adding a specific rule. The major disadvantage is that in some areas, it is not easy to decide on what the rules should be, i.e., how to define a good model. We also believe this same approach can be used to represent the termination processes of metabolism, namely excretion and incorporation.

CONCLUSION

XENO is an interactive computer-graphics program that accepts a drawing of the xenobiotic compound and then generates plausible metabolites and displays their structures on a CRT terminal along with a rating of potential biological activity. The program has numerous capabilities and advantages in assisting the metabolic analysis. It is capable of storing and retrieving chemical structure and relevant information of the xenobiotic compound and its computer-generated metabolites. The metabolic reactions and the stereochemical, electronic, and steric effects on the reactions can be represented by the program. The biological factors, such as species variations, can also be included in the reaction.

XENO's knowledge-based metabolism is mechanistically oriented, rather than rote-memory oriented and consequently is not limited to molecules whose metabolism is known. All plausible metabolites are created based on the knowledge the program has. Each metabolite will have its plausible biological activity in four categories evaluated, using a unique rule-based structure-activity prediction module.

We view XENO as a tool that can assist chemists, biochemists, and pharmacologists not only in evaluating and studying metabolism itself, but also in predicting the metabolite's potential biological activity.

REFERENCES

1 Low, L. K., and N. Castagnoli Jr. Drug biotransformations. In M. E. Wolff (ed.), *Burger's Medicinal Chemistry. Part I. The Basis of Medicinal Chemistry*, pp. 107–226. New York: Wiley (1980).

2 Williams, R. T. *Detoxication Mechanisms, the Metabolism and Detoxification of Drugs, Toxic Substances and Other Organic Compounds*. New York: Wiley (1959).

3 Parke, D. V. The impact of drug metabolism on medical research. Part 1. Survey of metabolic processes. *Chem. Ind.*, pp. 380–388 (1976).

4 Testa, B., and P. Jenner. *Drug metabolism: Chemical and Biochemical Aspects*. New York: Dekker (1976).

5 Wipke, W. T. Computer-assisted three-dimensional synthetic analysis. In W. T. Wipke, S. R. Heller, and K. J. Feldman (eds.), *Computer Representation and Manipulation of Chemical Information*, pp. 147–174. New York: Wiley (1974).

6 Ouchi, G. I. Computer-Assisted Prediction of Plausible Metabolites of Xenobiotic Compounds, pp. 75-80. Thesis, University of California (1978).

7 Wipke, W. T., H. Braun, G. Smith, F. Choplin, and W. Sieber. SECS—simulation and evaluation of chemical synthesis: strategy and planning. In W. T. Wipke and W. J. Howe (eds.), *Computer Assisted Organic Synthesis, ACS Symposium Series vol. 61*, pp. 97-127. Washington, D.C.: American Chemical Society (1977).

8 Nelson, S. D. Chemical and biological factors influencing drug biotransformation. In M. E. Wolff (ed.), *Burger's Medicinal Chemistry. Part I. The Basis of Medicinal Chemistry*, pp. 227-269. New York: Wiley (1980).

9 Spann, M. L., K. C. Chu, W. T. Wipke, and G. Ouchi. Use of computerized methods to predict metabolic pathways and metabolites. *J. Environ. Pathol. Toxicol.* 2:123-131 (1978).

10 Testa, B., and P. Jenner. A structural approach to selectivity in drug metabolism and disposition. In P. Jenner and B. Testa (eds.), *Concepts in Drug Metabolism, Part A*, pp. 53-176. New York: Dekker (1980).

11 Ullrich, V. Enzymatic hydroxylations with molecular oxygen. *Angew Chem. Int. Edit.* 11:701-712 (1972).

12 Daly, J. W., D. M. Jerina, and B. Witkop. Arene oxides and the NIH shift: the metabolism, toxicity and carcinogenicity of aromatic compounds. *Experientia* 28:1129-1149 (1972).

13 Daly, J. W., D. M. Jerina, and B. Witkop. Migration of deuterium during hydroxylation of aromatic substrates by liver microsomes: I. Influence of ring substituents. *Arch. Biochem. Biophys.* 128:517-527 (1968).

14 Creaven, P. J., D. V. Parke, and R. T. Williams. A fluorimetric study of the hydroxylation of biphenyl *in vitro* by liver preparations of various species. *Biochem. J.* 96:879-885 (1965).

15 Wheland, G. W. A quantum mechanical investigation of the orientation of substituents in aromatic molecules. *J. Am. Chem. Soc.* 64:900-908 (1942).

16 Ullrich, V., J. Wolf, E. Amadori, and H. Staudinger. The mixed-function oxygenation of 4-haloacetanilides in rat liver microsomes and model systems. *Hoppe-Seylers Z. Physiol. Chem.* 349:85-94 (1968).

17 Parke, D. V. Studies in detoxication. 84. The metabolism of [14C] aniline in the rabbit and other animals. *Biochem. J.* 77:493-503 (1960).

18 Acheson, R. M., and S. Gibbard. The hydroxylation of benzoic acid by rats and guinea pig. *Biochim. Biophys. Acta* 59:320-325 (1962).

19 Parke, D. V. Studies in detoxication. 68. The metabolism of [14C] nitrobenzene in the rabbit and guinea pig. *Biochem. J.* 62:339-346 (1956).

20 Crammer, J. L., B. Scott, and B. Rolfe. Metabolism of 14C-imipramine: II. Urinary metabolites in man. *Psychopharmacologia* 15:207-225 (1969).

21 Keeaghan, J. B., and R. N. Boyes. Tissue distribution, metabolism and excretion of lidocaine in rats, guinea pigs and man. *J. Pharmacol. Exp. Ther.* 180:454-463 (1972).

22 Mixich, G. Isolierung, struktur und synthese des metaboliten von azapropazon-dihydrat. *Helv. Chim. Acta* 55:1031–1038 (1972).
23 Horning, M. G., W. G. Stillwell, G. W. Griffin, and W. S. Tsang. Epoxide intermediates in the metabolism of naphthalene by the rat. *Drug Metab. Disposit.* 8:404–414 (1980).
24 Parke, D. V. *The Biochemistry of Foreign Compounds.* Oxford: Pergamon Press (1968).
25 Williams, R. T. The metabolism of certain drugs and food chemicals in man. *Ann N.Y. Acad. Sci.* 179:141–154 (1971).
26 Williams, R. T. Species variations in drug biotransformations. In B. N. LaDu, H. G. Mandel, and E. L. Way (eds.), *Fundamentals of Drug Metabolism and Drug Disposition*, pp. 187–205. Baltimore: Williams & Wilkins (1971).
27 DiCarlo, F. J. Interspecies comparisons of oxisuran metabolism and pharmacokinetics. *Drug Metab. Rev.* 10:225–237 (1979).
28 Weisburger, J. H., P. H. Grantham, E. Vanhorn, N. H. Steigbigel, D. P. Rall, and E. K. Weisburger. Activation and detoxification of N-2-fluorenylacetamide in man. *Cancer Res.* 24:475–479 (1964).
29 Miller, E. C., J. A. Miller, and M. Enomoto. Comparative carcinogenicities of 2-acetylaminofluorene and its N-hydroxy metabolite in mice, hamsters, and guinea pigs. *Cancer Res* 24:2018–2031 (1964).
30 Hansch, C. Quantitative structure-activity relationships in drug design. In E. J. Ariën (ed.), *Drug Design*, vol. I, pp. 271–342. New York: Academic Press (1971).
31 Free, S. M., and J. W. Wilson. A mathematical contribution to structure-activity studies. *J. Med. Chem.* 7:395–399 (1964).
32 Kier, L. B. *Molecular Orbital Theory in Drug Research.* New York: Academic Press (1971).
33 Richards, W. G., and M. E. Black. Quantum chemistry in drug research. *Prog. Med. Chem.* 11:67–90 (1975).
34 Stuper, A. J., W. E. Brugger, and P. C. Jurs. *Computer Assisted Studies of Chemical Structure and Biological Functions.* New York: Wiley (1979).
35 Kirschner, G. L., and B. R. Kowalski. The application of pattern recognition to drug design. In E. J. Ariën (ed.), *Drug Design*, vol. VIII, pp. 73–131. New York: Academic Press (1979).
36 Hansch, C., E. J. Lien, and F. Helmer. Structure-activity correlations in the metabolism of drugs. *Arch. Biochem. Biophys.* 128:319–330 (1968).
37 Testa, B., and B. Salvesen. Quantitative structure-activity relationships in drug metabolism and disposition: pharmacokinetics of N-substituted amphetamines in humans. *J. Pharmacol. Sci.* 69:497–501 (1980).
38 Loew, G. H., B. S. Sudhindra, S. Burt, G. R. Pack, and R. MacElroy. Aromatic amine carcinogenesis: activation and interaction with nucleic acid bases. *Int. J. Quantum Chem. Quantum Biol. Symp.* 6:259–281 (1979).

39 Loew, G. H., B. S. Sudhindra, and F. E. Ferrell, Jr. Quantum chemical studies of polycyclic aromatic hydrocarbons and their metabolites: correlations to carcinogenicity. *Chem.-Biol. Interact.* 26:75–89 (1979).
40 Dehn, R. L., and C. T. Helmes. *An Automatic Procedure for Assessing Possible Carcinogenic Activity of Chemicals Prior to Testing.* Prepared for National Cancer Institute Contract N01-CP-33285, NIH-NCI-71-2045 (1974).

Chapter 11

Computer Techniques for Representation of Three-Dimensional Substructures and Exploration of Potential Pharmacophores

Dennis H. Smith, James G. Nourse,
and Christopher W. Crandell

INTRODUCTION

Our research at Stanford is directed primarily at developing new techniques and algorithms for computer analysis of molecular structures. Our goal is to develop interactive computer programs that assist chemists and biochemists in solving structural problems. Until recently our focus has been almost exclusively on elucidation of unknown molecular structures (1-3). Now, however, we have a number of interactive computer programs the operation of which depends on characterization of the configurational stereochemistry of either known structures (4, 5) or sets of candidate structures for an unknown (6). As our computer techniques are extended to deal with conformational stereochemistry (the primary emphasis of this chapter), it is clear that they will have applications in several areas of structural chemistry beyond analysis of unknown structures. In this chapter we wish to present some recent work on development of algorithms for computer representation and manipulation of molecular stereochemistry, representations that include both configurational and conformational information.

Our intent is to develop methods for structure representation that capture the relationships of atoms in three-dimensional space, i.e., descriptions of the configuration and conformation not only of a complete structure but also of substructural fragments of a complete structure. These methods open the way for us to develop correlations between various structures and their properties. These correlations are often called structure-activity relationships. For our purposes we choose to define activity very broadly. The activity may be rate of reaction in a chemical synthesis, a characteristic fingerprint in spectroscopic analysis, or biological activity, including the focus of the present volume on toxicological properties.

We hardly need to emphasize the importance of the choice of structural representation in the study of structure-activity relationships. The activity of a compound may be influenced by many factors, including intrinsic activity, reactivity, bioavailability, and so forth. Analysis of these factors may require representations that capture electronic properties, hydrophobicity, and details of molecular geometry. These aspects have been discussed at length in this volume and in many other publications (7, 8); they need not be discussed further here. To the extent that activity is a function of molecular geometry (stereochemistry), there is a need for computational techniques that allow intercomparison of structures and their component substructures in three-dimensional space. This is the focus of our current work in structural representations; the current status of two aspects of this work is summarized in subsequent sections.

In reading the following sections, it must be kept in mind that this is a report of work in progress. Although there are many potential applications for our techniques, to this point our efforts have been directed at solving a number of problems related to the fundamental algorithms themselves. Thus, emphasis will focus on presenting methods for characterizing molecular stereochemistry that lead to specific computer programs. These programs should have significant utility in the area of structure-activity relationships, but we have so far only demonstrated this for the relationships between substructures with configurational stereochemistry and the chemical shifts of carbon atoms in ^{13}C nuclear magnetic resonance spectroscopy (NMR) (4, 5).

The following presentation is in two parts. Both deal with methods for representation of the configuration and conformation of substructural fragments of a larger structure so that: (*a*) the representations can be related to specific properties, or activities, of the structure and (*b*) substructures can be compared to determine equivalence, in three-dimensional space, wherever they occur in a large set of structures. The first part of our presentation describes a method that is applicable to structural representations wherein molecular connectivity is an essential requirement, for example, when the observed activity is the chemical shift of a hydrogen atom in ^{1}H NMR. The second part of our presentation describes a different approach to describing the geometry of a structure, one that is especially applicable to identification of common three-dimensional substructures of arbitrary size in a set of structures. In this approach we characterize the relationship of atoms in space independent of molecular connectivity.

REPRESENTATION OF SUBSTRUCTURES
WITH CONFIGURATION AND CONFORMATION

We have recently described and implemented a method for representing substructures using an atom-centered code that describes the substructural environment of the atom out to a specified bond radius, usually four bonds (4, 5). This representation captures all the constitutional and configurational stereochemical information in that environment (4). This is illustrated in Fig. 1, wherein the atoms of 1 and 3 that bear asterisks are the central atoms; the resulting substructure captured by a four-bond radius environment is shown as 2 and 4, respectively. Where configurations are specified in the original structure, configuration designations are also assigned to the substructure (4) (Fig. 1, 3 and 4).

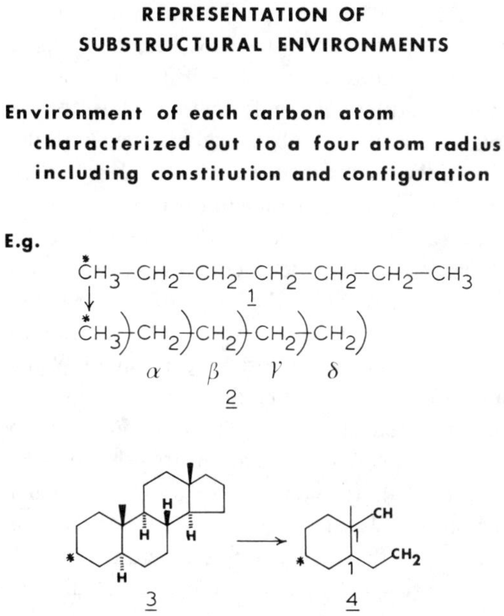

REPRESENTATION OF
SUBSTRUCTURAL ENVIRONMENTS

Environment of each carbon atom
characterized out to a four atom radius
including constitution and configuration

E.g.

Figure 1 Shell structure captured by the atom-centered code out to a four bond radius. 2 is the environment characterized for the methyl group (asterisk) of 1, while 4 represents the substructural environment characterizing the asterisked atom in 3. Relevant configurations of 3 are represented as part of the characterization of the substructure 4 (4).

We are extending this substructure representation to include conformations also. Such a representation could implicitly include all the geometric information about the substructure. However, this method is likely to be more useful in cases in which the constitution and configuration of the structure are important in addition to the actual position of atoms in space. Such would be the case if through-bond properties are important such as in ^{1}H NMR.

For the anticipated purposes [such as a large data base of substructures and their associated properties (4, 5)], it is important that efficient computer methods be used to characterize quickly and compactly the substructural environments of atoms in large numbers of structures. Based on our past experience, labeling algorithms (9) are nicely suited for this purpose. By labeling we mean that bonds in a substructure must be labeled with some discrete property that in some way designates the conformation. An obvious choice would be rotameric position (staggered, eclipsed, etc.). A somewhat less obvious choice might be torsional angle ranges. The point is that some discrete property must be chosen and it will be assumed one is in hand. For the purposes of this discussion the choice will be rotameric position (three staggered rotamers).

A suitably designed labeling procedure can be used as the basis for enumeration (counting) and generation (constructing) of possible conformations for a structure or substructure. In fact, we have recently illustrated how such a procedure can be used to enumerate conformations (10). However, the focus of this section is on the related problem of representation of substructures, which assumes some initial designation for the structure's conformation. Thus, for the purposes of this discussion, the bonds are assumed to be already labeled with the chosen designations for conformation. We assume this is a rational designation, one that corresponds to a realizable structure in three-dimensional space.

The specific problem here is the canonical or unique naming of a substructure with these conformation designations, because eventually substructures must be compared with one another and it is critical that the same substructure from a variety of different structures possess the same "name." Our solution to this problem differs substantially from the scheme proposed previously by Wipke (11) for developing canonical names for structures, including configuration and conformation designations. In our case, the shell structure imposed on our atom centered codes (see Fig. 1) imposes a numbering of the atoms in order to make the name canonical *at all shell levels* (4). It is extremely useful for many applications to have the configuration (4) and conformation designations separate parts of the canonical name so that when necessary either or both designations can be ignored, leaving the remaining name still in a canonical form at all shell levels. The naming procedure requires a renumbering of each substructure (originally numbered and assigned configurations as a portion of the complete structure from which it was obtained). As we discuss more completely below, neither configuration nor conformation designations are invariant to the renumbering, and this must be taken into account. In addition, as in most canonicalization methods, it is particularly important that symmetry be properly accommodated. This may sound like a trivial problem since so few chemical structures actually have any symmetry. However, it must be remembered that we are talking primarily about substructures that often possess symmetry. For example, the androstane skeleton (5) possesses no symmetry, yet the substructure 6, centered about C−8, is highly symmetrical considering both constitution *and* configuration.

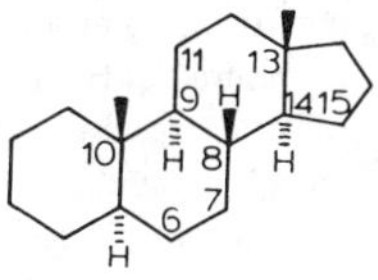

5

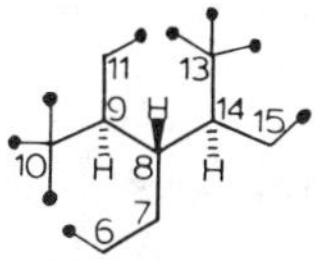

6

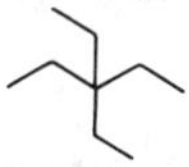

7

Assigning a canonical name would still be a fairly easy problem if the previously assigned labels could be freely permuted using the symmetry group of the substructure (9). However, in this case, as in the case of configurational stereochemistry (12), the symmetry operations affect the labels (rotameric states or positions), and these operations cannot be done in the easiest, independent manner. To visualize this consider the symmetrical structure 3,3-diethylpentane (7).

There are symmetry operations (remember this is the symmetry group based on the connectivity and stereocenter configurations, not the usual geometric point group) that simply exchange all the rotamers about any of the bonds to the central atom. Again this is a symmetric structure, but even this pathological case occurs in a substructure as simple as a quaternary carbon atom connected to four methylene groups.

To illustrate the method we are describing, refer to the conformation of 2,4-dimethylpentane (8) shown in Fig. 2. (Again this is a symmetrical molecule, but this is a prototype for a substructure as simple as a three-carbon chain of methylene groups, certainly a frequently occurring substructure.)

The labels (−), (+), and (T) assigned to the rotamers in Fig. 2 refer to the

Figure 2 Two conformations of $\underline{8}$, $\underline{A}$ and $\underline{B}$. Conformations are shown as Newman projections, looking down first the C—2, C—3 bond, then the C—4, C—3 bond. Each projection is named according to the relative positions of the lowest numbered substituents on opposite sides of the central bond, using — to indicate (−)-gauche, + to indicate (+)-gauche and T to indicate *trans*. Thus $\underline{A}$ corresponds to 1,4-(T), 2,5-(+) and $\underline{B}$ corresponds to 1,4-(−), 2,5-(−). The C_2 operation corresponds to that given in Table 1.

(−)-gauche, (+)-gauche, and *trans* rotamers about the indicated C—2, C—3 and C—4, C—3 bonds, based on the numbering of the substituents of $\underline{8}$.

The four symmetry operations applicable to this structure are shown as represented by their atomic permutations, geometric point group, and central bond permutations in Table 1.

Two possible conformations of $\underline{8}$, $\underline{A}$ and $\underline{B}$, are shown in Fig. 2 as Newman projections, looking down the C—2, C—3 bond and C—4, C—3 bond. Consider the effects on $\underline{A}$ and $\underline{B}$ of the atomic permutation (17)(24)(56) (Table 1). This permutation has the effect of interconverting $\underline{A}$ and $\underline{B}$. (Intuitively, the permutation is just a C_2 rotation although the computer representation does not "reflect" this intuitive picture.) As can be seen in Fig. 2, conformations $\underline{A}$ and $\underline{B}$ [which can be designated using the lowest substituent numbers across the central bond (11) as the 1,4-(T), 2,5-(+) conformation and the 1,4-(−), 2,5-(−) conformation, respectively] are equivalent. This can be viewed as a canonicalization step. If we were presented with the 1,4-(T), 2,5-(+) conformation and subjected it to the C_2 permutation, we would obtain the 1,4-(−), 2,5-(−) conformation. In our substructure representation method, one

Table 1 Symmetry Group for 2,4-Dimethylpentane ($\underline{8}$)

Atomic permutation	Point group operation	Central bond permutation
E	E	(23)(34)
(17)(24)(56)	C_2	(23 34)
(15)(24)(67)	σ_v	(23 34)
(16)(57)	σ_v	(23)(34)

Table 2   Effect (Column 3) of Application of the Symmetry Operation (17)(24)(56) (C2, Table 1) to the Conformation of 2,4-dimethylpentane (8) Given in Column 1

Initial conformation	Symmetry operation	Resulting conformation
[−−]	(17)(24)(56)	[T+]
[−T]		[++]
[−+]		[−+]
[T+]		[T−]
[TT]		[+−]
[+T]		[+T]

of these would be considered a "lower" designation; there would be an equivalent designation obtained by other symmetry operations, which would be "lowest," thus canonical. Using the compact notation of [−−] for 1,4-(−), 2,5-(−), Table 2 shows the effect of the C_2 symmetry operation on all the possible conformations (again, assuming just three possible torsional positions), with the lowest one in the first column based on the ordering $− < T < +$.

This method is applicable to the other symmetry permutations of this structure (Table 1). These are reflective operations and therefore collect mirror image conformations together. For some purposes this would be desirable, such as in NMR. For example, in our previous work on ^{13}C NMR (4, 5), enantiomeric substructures were not distinguished. In an application such as interpretation of chiroptical spectra, enantiomeric pairs would have to be distinguished. The method, described separately in more detail (10), is capable of differentiation of enantiomers if the application requires it.

Using this method, substructures can be canonically named with conformation designations. This scheme is eminently suitable for characterizing atom-centered substructures. Thus, substructures can be represented with a shell structure so that the substructure has a unique name that captures constitution, configuration, and conformation and is canonical at all shell levels.

THREE-DIMENSIONAL COMMON SUBSTRUCTURES

A frequently encountered problem in methods for comparison of chemical structures (for any purpose including structure-activity relationships) is to determine what structural features or substructures they have in common. In structure-activity studies, one hypothesis would be that three-dimensional common substructures, in a set of structures displaying similar biological activity, are responsible for the observed activity. A program to test this hypothesis would be useful even if no common substructures could be identified. Such an outcome would suggest that factors beyond the actual structures themselves had been overlooked.

We previously presented a solution to this problem for the case of constitutional representations of structures in which molecular connectivity was utilized as an integral part of the definition of commonality (13). This approach is not useful for structure-activity relationships based on three-dimensional representations of structure, although, as indicated below, there are key features of the algorithm (13) that find utility in the three-dimensional problem. In particular, molecular connectivity plays at best only a secondary role in that common substructures are sought by their relationships in space independent of the connectivity of the constituent atoms of the substructure. In other words, a pharmacophore may be a collection of atoms in the proper geometric relationship, independent of how the atoms are interconnected.

Several approaches to comparison of three-dimensional representations of structures to determine common features have been presented. One approach is to use computer graphics to superimpose manually two or more structures to determine commonality by direct overlap. This technique is limited because of the difficulty of visualizing multiple structures and quantitating the degree of overlap. Alternatively, procedures for computing the degree of overlap of several structures have been presented (14, 15). These methods are limited the total number of structures that can be compared and, most importantly, by initial assumptions on where each structure is placed in the coordinate system. A more general approach has been suggested, although not demonstrated, based on extensions of an algorithm for three-dimensional substructure searching (graph matching) (16).

We propose a more general approach to the problem of identifying three-dimensional common substructures. In particular, we propose a solution to the following, narrowly defined problem:

Given:

1 A set of molecular structures all of which possess the same "activity." We assume that the chemist or biochemist using the program has exercised his or her judgment of what constitutes similar activities.

2 A set of three-dimensional coordinates (X,Y,Z) for the position of every atom in every structure. We assume that other techniques, for example, x-ray crystallography or quantum mechanical or empirical forcefield energy minimization procedures, exist to define the geometry of each structure precisely.

3 A set of constraints supplied to the program on atom and substructural properties deemed relevant to the search for common substructures. These constraints are supplied by the person using the interactive program and represent his or her best judgments on criteria for commonality.

Find: three-dimensional substructures of a given size, largest size, or "maximal" (13) common to the set of structures.

This program assumes that considerable chemical, biological, and structural data are available and that the chemist has exercised good judgment on the similarity of activities and criteria for commonality. Given such information, the program is designed to locate common three-dimensional substructures under a variety of constraints.

Method

This problem is one of a large class of combinatorial problems for which all known algorithms are exponential in some key element of the computations, in this case the number of possible substructures for a given structure, which is directly related to the number of atoms in the structure. Therefore, every effort must be made to constrain the search for common substructures and to employ efficient computational methods for making the search efficient.

We summarize in Fig. 3 the major steps in our method. In the following sections we discuss several elements of Fig. 3, assuming that structures are input and that there is some method such as interactive graphics to aid in the interpretation of the summary output.

Representation The first step in the program is to transform the representation of structure from X,Y,Z coordinates to interatomic distances from every atom to every other atom in the structure. Because connectivity is unimportant in this approach (and can in any case be determined at any point by reference to a connection table or an examination of the distances themselves) the distances are merely stored in an n by n array, subsequently referred to as a *distance matrix*, where n is the number of atoms. The distance matrix for the chair conformation of cyclohexane (9) is given in Fig. 4. In Fig. 4, only the top half of what is a symmetrical matrix is filled in to emphasize that it is a symmetrical matrix. The diagonal elements (n1, n2, etc., can be used to store the name of atom n.

The distance matrix representation has two primary advantages: (a) the necessary computations are far simpler to carry out in "distance space" than in "coordinate space," and (b) the distance matrix is one representation of a special kind of graph called a "general graph" (17) in which every atom can be considered "connected" to every other atom. [In our case the general graph is augmented with various atom ("node") properties and the "connections" ("edges") are augmented with the distance information.] The general graph is attractive because (a) it has chemical significance in that any

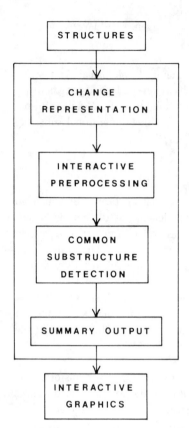

Figure 3 Block diagram indicating the major steps in the procedure for finding three-dimensional common substructures.

REPRESENTATION

X, Y, Z Coordinates ➡ Distance Matrix

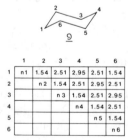

Figure 4 The distance matrix representation for the chair conformation of cyclohexane (9). The diagonal elements contain designations for the atom name. The lower half of the matrix is not filled in to emphasize that it is a symmetrical matrix and only the top, right half need be kept for computer processing.

combination of atoms, whether connected in the original structure or not, can participate in a common substructure that might be the putative pharmacophore, and (*b*) the characteristics of general graphs simplify subsequent computations, particularly construction of canonical names used in comparisons of substructures.

Preprocessing There are several preprocessing steps that serve to constrain the program prior to the actual search for common substructures. It is critical to the success of such a search that the problem be constrained as much as possible. The scope of the problem without constraints is indicated in Fig. 5. For a reasonably sized structure (e.g., 30 atoms, Fig. 5), the number of substructures of a specified size *m* quickly becomes astronomical as *m* increases.

In an interactive session with the program the chemist will be asked to supply information summarized in Table 3. The first set of constraints (substructural constraints) concerns portions of the structures that the chemist wishes to regard as common from the outset. For example, if a set of steroids that share a geometrically equivalent steroid nucleus is analyzed, it is pointless to perform a vast number of computations merely to discover that commonality. Such a nucleus can be defined to be common from the beginning. These substructures, which may be of arbitrary complexity, can be defined using Editstruc, our structure editor (1), and located within each structure using existing graph matching routines (18). Once located, the constituent atoms are collapsed to a single point resting at the center of mass (in coordinate space), and distances from this point to all other atoms are adjusted accordingly. This is illustrated in Fig. 6 for the androstane skeleton substituted with four substituents R_1-R_4 (10). If this skeleton were defined to be in common, the transformation indicated in Fig. 6 would take place,

SCOPE OF PROBLEM

For $\underline{n}$ atoms,
number of substructures
of size $\underline{m}$ =

$$\frac{n!}{m!\,(n-m)!}$$

For n=30,

m	Number
2	435
3	4060
4	27405
8	5.85×10^6
10	3.00×10^7
15	1.55×10^8

Figure 5 The number of possible substructures of size *m* for selected values of *m*, for a 30-atom structure.

Table 3   Constraints Available on the Program that Finds Three-Dimensional Substructures

Constraint	Description
Substructural	Substructures defined as common to all structures
Atom Properties	Selected properties of atoms to be used in deriving atom names
Distances	Distance ranges to be used in comparing interatomic distances
Control	Parameters to control the search procedure

with S_1 becoming a new "atom" located in coordinate space at the center of mass of the unsubstituted skeleton. The advantage of substructural constraints is that they reduce the number of atoms in each structure and thus reduce the combinatorial search.

The second type of constraint (Table 3) deals with atom properties that are deemed important during the subsequent search procedure. A variety of atom properties can be selected, including those that differentiate atoms by name, hybridization, degree of substitution, electronegativity, charge, and so forth. In this way, the effective name of an atom used in the search procedure can be of any specificity, ranging from regarding all atoms as having the same name to having very detailed names that include several of the above properties. After selection of the properties, every atom in every structure is renamed according to the selections.

The third type of constraint (Table 3) deals with specification of what interatomic distances are to be regarded as the "same." Not only do we have to allow for experimental error and for the possibility of some flexibility in the structures, we also want to allow for varying levels of search. In this way, very coarse ranges on distances can be used to see if there are any gross similarities in constituent substructures. Finer ranges can be used to select any

**INTERACTIVE
PREPROCESSING**

1) Substructural Constraints

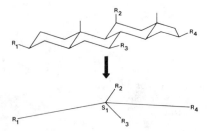

Figure 6 An illustration of the use of substructural constraints. The androstane nucleus, previously identified as a common substructural element, is collapsed to its center of mass (S_1), with distances for substituents R_1–R_4 now referenced to S_1.

desired degree of commonality in interatomic distance. Currently we are experimenting with different methods for representing distance ranges. Once these ranges are specified, an internal look-up table is built, which associates each range with a specific designation. Subsequently, distances retrieved from the distance matrix will be compared to the table to determine the proper range and designation.

The fourth type of constraint (Table 1) deals with actual controls on the search procedure itself. The program can be instructed to find all common substructures, the largest common substructure, the maximal (13) common substructure, or substructures of size n, in which n is the number of atoms. To allow for inadequacies in the data set of structures or coordinates, the scientist can require that only a specified percentage of structures possess substructures in common. Finally, one structure can be identified as a "key" structure (for example, the parent compound of a series of compounds) to which all other structures are to be compared, and the search for common substructures will continue as long as at least one other structure possesses a substructure common to the "key."

Algorithm The algorithm for identifying three-dimensional common substructures for a set of structures has several goals in common with the algorithm for finding two-dimensional common substructures (13), although the operational procedures are quite different. In particular, the first goal is to begin by finding all common substructures of the smallest size of interest, i.e., two atom substructures in our case. The algorithm then proceeds by finding all common substructures of size three based on those that were common at size two and continues in this fashion until a terminating condition specified by the control constraints (Table 3) is reached. At each step in the procedure the goal is to remove from further consideration any substructures that were not found to be common to the set of structures.

Major steps in the algorithm are summarized in Fig. 7. As shown in Fig. 7, common substructures of $SIZE = 2$ are first found. Each structure (STRUC) is processed in turn. Substructures are located and assigned canonical names [in GROWSUBS(STRUC,SIZE)]. The procedure for assigning names is discussed in the next section. A history list (Fig. 7) is maintained as each structure is processed, keeping a record of which substructures were located in which structures. When all structures have been processed for $SIZE = 2$, the history list is used to update the distances matrix (DM) for each structure, removing pairwise distances (see Fig. 4) that were found not to be in common from further consideration. Terminating conditions (the control constraints, Table 3) are tested. If there are none, the procedure is repeated for $SIZE = 3$ and subsequently larger sizes.

As the size of substructures increases linearly in the procedure, the number of possible substructures of that size increases exponentially (until the

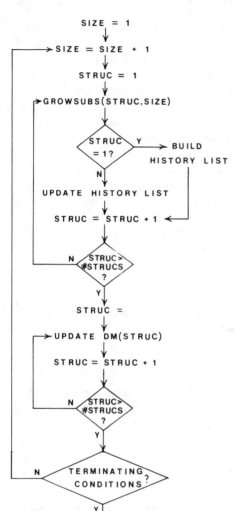

Figure 7 A flow chart of the algorithm for finding three-dimensional common substructures. SIZE refers to the number of atoms in the substructure, STRUC is the structure number in the set of structures #STRUCS, and DM is the distance matrix of the associated structure. GROWSUBS(STRUC,SIZE) is the routine that finds all substructures of given SIZE in the given STRUC, and assigns canonical names to each substructure.

size of the substructure reaches half the number of atoms in a given structure). However, because a substructure is "grown" to larger size only if the substructure of one fewer atoms on which it is based was found to be common to the set of structures, it is possible to limit severely the potential exponential growth. The algorithm will have to perform large numbers of computations only if the structures are *very* similar, and this can be controlled by reducing the search by prior specification of substructural constraints (Table 3).

A detailed description of the algorithm is inappropriate because experience will no doubt lead to program modifications. The basic goals and algorithmic descriptions are presented in more detail for the problem of two-dimensional common substructures (13). The primary differences in the procedures are concerned with deriving canonical names for substructures so that they can be compared for identity and the necessity for treatment of stereochemistry. These interrelated topics are discussed briefly below.

Canonical Names for Substructures Consider the possible substructures of size 2 for cyclohexane (9) (chair conformation), based on the distance matrix of Fig. 4, as shown in Fig. 8. If all the atoms of 9 were different there would be 15 possible substructures of size 2. However, there are only three unique substructures representing six occurrences of $CH_2 - CH_2$, with a 1-2 distance of 1.54 A; six occurrences of $CH_2 - CH_2$, with a 1-3 distance of 2.51 A; and three occurrences of $CH_2 - CH_2$, with a 1-4 distance of 2.95 A (Fig. 8). A canonical naming procedure has been devised that allows rapid construction and comparison of names so that only unique substructures, such as those shown in Fig. 8, are retained in the history list (Fig. 7). This procedure is of necessity very different from the procedure described in the first part of this Chapter. The former is applicable to atom-centered codes for connected atoms. Here we have no such "focus" for a substructure, nor is connectivity an important controlling factor.

At each step in the procedure, a substructure that is a candidate for a substructure common to the set of structures must be named in order to identify it and to allow it to be compared with other substructures of the same size to determine equivalence. In our procedure, any two substructures comprised of the same atoms and interatomic distances (subject to distance constraints, Table 3) will be given the same name. Once this is accomplished, it is an easy matter to compare the names in the computer.

Substructures are named in the following way. Each constituent atom has a name, assigned in the preprocessing step based on atom constraints (Table

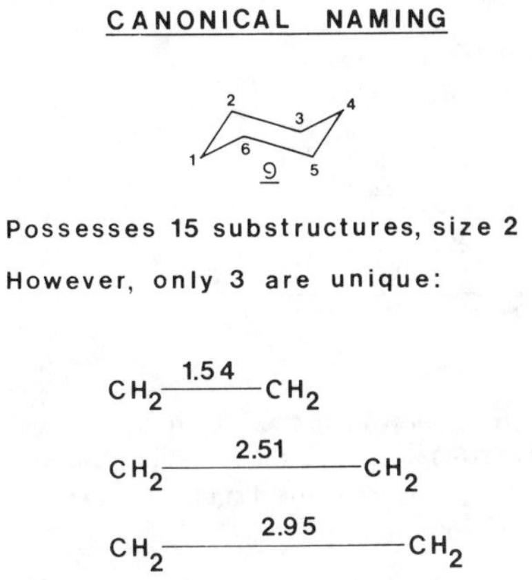

CANONICAL NAMING

Possesses 15 substructures, size 2

However, only 3 are unique:

Figure 8 The three unique substructures of size 2, of the 15 possible two-atom substructures, for the chair conformation of cyclohexane (9) (see Fig. 4).

3). Each atom pair is characterized by two atom names and a designator for the interatomic distance (assigned based on distance constraints, Table 3). The atom names are lexicographically ordered so that every two-atom substructure of the same atom names and distance designator possesses the same name. This ordering is possible because we are dealing with *undirected* graphs (17), i.e., atoms are simply "connected" in the general graph and the connection implies no direction from atom 1 to atom 2. Canonical names so constructed are sufficient for the first pass through the program to determine common substructures of size 2 (Fig. 7). Treatment of substructures of size 2 is summarized in Fig. 9. From ATOM-2, ATOM-1, and the interatomic distance D-1,2, we construct a lexicographically ordered name consisting of NAME1 and NAME2, together with a distance designation ND12. This is abbreviated for simplicity in Fig. 9 as NAME12.

For substructures of size 3, selected as outlined above (Fig. 7), canonical names are constructed using three two-atom pairs*. In other words, given three atoms *a,b,c*, the lexicographically ordered pairs *ab*, *bc*, *ac* are used to construct a new name in which an additional lexicographical ordering is imposed to determine the sequence of the three pairs, thereby arriving at a canonical name for substructures of size 3. This is illustrated for $a = 1$, $b = 2$, and $c = 3$ in Fig. 9, in which the resulting canonical name (in abbreviated form, see above) for the substructure is as given. Again, this ordering, now of sets of pairs, is proper because we are dealing with general graphs (17). Because all atoms are "connected" to all other atoms, a substructure is defined explicitly, taking the set of pairs in any order. Thus we can impose any reordering scheme on the set and still refer to the same substructure.

For substructures of size 4 atoms (and higher) the canonical naming procedure is modified both to take into account stereochemistry and to reduce the computer memory required to store the name*.

*See footnote on page 188.

Method: Derive names from component substructures
of size 2, supplemented with stereochemistry

Size

2   ATOM-2, ATOM-1, D-1,2 ⟶ (NAME1 NAME2 ND12) ⟶ ⌐(NAME12)⌐

3   ⌐((NAME12) (NAME13) (NAME23))⌐

4   ⌐((NAME12) (NAME13) (NAME23) (NAME4 STEREO4 ND14 ND24 ND34))⌐

5   ⌐((NAME12) (NAME13) (NAME23) (NAME4 STEREO4 ND14 ND24 ND34)
              (NAME5 STEREO5 ND15 ND25 ND35))⌐

Figure 9 Canonical substructure names, abbreviated as shown for the substructure name for size = 2, for substructures of increasing size. STEREOn refers to the stereo designation for the fourth, fifth, . . . atoms in the substructure. NDnm refers to the distance designation for the n,m interatomic distance. See text for further explanation.

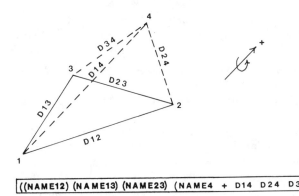

((NAME12) (NAME13) (NAME23) (NAME4 + D14 D24 D34))

Figure 10 Illustration of construction of the canonical name for a four-atom substructure. Assuming that atom 4 lies above the plane formed by atoms 1,2,3 (not behind, into the plane of the figure), the stereo tag for atom 4 is +.

Stereochemistry Stereochemistry often plays an important role in determining the activity of a molecule. However, in transforming the structural representation from X,Y,Z coordinates to distance space we have discarded stereochemical information. The substituents about the R and S forms of a given chiral center have the same distance relationships among themselves and the chiral center. Consideration of stereochemistry must take place in our procedure when sufficient atoms are included in a substructure to differentiate mirror image occurrences of two substructures that are otherwise the same. In general, this occurs with substructures of size 4 atoms (exceptions are discussed below).

Given four atoms, three may be chosen to specify a plane. The stereochemical differentiation must be on the basis of the location of the fourth atom with respect to that plane, i.e., it lies on one side of the plane or the other in three-dimensional space. Therefore, we must return to the set of X,Y,Z coordinates in order to determine a parity designation that specifies on which side of the plane lies the fourth atom. This is accomplished by choosing a set of three atoms for a reference plane and assigning parity based on the sign of the vector pointing to the fourth atom using the right-hand rule. This is illustrated for the four atoms labeled 1–4 in Fig. 10 (assume that atom 4 lies above the plane specified by 1–3 because it is not clear from the actual drawing). Following the right-hand rule, the sign of the vector is designated as +. Therefore, the name associated with the four-atom substructure (see Fig. 9 for the form of the canonical name and the location of the stereo tag in the name itself) is as given in Fig. 10, with the stereo tag +.

This procedure is general to four, five, six, etc., atom substructures. The steps in deriving a canonical name for any size are the following:

1 Given n atoms, $n > 3$, choose a set of three atoms for the reference plane. This is accomplished by selecting the lexicographically "least" name from the set of all possible "legal" (see below) three-atom substructure names, wherein the names themselves are canonical based on the same procedure used for treating substructures of size 3 atoms, above.

2 For every other atom, determine the parity designation for stereochemistry.

3 Associate with each atom from step 2 a name that consists of its atom name, selected by atom constraints (Table 3), the parity designation, and the set of distances to the three atoms selected for the original plane.

4 Build the canonical name by extending the name assigned to the three atoms in the plane with a lexicographically ordered list of names for additional atoms (each name assigned in step 4).

The names constructed in this fashion for substructures of size 4 and 5 are summarized (again in abbreviated form) in Fig. 9. Canonical names derived in this way are then used for subsequent comparisons. This procedure involves recomputation of the names at every increase in size of the substructures, as would any other procedure, in order to guarantee that the same substructure found in another structure possesses precisely the same name. The storage requirement for names is, however, reduced significantly,* as is the effort required to compare names for equivalence.

There are three special cases in assigning stereochemistry. The first two special cases bear on selection of a "legal" reference plane:

1 If a three-atom substructure that is a candidate for the reference plane possesses two (or more) atom pairs of exactly the same name it must be rejected as a legal candidate. Stereochemical designations would make no sense in this case because the right-hand rule for assigning a parity designation could be applied in two ways. This situation is related to the fact that a tetra-substituted carbon atom is not a chiral center unless there are four nonequivalent substituents at that center. If all three-atom substructures are rejected by this test, there is no basis for assigning stereochemistry. The canonical name becomes that shown in Fig. 9 for sizes 4 and 5, with the stereo tag set to O, indicating undifferentiated.

---

*The number of atom pairs, or the number of distances, required to specify completely an n atom substructure is $n(n-1)/2$. This number is proportional to n^2, while the number of X,Y,Z coordinates required to specify the same substructure in coordinate space is only $3n$, which becomes fewer than the number of distances at $n = 8$. However, we reduce the amount of information necessary to characterize the substructure uniquely by considering the stereochemistry of the substructure. Three distances for the three atoms in the plane are required, plus a parity designation and three additional distances for each additional atom, or $3 + 4(n-3)$, or $4n - 9$ pieces of information. At $n > 6$ this procedure requires less storage space than the raw distances, plus the stereochemistry is preserved.

2 If a three-atom substructure is legal (see case 1), then it must be checked to see if it is unique. Often the situation arises in which there is more than one three-atom substructure, each composed of precisely the same three atom pairs (names and interatomic distances) and, thus, canonical names for size 3. Such substructures cannot be used for the reference plane in the above procedure; there is ambiguity in which should be chosen and, thus, in the resulting parity designations. Therefore, the actual search for candidates for the reference plane must select the "best" candidate, best being defined as a three-atom substructure that is legal according to case 1 above, that is lexicographically least, *and that is unique to the set of three-atom substructures.* If no three-atom substructure meets these criteria, the name is simply constructed as in 1, with O assigned to the stereo tags.

3 The geometric relationship of the atoms place them all in the same plane. This situation will often occur, particularly for planar molecules. In this case, as above, the stereo tag must be assigned as O.

CONCLUSIONS

We have presented two methods for detecting and characterizing substructures in three-dimensional representations of structure. The choice of method depends strongly on the application. The first method assumes that one is characterizing the local substructural environment of an atom (or functionality), wherein atom connectivities play a crucial role in the associated "activity." Further, this method is of utility in building a data base of structures together with their component substructures and activities because proper account is taken of the local substructural configuration and conformation so that unique or canonical names can be assigned to the substructures.

The second method is applicable to structure-activity relationships in which atom connectivities play a secondary role; the relationship of atoms in three-dimensional space independent of connectivity is important. This method places a significant burden on the chemist or biochemist because he or she must determine whether or not the "activity" is indeed similar for a set of structures. In addition, the conformation of each structure must be designated. Although the method is potentially applicable to intercomparison of structures, each with several possible conformations, the combinatorial problem of picking one conformation for each structure and repeatedly applying the program introduces another exponential factor in an already very large computational problem.

Both methods are currently under development. We are designing both methods so that they can be accessed as interactive computer programs by those persons with actual biochemical problems who wish to collaborate with us on further development. Please contact the authors for additional information.

REFERENCES

1 Carhart, R. E., D. H. Smith, H. Brown, and C. Djerassi. Applications of artificial intelligence for chemical inference. XVII. An approach to computer-assisted elucidation of molecular structure. *J. Am. Chem. Soc.* 97:5755-5762 (1975).

2 Djerassi, C., D. H. Smith, and T. H. Varkony. A novel role of computers in the natural products field. *Naturwissenschaften* 66:9-21 (1979).

3 Carhart, R. E., D. H. Smith, N. A. B. Gray, J. G. Nourse, and C. Djerassi. GENOA: A computer program for structure elucidation based on overlapping and alternative substructures. *J. Org. Chem.* 46:1708-1718 (1981).

4 Gray, N. A. B., J. G. Nourse, C. W. Crandell, D. H. Smith, and C. Djerassi. Stereochemical substructure codes for 13C spectral analysis. *Org. Magn. Reson.* 15:375-389 (1981).

5 Gray, N. A. B., C. W. Crandell, J. G. Nourse, D. H. Smith, M. L. Dageforde, and C. Djerassi. Computer-assisted structural interpretation of C-13 spectral data. *J. Org. Chem.* 46:703-715 (1981).

6 Nourse, J. G., D. H. Smith, R. E. Carhart, and C. Djerassi. Computer-assisted elucidation of molecular structure with stereochemistry. *J. Am. Chem. Soc.* 102:6289-6295 (1980).

7 Stuper, A. J., W. E. Brugger, and P. C. Jurs. *Computer Assisted Studies of Chemical Structure and Biological Function.* New York: Wiley (1979).

8 Olson, E. C., and R. E. Christoffersen. *Computer-Assisted Drug Design.* Washington, D.C.: American Chemical Society (1979).

9 Masinter, L. M., N. S. Sridharan, R. E. Carhart, and D. H. Smith. Applications of artificial intelligence for chemical inference. XIII. Labeling of objects having symmetry. *J. Am. Chem. Soc.* 96:7714-7723 (1974).

10 Nourse, J. G. Specification and unconstrained enumeration of conformations of chemical structures for computer-assisted structure elucidation. *J. Chem. Inf. Comp. Sci.* 21:168-172 (1981).

11 Wipke, W. T., and T. M. Dyott. Stereochemically Unique Naming Algorithm. *J. Am. Chem. Soc.* 96:4834-4842 (1974).

12 Nourse, J. G. The Configuration Symmetry Group and Its Application to Stereoisomer Generation, Specification, and Enumeration. *Am. Chem. Soc.* 101:1210-1216 (1979).

13 Varkony, T. H., Y. Shiloach, and D. H. Smith. Computer-assisted examination of chemical compounds for structural similarities. *J. Chem. Inf. Comp. Sci.* 19:104-111 (1979).

14 Rohrer, D. C., and H. Perry. FITMOL. In J. J. Wood (ed.), *Public Procedures: A Program Exchange for PROPHET Users.* Cambridge, MA: Bolt, Beranek and Newman (1978).

15 Cohen, N. C. Beyond the 2–D chemical structure. In E. C. Olsen and R. E. Christoffersen (eds.), *Computer Assisted Drug Design*, pp. 371–381. Washington, D.C.: American Chemical Society (1979).

16 Lesk, A. M. Detection of three-dimensional patterns of atoms in chemical structures. *Communications of the ACM* 22:219–224 (1979).

17 Harary, F. *Graph Theory*. Reading, MA: Addison Wesley (1971).

18 Carhart, R. E., and D. H. Smith. Applications of Artificial Intelligence for Chemical Inference. XX. "Intelligent" use of Constraints in Computer-Assisted Structure Elucidation. *Computer Chem.* 1:79–84 (1976).

Chapter 12

QSAR, PROPHET,
and Environmental Toxicology

STRUCTURE–ACTIVITY CLASSIFICATION
OF CHEMICALS IN TERMS OF FISH
REPRODUCTIVE TOXICITY

Howard L. Johnson, Caroline C. Sigman,
Howard C. Bailey, and Karl Kuhlmann

The primary purpose of this presentation is to illustrate the use of a powerful interactive computer system in the area of environmental toxicology. PROPHET is one of several such systems available; its development has been sponsored by NIH (the Division of Research Resources), and there are currently more than 30 sites within the United States that subscribe to this time-share system. PROPHET software was developed and is maintained by Bolt, Beranek and Newman, Inc. and runs on a large government-owned Digital Equipment Corporation KL-10. Software is designed specifically for ease of use by the community of chemical-biological scientists in familiar terms of data tables, graphs, and molecular structures.

The two examples chosen as illustrations of the use of PROPHET software for QSAR analysis in environmental toxicology are rather distinct. The first deals with the problem of predicting the potential hazards of environmental chemicals in terms of reproductive toxicity in fish. The second example deals with the problem of anticipating the degree of hazard of environmental chemicals relative to potential carcinogenic effects in humans. Both cases, however, are typical with respect to a major current problem in environmental toxicology; the quantity and quality of standardized quantitative biological data are seldom adequate.

The study of fish reproductive toxicity was sponsored by the EPA and centers on data mostly extracted from the open literature; it pertains to 72 organic chemicals of widely varying structure as summarized in Table 1. The total number of literature citations that provided minimal toxic concentration values for these 72 compounds was 106. In some cases the variation in such concentration values for a single compound was more than 50 percent of the range of minimal toxic concentrations for the entire data base; in many other cases only a single toxicity value was available, with no indication of the reliability of the value. Structural classification was manual (Table 1), and multiple linear regression analysis was limited to gross parameters (molecular weight and log P) due to the inherent structural diversity and variability of the data base.

Figure 1 is a PROPHET graph of toxicity (potency, log $1/c$) versus molecular weight. While the linear correlation (solid line) was rather poor, the graph suggested a relationship (dashed line) that is perturbed by specific outliers of relative low toxicity.

Table 1 Characterization of Fish Reproductive Toxicity Data Base

Class code	Definition	Number of citations	Number of chemicals
! ARX	Halogenated aromatics	8	7
2 ARNO2	Nitro aromatics	5	5
3 ARALP	Alkyl & polycyclic aromatics	2	2
4 XAL	Halogenated alkyl aliph. & alicyclic	14	12
5 XALAR	Halogenated arylalkyl aliph. & alicyclic	6	2
6 XBI	Halogenated bicyclic aliph. & alicyclic	18	6
7 CON	Carbamates	3	2
8 OHAR	Phenols	9	8
9 POS	(Thio)phosphates	11	6
10 COAR	Phthalates, aromatic lactones	2	2
11 UCON	Ureides	2	2
12 NAR	Aromatic & heterocyclic amines	6	4
13 MC	Organometallics	5	4
14 MIS	Miscellaneous	15	10

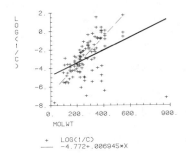

Figure 1 Relationship of potency to molecular weight.

Log P data were available for 62 of the compounds and appeared to be related to molecular weight in a fairly consistent manner (Fig. 2, solid line) except for certain ionic compounds and a highly polar subset (Fig. 2, dashed line). The dashed line of Fig. 2 suggested a basis for a binary "polarity parameter" (2 log P units; $FP-$) to charactize this unusually polar subset as shown in Table 2. Similarly, the unusual polarity of an additional six ionic compounds could be described in terms of their unique propensities for ionization (Table 2; $FI = F_0(N)$, where F_0 is a function of pK_a or pK_b). These unusually polar compounds are identified by number symbols in Fig. 3, which otherwise shows the same relationship as in Fig. 1.

Together with molecular weight, the polarity parameters (FP and FI) proved to be significant in accounting for the potency of the entire data set. The results of stepwise linear multiple regression are shown in Fig. 4. The three included parameters accounted for approximately 60 percent of the variation in potency ($R^2 = 0.59$). The remaining variation is substantially experimental as illustrated by the wide variations in potency values for individual compounds in Fig. 3.

One of the convenient interactive graphics features of a system such as PROPHET is the ability to immediately identify specific data points on a graphic display in terms of any of the data associated with those points. The display may be "queried" for instant graphic identification of outliers or other specific points in terms of, for example, compound number, name, or any other property. This feature results in a display such as Fig. 3.

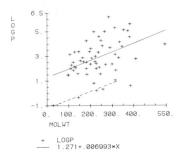

Figure 2 Relationship of log p to molecular weight.

Table 2   Polarity Parameters

Parameter	Function
1 *FP*	Binary polarity parameter (graphic; 0 or 2)
2	
3 *FI*	$F_0(N); F_0 = F(pK_a$ or $pK_b)$ (Range = 0 to 4)
4	—SO_3 (—) (benzenesulfonic acid, $pK_a = 0.7$) $F_0 = 4$
5	—COO(—) (Phenoxyacetic acid, $pK_a = 3.1$) $F_0 = 2$
6	—COO(—) (Picolinic acid, $pK_a = 4.7$) $F_0 = 0$

N = No. of such groups in mol. (range = 0 to 4).

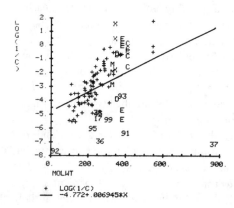

+   LOG(1/C)
——   -4.772+.006945*X

Figure 3 Polar compounds and data variability in the potency-molecular weight relationship. E = endrin, C = chlordane, D = diazinon, M = malathion.

```
VARIABLE X ( 3) ENTERED AT F=  13.211

MULTIPLE CORRELATION COEFFICIENT         R= 0.76691
   CORRECTED FOR DEGREE OF FREEDOM     R(C)= 0.75897
STANDARD ERROR OF ESTIMATE                = 1.2568
DEGREES OF FREEDOM                        =102

VARIABLE                     CONTRIB.   REGRESSION    STANDARD    T TEST OF
                             TO RSQ     COEFF. (B)   ERROR OF B   B COEFF.

1 MOLWT              *       -0.39004    .1209E-01   .1231E-02    9.828
2 FI                 *       -0.34630   - .8025      .8665E-01   -9.261
3 FP                 *       -0.05334   -1.058       .2912       -3.635
4 LOG(1/C)         DEPENDENT VARIABLE
* VARIABLE IN EQUATION

CONSTANT =      -5.8468
OVERALL F=  48.553


DO YOU WISH TO SEE THE RESIDUALS ?

N

PLEASE SAY WHETHER TO ENTER A VARIABLE I (+I), TO REMOVE IT (-I),
   OR TO EXIT (0).   STEPWISE SOLUTION SUGGESTS    0
```

Figure 4 Three-parameter potency correlation.

```
VARIABLE X ( 2) ENTERED AT F=   101.56

MULTIPLE CORRELATION COEFFICIENT           R= 0.76508
   CORRECTED FOR DEGREE OF FREEDOM     R(C)= 0.75980
STANDARD ERROR OF ESTIMATE                 = 1.2550
DEGREES OF FREEDOM                         =103

VARIABLE                 CONTRIB.    REGRESSION    STANDARD    T TEST OF
                         TO RSQ      COEFF. (B)    ERROR OF B  B COEFF.

1 MOLWT            *     -0.44358     .1238E-01    .1180E-02    10.50
2 PF               *     -0.40886    - .8257       .8193E-01   -10.08
3 LOG(1/C)               DEPENDENT VARIABLE
* VARIABLE IN EQUATION

CONSTANT =          -5.9401
OVERALL F=   72.699


DO YOU WISH TO SEE THE RESIDUALS ?

N

PLEASE SAY WHETHER TO ENTER A VARIABLE I (+I), TO REMOVE IT (-I),
  OR TO EXIT (0).  STEPWISE SOLUTION SUGGESTS   0
```

Figure 5 Two-parameter potency correlation.

Two-dimensional illustrations of relationships involving three or more independent variables are impractical. In order to facilitate a two-dimensional illustration, the polarity parameters (*FP*, *FI*) were combined into a single parameter (*FP*). The resulting two-parameter correlation is shown in Fig. 5, and its correlation surface is shown in the three-dimensional perspective graph of Fig. 6.

An alternative representation of the graph is made up of equally spaced "needles" projecting from the *X*, *Y* plane of Fig. 6 to the correlation surface (Fig. 7). It is instructive to compare the latter with a corresponding representation of the actual data points (Fig. 8). This dramatizes the differences between the derived theoretical correlation and the nature of the actual data on which the correlation is based. At the very least, the graphic comparison emphasizes areas of maximum uncertainty and suggests areas in parameter space that should be examined for validation or better definition of structure-toxicity relationships by selection of appropriate structures for experimental evaluation.

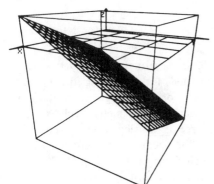

Figure 6 Two-parameter   correlation surface in perspective. *Z* = potency; *X* = molecular weight, *Y* = polarity.

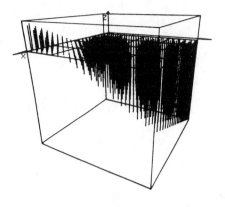

Figure 7 Two-parameter correlation surface in perspective: potency projections from the *X-Y* (molecular weight — polarity) plane.

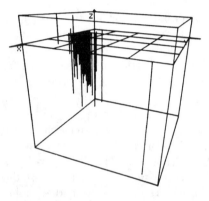

Figure 8 Actual data points in perspective as potency projections from the *X-Y* (molecular weight — polarity) plane.

II. STRUCTURE–ACTIVITY CLASSIFICATION OF CHEMICALS AS CARCINOGENS: APPLICATION OF AN ACTIVITY TREE AND THE PROPHET COMPUTER SYSTEM

Caroline C. Sigman, Karol L. Thompson, and C. Tucker Helmes

At SRI, we are in the process of developing a structure-activity tree as the primary component of a systematic method for evaluating the potential carcinogenicity of untested chemicals and for analyzing the relationships between the structures of chemical carcinogens and parameters such as species affected and tumor site. The activity tree is developed, maintained, and applied to the evaluation of chemicals via the chemical structure analysis and data management capabilities of the PROPHET computer system (1, 2).

The concept of the activity tree was first described by SIR in 1974 (3). It is designed to be an index to the structural features of chemicals associated with carcinogenicity. This index has as its basic units rather broad chemical structure classes known to contain carcinogens (e.g., alkyl halides). The

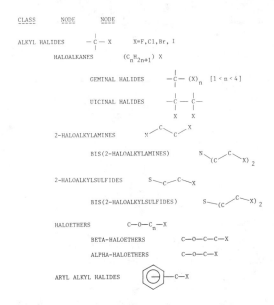

Figure 9 Structure-activity tree for carcinogenesis. Organization of activity tree illustrated by the alkyl halides carcinogen class and its nodes.

carcinogen classes are branched into subclasses by specific structural features. The subclasses, known as nodes, represent structural groups for which carcinogenicity data are available and, in most cases, reflect expected differences in carcinogenic behavior among chemicals belonging to the class. The organization of the activity tree is depicted in Fig. 9, using the alkyl halides carcinogen class and its nodes as an example. Assignments of activity tree classes and nodes are based on expert evaluation of chemical carcinogenicity test data and are made when the available data are judged to reflect a significant association between a chemical structure and carcinogenicity.

Chemicals may fall into more than one class, node, or both. When a significant number of carcinogens are found to fall into the same combination of multiple classes/nodes, a new node may be assigned to represent the structural features of the combination. This new node is then linked to all of its parent classes/nodes. For example, amino/nitroquinolines is a node on the activity tree. It is derived from both the aryl amino/nitro/azo compounds and the quinolines carcinogen classes and from nodes therein (Fig. 10). Currently there are 15 carcinogen classes (Table 3) and 54 nodes on the activity tree.

Chemical Classification Procedures

Associated with each carcinogen class/node in PROPHET is a set of chemical structure fragments that may be used in combination with a set of search

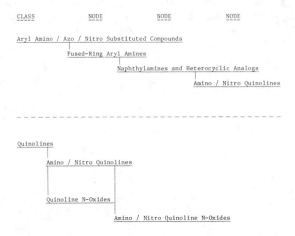

Figure 10 Structure-activity tree for carcinogenesis. Assignment of nodes to structures represented by more than one class/node. Illustrated by the node for amino/nitro quinolines.

procedures to identify chemicals belonging to the specified class/node. These procedures take advantage of the chemical substructure search capabilities of PROPHET to match the structural fragments with the structures of chemicals of interest that are also entered and stored in PROPHET. These procedures are applied both in the evaluation of the potential carcinogenicity of untested chemicals and in the analysis of chemicals of known carcinogenicity for developing and refining the activity tree.

**Table 3   Structure-Activity Tree
for Carcinogenesis: Carcinogen Classes**

Alkyl halides
Vinyl halides
Aryl halides
Alkyl sulfates/sulfonates
3-Atom heterocycles
Lactones
Aryl amino/nitro/azo substituted compounds
Quinolines
Acridines
Polycyclic aryl *N*-heterocycles
Benzodifurans
Dioxanes
Polycyclic aryl hydrocarbons
Hydrazines
N-Nitroso compounds

```
PROPHET 56        CAROLINE SIGMAN    11/4/88
CHM/SITE:  ACTIVITY TREE FOR CARCINOGENESIS
           CLASS ANALYSIS OF CHEMICALS FROM NCI TECHNICAL REPTS
           CHEMICALS CLASSED ONLY AS VINYL HALIDES
           THAT ARE CARCINOGENS--TUMOR SITE ANALYSIS          3R X 15C
```

0 CAS NO.	1 REPT NO	2 CHEMICAL NAME	3 ACTIVITY R/M
1 000000079-01-6	2	TRICHLOROETHYLENE	IS/C
2 000000127-18-4	13.	TETRACHLOROETHYLENE	IA/C
3 000000095-06-7	115.	SULFALLATE	C/C

0 CAS NO.	4 RAT,MALE ACTIVITY	5 RAT,MALE ROUTE	6 RAT,MALE SITE	7 RAT,FEMALE ACTIVITY
1 000000079-01-6	NS	IG	MU	NS
2 000000127-18-4	NA	PO		NA
3 000000095-06-7	C	PO	FS	C

0 CAS NO.	8 RAT,FEMALE ROUTE	9 RAT,FEMALE SITE	10 MOUSE,MALE ACTIVITY	11 MOUSE,MALE ROUTE
1 000000079-01-6	IG	MU	C	IG
2 000000127-18-4	PO		C	PO
3 000000095-06-7	PO	MG	C	PO

```
PROPHET 56        CAROLINE SIGMAN    11/4/88
CHM/SITE:  ACTIVITY TREE FOR CARCINOGENESIS
           CLASS ANALYSIS OF CHEMICALS FROM NCI TECHNICAL REPTS
           CHEMICALS CLASSED ONLY AS VINYL HALIDES
           THAT ARE CARCINOGENS--TUMOR SITE ANALYSIS          3R X 15C
```

0 CAS NO.	12 MOUSE,MALE SITE	13 MOUSE,FEMALE ACTIVITY	14 MOUSE,FEMALE ROUTE	15 MOUSE,FEMALE SITE
1 000000079-01-6	LI	C	IG	LI
2 000000127-18-4	LI	C	PO	LI
3 000000095-06-7	PU	C	PO	MG

Figure 11 Structure-activity tree for carcinogenesis. Data base of carcinogens associated with activity tree illustrated by carcinogens classified on the tree only as vinyl halides.

Data Base of Carcinogens

Also associated with the activity tree in PROPHET is a data base of carcinogens classified by the appropriate classes/nodes along with biological parameters such as species, sex, route of administration, and tumor sites (Fig. 11). These data can be analyzed in several ways useful in the evaluation of the relationships between chemical structure and carcinogenicity. Two examples are the identification of (a) major tumor sites by species and route of administration for carcinogens belonging to a given node and (b) the structural types of chemicals causing tumors at a specific site.

Estimates of the strength of evidence associating the chemical structure with carcinogenicity are tabulated for each class/node. These estimates are based on the best tested chemicals in each structural group and consider such factors as the number of test conditions under which the chemicals are carcinogenic, the multiplicity of sites at which tumors are observed, the number of species/strains in which the chemicals are carcinogenic, and the quality of the available test data. Such estimates are useful in many of the studies we carry out that require prioritizing untested chemicals on the basis of suspicion of carcinogenicity; however, we have not yet found a set of criteria that is totally adequate for characterizing the strength of evidence for carcinogenicity. We expect that the estimates will be continually reevaluated as the carcinogens data base and the applications of the activity tree expand.

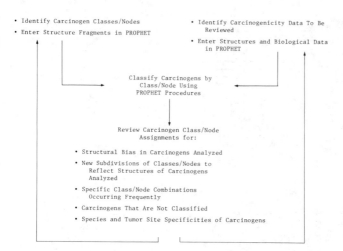

Figure 12 Structure-activity tree for carcinogenesis. Schemata of procedure for developing and refining activity tree.

Development of the Activity Tree

The steps in developing and refining the activity tree are as follows (Fig. 12):

1 *Identify initial set of carcinogen classes and nodes.* The chemical classes/nodes chosen for the current activity tree were drawn primarily from recent reviews on carcinogens (e.g., 4) and from those identified in the original description of the activity tree concept (3). As is evident in the list of classes in Table 3, we have not yet evaluated all the structural classes known to be associated with carcinogenicity. The classes on the activity tree thus far are those we have encountered most frequently in studies in which the activity tree has been applied to evaluation of untested chemicals. Also, nodes have not yet been developed for all of the classes in the activity tree (e.g., *N*-nitroso compounds). Fragment structures corresponding to the chosen classes and nodes are entered in **PROPHET**.

2 *Identify carcinogenicity data to be reviewed.* The carcinogens reviewed thus far in the development of the activity tree are those identified in the National Cancer Institute Carcinogenesis Bioassay Program Technical Report Series (5). This set of carcinogenicity data, as well as other sets that will be added, presents significant results of well-documented tests that have been carried out by protocols judged to be adequate by experts in carcinogenicity testing. The structures, names, and associated biological data (species/sex, route of administration, and major tumor sites) for all of the carcinogens to be reviewed are entered in **PROPHET**.

3 *Classify carcinogens by class/node.* The carcinogens are analyzed using the activity tree structural fragments from step 1 and the substructure search capabilities of PROPHET to group them into the appropriate classes/nodes. Results are presented as a matrix listing of the carcinogens versus all the appropriate class/node assignments and as listings of the carcinogens by class and node.

4 *Review carcinogen class/node assignments.* For all of the carcinogens, the class/node assignments are evaluated. Considerations include (*a*) structural bias indicating the need for additional data on chemicals better representing the variation within a class or node (e.g., currently, the majority of the alkyl halides carcinogens reviewed are chlorides; more data on bromides, iodides, and fluorides are needed to develop the class/node structure adequately), (*b*) new subdivisions of current classes/nodes that better reflect the structures of the carcinogens reviewed (e.g., an initial review of the haloalkane carcinogens led to the assignment of *gem* and *vic* haloalkanes as nodes), and (*c*) frequently occurring combinations of class/node assignments that may warrant new node assignments (e.g., a new node may be assigned to represent the five carcinogens that now fall into both the aryl halides class and the aniline node; chlordane and analogous pesticide carcinogens also represent a distinct structural group that now falls under several nodes). Also, carcinogens that cannot be classified on the activity tree are prime candidates to be the bases for new carcinogen classes. A currently unclassified carcinogen is trimethylphosphate.

The biological data incorporated into the activity tree are expected to be useful in identifying structural groups (i.e., new nodes), both within existing nodes and across classes and nodes, that are associated with specific species, routes of administration, and tumor sites. Analyses to evaluate these relationships have not yet been undertaken.

As indicated in Fig. 12, the development of the activity tree is iterative. During each round of the evaluation process, attempts are made to remedy both gaps in the structure of the carcinogens reviewed and in the class/node assignments.

Future Developments and Applications

As is evident, the process of developing and applying the activity tree for carcinogenicity has just begun, and its success as a tool for evaluating structure-activity relationships in carcinogenicity has yet to be proved. There are numerous possibilities, however, that can be envisioned for extending the applications of the activity tree. One such application is using the carcinogens in nodes as the basis for more quantitative structure-activity analysis, perhaps as part of a program for evaluating carcinogenic hazards such as that outlined

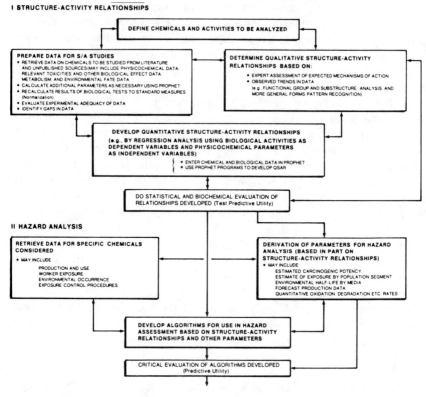

Figure 13 Structure-activity tree for carcinogenesis. Integration of activity tree (qualitative structure-activity relationships) into model for prediction of potential carcinogenic hazards of chemicals.

in Fig. 13. Another extension would be incorporation of other than carcinogenicity data (e.g., mutagenicity data) in defining and refining the activity tree. Finally, there is the possible application of the activity tree concept to other toxic effects.

REFERENCES

1 Wood, J. J., and C. Hollister. *User's Manual for the PROPHET System*, version 3.6. Prepared by Bolt, Beranek, and Newman, Inc. under NIH Contract N01-RR-8-2118.
2 Rindone, W. P., and T. Kush (eds.). *PROPHET Molecules—A User's Guide to the Molecule Facilities of the PROPHET System*. Prepared by Bolt, Beranek, and Newman, Inc. under NIH contract N01-RR-8-2218 (April 1980).

3 Dehn, R. L., and C. T. Helmes. *An Automatic Procedure for Assessing Possible Carcinogenic Activity of Chemicals Prior to Testing.* Prepared for the National Cancer Institute by SRI under Contract No. N01-CP-33285 (June 1974).

4 Searle, C. E. (ed.). *ACS Monograph 173: Chemical Carcinogens.* Washington, D.C.: American Chemical Society (1976).

5 NCI Technical Report Series: Bioassay of chemicals for carcinogenicity. National Cancer Institute, National Institutes of Health, U.S. Department of Health, Education and Welfare, Bethesda, Maryland (1977–1979).

Chapter 13

Relating Bacterial Mutagenesis Activity to Chemical Structure

John F. Tinker

INTRODUCTION

The computerized structure-activity program described herein for relating bacterial mutagenesis activity to chemical structure employs a substructure recognition process based on the procedure of Hodes (1, 2). Structural information is accepted from connection tables (Chemical Abstracts Registry II or III) or mechanical chemical code topological screen system (MCC-TSS) ciphers of Lefkowitz (3). Typically in this program the basic substructure unit (ganglion) is an atom triplet. Data for correlation are provided by over 1800 results from mutagenesis test run in the Ames *Salmonella typhimurium* test, obtained from the literature. Statistical weights for ganglia are calculated from the program of Hodes (1, 2). The program calculates the level of activity to be expected of an unknown structure, with an estimate of confidence (4).

Results from operation of the program over several years have revealed the correlation of biological data with chemical structure and the self-consistency of the data. Factors and decisions affecting the acceptance of

The lists on p. 210 and Fig. 5 were reprinted with permission from *J. Chem. Inf. Comput. Sci.*, 21:3–7, 1981. Copyright © 1981 American Chemical Society.

results are presented as are new program facilities—list processing, similarity index, and listing. The rationale for including a factor, related to the test protocol and the purity of the substance, and the way of employing it are reviewed. Also considered are possible applications of this program to other types of data.

INPUT

Input to the program consists of data, structures corresponding to the data, and structures to be estimated (Fig. 1).

TREATMENT OF ACTIVITY DATA

The program begins by categorizing the activity data according to levels of activity, e.g., low, medium, high (Fig. 1). Estimates are made in terms of the same levels. The number of levels, or categories of activity intensity, can vary from as few as two to as many as eight, as desired. For data expressed in quantitative terms, a category is defined as a range of values. For example, high acute oral toxicity is defined as an LD_{50} smaller than 50 mg/kg. The definitions of activity categories can be changed from run to run.

STRUCTURAL FEATURES

Many structure-activity correlation programs require the editor to identify the important structural features, either before or during the analysis. For this program, however, it is sufficient to choose an algorithm that will derive from the complete structure a set of structural features, provided that the important features are included (Fig. 2). The lower right-hand box of Fig. 2 indicates that the program derives automatically such a set.

CHOOSING THE ALGORITHM

An effective set of substructure units that serves to distinguish among groups of structures is the set of triplet ganglia; each is a unit of three connected

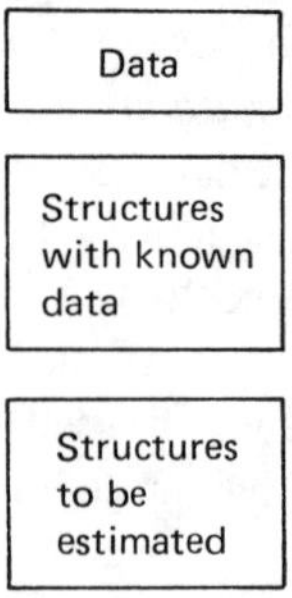

> Data

> Structures
> with known
> data

> Structures
> to be
> estimated

Figure 1 System organization: input.

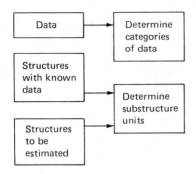

Figure 2 System organization: structural features.

nonhydrogen atoms together with the terminal bonds. In addition to the triplet ganglia, Hodes (1, 2) and the present system use subunits for rings: one subunit for each ring and one for each ring system consisting of two or more fused rings. To avoid redundant subunits, both systems have eliminated the linear subunits that are derived exclusively from ring carbon atoms. Assignment of weights to each substructure unit (Fig. 3), and summing these for a structure, is done exactly as described (1, 2). This procedure reduces the large and variable dimensionality to a small one.

PROGRAM CAPABILITIES

As part of the next step, regression analysis, the program calculates the degree to which the activity depends on a structure, averaged over all data. It first calculates the confidence limit at which each category is statistically distinct from each of the other categories; significant limits imply good dependence of activity on structure. Then, for every structure submitted to the program, the activity category is calculated based on the entire set of data whether or not its activity is known. In addition, the probability of the correctness of assigning a structure to other categories of activity is calculated, based on the sample size (5) in the categories. This value is an indication of the reliability of the activity prediction for each structure.

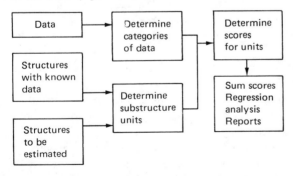

Figure 3 System organization: assignment of weights and summing of these for a structure.

Any sort of data may be used. Data may be qualitative or quantitative and may be expressed in different ways. For each run, the way each kind of expression is to be categorized must be explained.

Structures are accepted by the program if expressed as Chemical Abstracts connection tables, mechanical chemical code (3) ciphers, or a mixture of both.

In summary, the program is exactly like the one developed at the National Cancer Institute to estimate antitumor activity, except for the use of other data and the following program modifications:

1 As many as eight activity categories may be specified.

2 Categories may be defined separately for various activity codes and various types of data and may be combined for an analysis.

3 Confidence limits for statistically significant differences between each pair of categories are calculated.

4 For each substance, the input category, the calculated category, the distance in arbitrary units from the mean of each category, and the probability of classification in other significant categories are reported. The reports are sorted in several ways, so that a substance can be located easily if its registry number is known or if its position is inconsistent with the rest of its category.

5 Data can be traced through the program. For each structure, it is easy to find the substructures that contribute to its categorization and to locate the references that contain the test results pertinent to that estimation. Thus, the resemblance of unknown to known structures, deduced by the program, is exactly laid out for consideration by the users of the program.

ADVANTAGES OF THE PROGRAM

1 All of the activity data may be used. This includes mixed quantitative and qualitative data. They need not be perfectly consistent nor statistically separated. Wrong data are tolerated and can be detected as described later.

2 The structures need not be closely related. A wide variety of structures can be used in a run, both with known results and with results to be estimated.

3 Several thousand structures can be used in a run, and several hundred can be estimated at the same time, at a reasonable cost.

4 Editorial effort is minimized. The program is tolerant of moderately inconsistent data and can make many estimates in a single run without recursive analysis, so it is easy to use.

5 There is no need to discard data, and there is no way to modify or alter the results by changing substructures or adjusting activity data.

VALIDATION OF THE PROGRAM

One measure of validity is the degree of internal consistency indicated by the program. Thus if knowns were re-entered as unknowns and the predictions were the same as the actual values, the internal consistency would be perfect. The program always predicts each known, using not only the single datum for it but all the appropriate data from the other knowns. Each prediction of a known, or reclassification of a known, makes use of more than one input datum point. Thus one can use the reclassification of the data both as a measure of internal consistency of the data and as an indication of the successful correlation of structure with data.

Several runs, using data on bacterial mutagenic potential, illustrate the internal consistency and its variation when the length of the linear-sequency subunits is changed. The separation between four of the five activity groups is statistically significant at better than 99.999 percent confidence. In the run presented in Fig. 4 the potent and strong activity groups are not distinct.

The statistically significant differences between each pair of groups, and their good separation, are evidence for accepting two hypotheses: these data depend on structural similarity; the substructural units successfully reflect structural similarity.

In addition, 70 percent of the data was reclassified exactly as it was reported. This result gives us confidence that on the whole the data as categorized by the assigned fences are internally consistent to an acceptable degree.

The summary of reclassificaton shown in Fig. 5 indicates that for many of the structures there are enough data to give a satisfactory classification, but for many, the probability is not as great as one might wish. This situation can be improved by adding more data.

Eight substances were added to these runs before the corresponding data were added, so they were automatically estimated. All were inactive; in each of the runs, seven were estimated to be inactive and one (the same for all runs) to be moderately active. This corresponds to 87.5 percent agreement.

The program calculates a function that can be regarded as a degree of similarity, which is illustrated by an example. Structures II, III, and IV in Fig. 6 were used, among others, by the program to reclassify I. The degree of similarity between two structures can be expressed as the ratio of the number

THE DIFFERENCES (95% LEVEL) ARE				
	1 WEAK	2 MODERATE	3 STRONG	4 POTENT
0 LOW	SIGNIFICANT	SIGNIFICANT	SIGNIFICANT	SIGNIFICANT
1 WEAK		SIGNIFICANT	SIGNIFICANT	SIGNIFICANT
2 MODERATE			SIGNIFICANT	SIGNIFICANT
3 STRONG				NOT SIGNIFICANT

Figure 4 Sample run.

| NUMBER OF CASES CLASSIFIED INTO GROUP | | | | |
0 LOW	1	2	3	4
GROUP				
0 LOW				
222	39	44	11	4
26	117	16	6	3
71	43	254	30	9
10	3	15	66	9
2	0	3	3	13
17	9	17	1	0

Figure 5 Summary of reclassification.

of common subunits to the sum of that number plus the number of subunits not common from both structures. This ratio varies from zero (for no common subunits) to 1 (for all subunits in common). For the four structures, the results using triplet ganglia are shown in Fig. 6. The similarity index changes when the length of the linear substructure units changes. For a high degree of similarity, this index increases from doublet ganglia to quadruplet ganglia, as the values for III and IV show (Fig. 7). For intermediate degrees, the index decreases. Using triplet ganglia, the degree of similarity agrees satisfactorily with subjective judgment of similarity.

Validation of the program was also tested using compounds simultaneously submitted for bacterial mutagenesis testing and structure-activity correlation. Results are presently available for 34, using 1019 known data points. Of these, 74 percent agree exactly with the predicted category, and 88 percent agree within one category. Of the estimates that were one category away, one was high and four were low.

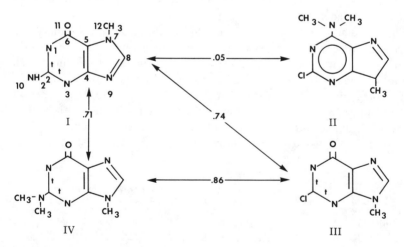

Figure 6 Similarity index based on triplet ganglia.

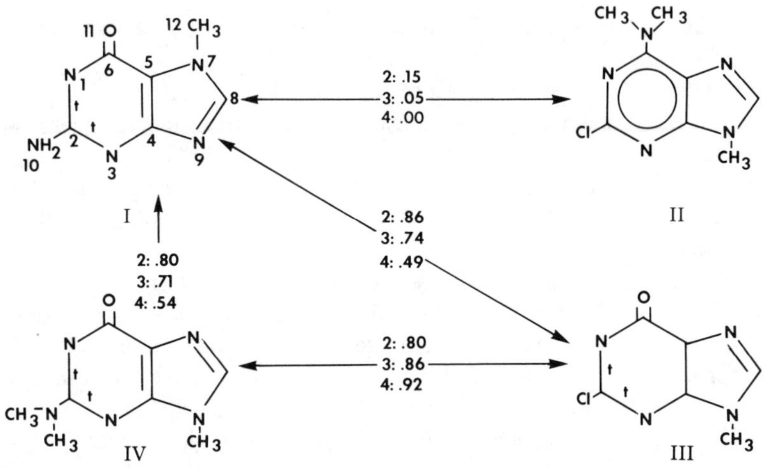

Figure 7 Similarity index based on double, triplet and quadruplet ganglia.

IDENTIFYING CONTRIBUTING STRUCTURES

A particular value of the program is that structures contributing to an activity or inactivity finding in the analysis can be located and identified. Thus, 7-methylguanine (I) was incorrectly entered as a moderate bacterial mutagen (6), but the program correctly predicted that it should be inactive. 7-Methylguanine is a normal constituent of transfer RNA (7) and is itself probably not mutagenic; however, when formed in DNA by methylation by carcinogens, although it is rapidly removed (7) it apparently leads to abnormalities (6). The structural analogy that the program locates is shown in part in Fig. 7. In addition, the program lists a large number of similar structures, most of them inactive. We would agree with its estimate that, on this basis, 7-methylguanine be inactive, contrary to the manner in which it was inadvertently entered. The results summarized here are discussed in detail elsewhere (4).

FACTORS INFLUENCING THE ACCEPTABILITY OF CALCULATED BIOLOGICAL PROPERTIES

The purpose of this program and others (8–15) is to predict the activity from known biological properties. Several factors influence the accuracy of these predictions in ways that are sometimes obvious and sometimes subtle. These factors are associated with the data and with the program.

Data

1 Selection. What is the basis for choosing the data used in the calculation? What is the rationale for the rejection of a class of data and of each individual

datum? Probably, the best estimation is made on the basis of the largest collection of reliable data.

2   Reliability. Many factors influence the reliability of a test.

   a. Identity and Purity. What means was used to assure the identity and purity of the material tested? Can the test result be ascribed to a single structure? Mixtures are often tested to assess the hazards associated with them, but these results are not often useful for correlating structure and activity.

   b. Test Performance. What is the history of the test in terms of consistency or variability of results and of correlation with the phenomenon of interest? For example, some tests are not well correlated with human reactions. The chick embryo test is now considered to be much too sensitive to predict teratogenic response in humans (16). Again, animal tests designed to predict human carcinogenic response have used a wide variety of protocols of varying reliability.

   c. Physical Properties. In the Ames test, unreliable results can result if the test compound has a low solubility in water, resulting in a precipitate that is physically unable to induce reversion. If the substance evaporates readily, the test may give an unreliable negative result. For example, ethylene bromide produces 50 times as many reversions when the incubation is done in a sealed vessel (Barber, E. D., Personal communication).

   d. Reactivity. If the substance reacts with itself or with some component of the test system, and if it is changed in an important way, the result is unreliable. A vinyl monomer, for instance, might be a mutagen, but it might polymerize rapidly to an innocuous substance.

   e. Toxicity. There are examples of chemicals that induce reversion only within a narrow concentration range near the toxic limit (Barber, E. D., Personal communication). Results of this sort are tedious to obtain and difficult to interpret.

   f. Chemical Substructure. Some tests may show an unexpected sensitivity to certain functional groups. For instance, most bacteria are highly sensitive to aromatic nitro compounds. These idiosyncrasies must be considered when extrapolating results, both estimated and determined, to other chemical species.

   g. Clerical Reliability. Besides the subtle factors, the more obvious ones must be considered. Adequate procedures for transcription of data are needed. Means of identifying data points that are inconsistent with the entire body of data are helpful and should be followed by careful examination and correction of errors and inconsistencies.

   h. Negative Results. Are there enough negative results? If the program or a human judge knows only of positive results, all estimates of unknowns will be positive. We have found it useful to test many relatively simple compounds, for instance syringaldehyde, to provide more data for inactive structures. In addition, we have included as inactive many compounds that are constituents of normal cells. These compounds, if they are not genuinely inactive, represent an inescapable minimum exposure to the normal cells.

Program

What is the rationale of the logic: why should this approach work? What are the limits of applicability in general and the scope of the calculation for a particular example? What is the history of the use of the program? What successful examples, and unsuccessful ones, have been reported? Is there a concise report of the validation of the program? If the computer implementation has changed, are there volume test results and parallel before-and-after examples? Do different models or different programs give the same calculated results?

Satisfactory answers to most of these questions, together with other data on the substance and on similar substances, can lend credence to calculated results. In any case, calculated results should not be considered in isolation; rather, all data on the substance of interest and related substances should be collected and judged as a unit.

COMPENSATION FOR INCOMPLETE PROTOCOL

Many data exist that cannot be ignored but do not meet the most strict requirements for greatest reliability. Besides, a positive result in one test is more convincing than many negative results.

The program described here allows the data editor to express his or her degree of acceptance by assigning a reliability factor. This factor can vary according to chemical class—the editor must define these classes—and can be different for differing results and protocols. The editor may consider, for instance, that a positive result in the Ames test with the most sensitive strain for a particular class of chemicals is approximately 40 percent as reliable as the test with all five of the usual strains and thus assigns the reliability factor of 0.40 for positive results with that one strain. If the editor considers a negative result in a test with only that one strain about 30 percent as conclusive as the full test, he or she then assigns a factor of 0.30 to the negative one-strain results.

These weights are counted like separate tests. A test with reliability of 2 counts the same as two independent tests of standard reliability (1).

Replicate tests increase the reliability; doubtful purity decreases it. All of these factors are set at run time and thus can be changed at the convenience of the editor.

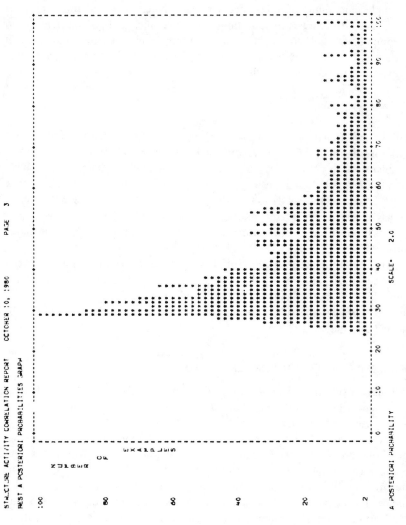

Figure 8 Summary of probability of correct classification.

216

The reliability factor has been implemented only recently. The use of the factor by the program is similar to the use by humans in taking more or less notice of better or poorer data. On this account, it tends to increase the acceptance of the program and its calculated results. Good choices of the factors should increase the consistency of the data as a whole. The detailed effect of the factor will be reported in a later presentation.

Some other program modifications include the following

1 Using the same data and the same hardware, a direct access file step required 8 min, while the list-processing equivalent implementation required $6\frac{1}{2}$ min. The list processing however was doing more work, and the time difference is accordingly greater for identical work.

2 The triplet ganglia were generated in 2 min by a program with straight-through coding, while a program with a recursive subroutine, calling itself twice, needed $3\frac{3}{4}$ min, nearly twice as long.

3 The calculated results are listed in a few new ways. A new graph (Fig. 8) shows a summary of the probability of correct classification, calculated from the ratio of distances to the closest mean and the next closest mean. In this run, relatively few substances have been classified securely and most lie within 25–60 percent probability.

A list has been added (Fig. 9) that shows explicitly the same data that were present before but difficult to assemble. For each substance in the run, 50 similar substances are listed. The document number, the registry number, and the activity class are given for each substance. For each similar substance the similarity index is calculated in two ways, once using the weights of the structural units and again using only the counts of the units. These calculations allow the data editor to include in the run a structure with unreliable data and to read from this list the 50 other substances in the same run most similar to it.

The final reports have been changed so that the activity class is named "inactive," "moderate," and so on (Fig. 10). The activity class is listed as originally entered, as found by the highest score, and as calculated finally by stepwise discriminant analysis, which considers the complete vector of scores. Structures for which these three scores do not agree are listed separately for the editor to review in detail. One tenth of the structures that are farthest from their closest mean are also listed separately. We have not yet had enough experience with examples to discuss them.

REFERENCES

1 Hodes, L., G. F. Hazard, R. I. Geran, and S. Richman. A statistical-heuristic method for automated selection of drugs for screening. *J. Med. Chem.* 20:469 (1977).

```
578-76-7 2 NEW CLASS:0 SCORE: +0.834003
0  96.2%( 81.8%)    146-91-8 DOC    233
0  96.2%( 81.8%)    118-00-3 DOC    233
0  96.2%( 81.8%)     86-01-1 DOC    233
0  96.2%( 81.8%)     85-32-5 DOC    233
0  96.2%( 81.8%)   3433-09-2 DOC    233
0  96.2%( 81.8%)   2564-35-4 DOC    233
0  96.2%( 81.8%)    961-07-9 DOC    233
0  96.2%( 81.8%)    902-04-5 DOC    233
0  81.9%( 81.8%)  36323-96-3 DOC     24
0  81.9%( 81.8%)  36323-92-9 DOC     24
2  70.5%( 59.0%)   2311-81-1 DOC    233
0  66.2%( 50.0%)    134-58-7 DOC   4965
0  66.2%( 50.0%)     73-40-5 DOC    233
0  66.2%( 50.0%)  18632-03-6 DOC    233
2  66.2%( 50.0%)  10360-12-0 DOC    233
2  66.2%( 50.0%)   2800-34-2 DOC    233
0  65.8%( 59.0%)    131-99-7 DOC    233
0  65.8%( 59.0%)     58-63-9 DOC    233
2  55.4%( 59.0%)     58-08-2 DOC   8409
?  55.4%( 59.0%)     58-08-2 DOC      1
0  41.8%( 27.2%)  36324-02-4 DOC     24
0  41.8%( 27.2%)   3977-29-5 DOC     24
0  41.8%( 27.2%)    674-97-5 DOC     24
0  35.8%( 27.2%)     68-94-0 DOC    233
0  35.7%( 31.8%)     69-89-6 DOC    233
2  33.1%( 22.7%)   6340-72-3 DOC    447
0  33.1%( 22.7%)   6340-69-8 DOC    447
0  29.5%( 22.7%)  13479-23-3 DOC      3
2  27.0%( 27.2%)    577-66-2 DOC    441
0  26.2%( 27.2%)   1110-93-2 DOC    233
0  24.5%( 18.1%)  36324-01-3 DOC     24
0  24.5%( 18.1%)  34415-10-6 DOC     24
0  23.9%( 22.7%)  30315-22-3 DOC      3
0  21.6%( 13.6%)     63-93-2 DOC    233
0  20.3%( 18.1%)  18905-27-8 DOC      3
```

Figure 9 Similarity index.

```
580-51-8   ORIGINAL GROUP: INACTIVE, (CASE #350)
           SCORE GROUP:      MODERATE, (SCORE RATIO 0.922356)
           ANALYSIS GROUP: WEAK
                1,020  0          1292-36  0:  4.200 0.158  1:  1.709 0.552  2:  3.640 0.209  3:  5.704 0.074
  (   -0.057,  -1.162,  +0.448)  4:  12.188 0.002
PROBABILITY OF CLASSIFICATION VERSUS GROUP 2  45.8% (OPTIMAL 49.1)
```

Figure 10 Final structure correlation report: activity class.

2 Hodes, L. Computer-aided selection of novel antitumor drugs for animal screening. In: *Computer-Assisted Drug Design*. E. C. Olson and R. E. Christofferson (eds.), ACS Symposium Series No. 112, pp. 583–602. Washington, D.C.: American Chemical Society (1979).

3 Lefkovitz, D., and A. R. Gennaro. Utility analysis for the MCC (mechanical chemical code) topological screen system. *J. Chem. Doc.* 10:86 (1970).

4 Tinker, J. F. A computerized structure-activity correlation program for relating bacterial mutagenesis activity. *J. Comp. Chem.* 2:231 (1981).

5 Lachenbruch, P. A. On expected probabilities of misclassification in discriminant analysis, necessary sample size, and a relation with the multiple correlation coefficient. *Biometrics* p. 823 (1968).

6 Kononova, S. D., A. M. Korolev, L. T. Eremenko, and L. L. Gumanov. Mutagenic effect of some esters of nitric acid on bacteriophage T4B. *Genetika* 8:101 (1972).

7 Lakings, D. B., T. P. Waalkes, E. Borek, C. W. Gehrke, J. E. Mrochek, J. Longmore, and R. H. Adamson. Composition, associated tissue methyltransferase activity, and catabolic end products of transfer RNA from carcinogen-induced hepatoma and normal monkey livers. *Cancer Res.* 37:285 (1977).

8 Olson, E. C., and R. E. Christofferson (eds.). *Computer-Assisted Drug Design*. ACS Symposium Series No. 112. Washington, D.C.: American Chemical Society (1979).

9 Stuper, A. J., W. E. Bruegger, P. C. Jurs. *Computer Assisted Studies of Chemical Structure and Biological Function*. New York: Wiley (1979).

10 Grund, P., J. D. Andose, J. B. Rhodes, and G. M. Smith. Three-dimensional molecular modeling and drug design. *Science* 208:1425–1431 (1980).

11 Lykos, P. (ed.). *Computer Modeling of Matter*. ACS Symposium Series No. 86. Washington, D.C.: American Chemical Society (1978).

12 Wipke, W. P., and W. J. Howe. *Computer Assisted Organic Synthesis*. ACS Symposium Series No. 61. Washington, D.C.: American Chemical Society (1977).

13 Smith, D. H. *Computer Assisted Structure Elucidation*. ACS Symposium Series No. 54. Washington, D.C.: American Chemical Society (1977).

14 Kowalski, B. R. *Chemometrics: Theory and Application*. ACS Symposium Series No. 52. Washington, D.C.: American Chemical Society (1977).

15 Howe, W. J., M. M. Milne, and A. F. Pennell. *Retrieval of Medicinal Chemical Information*. ACS Symposium Series No. 84. Washington, D.C.: American Chemical Society (1978).

16 *Principles for the Testing of Drugs for Teratogenicity*. World Health Organization Technical Report Series No. 364, p. 7. Geneva: World Health Organization, (1967).

Chapter 14

Quantitative Structure-Mutagenicity Relationships

William Paul Purcell

INTRODUCTION

Because of rather obvious practical implications, QSAR (1-4) technology was developed jointly among academicians, government researchers, and industrialists. The arm of application includes pharmaceutical, agricultural, chemical, cosmetic, and food chemistry. In essentially all areas of research, QSAR has been used as an aid in the design of molecules for specific purposes. The selectivity problem continues to be to maximize the desired response while minimizing the deleterious side effects. This general problem has become more acute as government regulatory controls require more and more demonstration of safety. Figure 1, for example, gives a schematic representation of the idealized molecule, which performs selectively by giving the maximum desired biological effect while maintaining maximum safety. One might generalize by saying that most research emphasized efficacy (ordinate, Fig. 1) prior to 1962,

The author would like to thank his scientific colleagues at L'ORÉAL in Paris, Drs. D. Bauer, J. P. Beck, A. Bugaut, G. Kalopissis, and M. M. Shahin, for their comments and discussions regarding the mechanism of mutagenicity. He would also like to thank Drs. C. Hansch and A. Leo for permission to discuss their unpublished work.

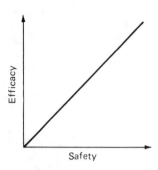

Figure 1 Plot of efficacy against safety for biologically interesting compounds.

when Congress passed amendments to the Food, Drug, and Cosmetic Act, and since 1962 trends are shifting to concentrate on maximizing safety (abscissa, Fig. 1).

As the search for new commercial compounds continues with increasing emphasis on safety, it is only natural that some work has begun on the application of QSAR to structure-mutagenicity data. It is beyond the scope of this paper to discuss the Ames test, its usefulness, its limitations, and its interpretation. The facts are that until something better comes along, the test will be used as one criterion for safety. Therefore, we need to deal with it on a scientific basis.

The purpose of this paper is (a) to examine the QSAR-mutagenicity work already reported and (b) to discuss the feasibility of predicting mutagenicity.

QSAR-MUTAGENICITY

Perhaps the most thorough QSAR work reported on mutagenicity data comes from Hansch's laboratory. In a study of seventeen 1-(X-phenyl)-3,3-dialkyl-triazenes of type I,

$$N = NN \diagup{CH_3} \diagdown R$$

I

Hansch and co-workers (5) derived Eq. 1:

$$\log \frac{1}{c} = 1.09 \log P - 1.63\ \sigma^+ + 5.58 \tag{1}$$

in which c is the molar concentration necessary to give 30 revertants per 10^8 *Salmonella typhimurium* TA92 in the Ames test, P is the octanol:water partition coefficient, and σ^+ is the "through resonance" electronic parameter (4). Equation 1 shows that increasing lipophilicity and increased electron release via through resonance increase mutagenicity. At this point it is appropriate to introduce and emphasize the point that the desired biological response parameter in QSAR-mutagenicity work should be the concentration of compound necessary to give a certain number of mutations per given number of bacteria. Also, the concentration should fall below the level of compound that is toxic to the bacteria.

Equation 1 was compared with the antitumor activity (6) of the triazenes against L1210 leukemia (Eq. 2).

$$\log \frac{1}{c} = 0.01 \log P - 0.042 \, (\log P)^2 - 0.31 \, \sigma^+ - 0.18 \, MR^{2,6}$$

$$+ \, 0.39 \, E_s - R + 4.12 \tag{2}$$

It appears from Eqs. 1 and 2 that mutagenicity is much more sensitive than antitumor activity to the electronic effect of substituents.

The general toxicity of the triazenes is correlated by Eq. 3 using LD_{50} for mice (7):

$$\log \frac{1}{c} = -0.024 \, (\log P)^2 - 0.26 \, \sigma^+ + 3.49 \tag{3}$$

From inspection of Eqs. 2 and 3, one would conclude that both gross toxicity and antitumor activity in mice show the same dependence on the electronic effects of substituents.

The practical application of this analysis is to manipulate the electronic and lipophilic character of the substituents in order to decrease the mutagenicity without destroying the antileukemia action of the compounds. Therefore, Eqs. 1 and 2 were used to illustrate how this could work. Table 1 gives the calculated log $1/c$ values for the Ames test (Eq. 1) and the antitumor potencies (Eq. 2) for two congeners. Antitumor potency is only reduced by a factor of 1.2, while mutagenicity decreases by a factor of 400.

Dacarbazine, a drug used clinically in cancer treatment, and aflatoxin B

Table 1 Comparsion of Mutagenic and Antitumor Activity of Two 1-(X-Phenyl)-3,3-dimethyltriazenes

4-X	log 1/c (mutagenicity)	log 1/c (antitumor)
H	5.75	3.58
SO$_2$NH$_2$	3.15	3.48

were assayed for mutagenicity as benchmarks for comparison. Aflatoxin B, one of the most carcinogenic compounds known, was found to be 10^7 times more mutagenic than dacarbazine.

Hansch and co-workers applied QSAR methodology to the structure-mutagenicity data of some platinum compounds of type II because of their importance as antitumor drugs (8).

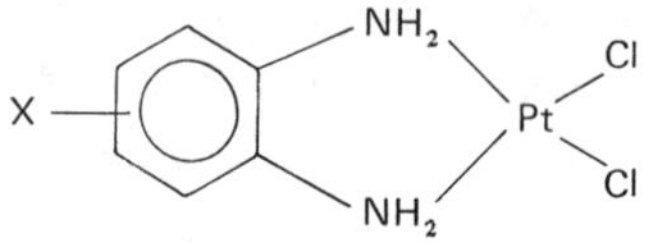

II

Equation 4 was reported in which σ^- is a more suitable electronic parameter (4) when substituents are in conjugation

$$\log \frac{1}{c} = 2.2 \sum \sigma^- + 5.8 \tag{4}$$

with a reaction center in which delocalization of a developing negative charge in the transition state is crucial in the rate-limiting step. The positive coefficient in Eq. 4 for this electronic term indicates that electron-withdrawing groups promote mutagenic activity. It is interesting to note that this is just the opposite result from Eq. 1.

Adding π and/or π^2 does not improve the correlation significantly in Eq. 4, which indicates that hydrophobic effects are not important or that there is not a significant lipophilic barrier between the mutagen in solution and its point of action in the bacterium.

Leo and others (personal communication) have conducted a comparison of mutagenic and carcinogenic activities of aniline mustards (III).

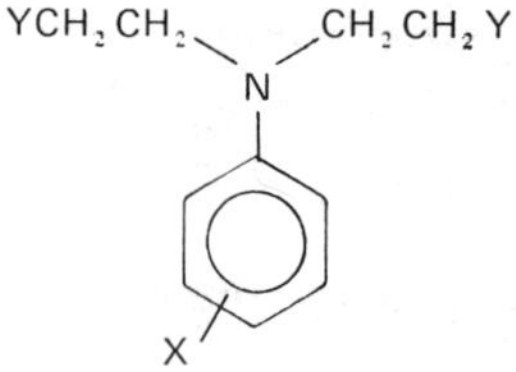

III

Fifteen derivatives were selected to minimize collinearity among hydrophobic, electronic, and molar refractive properties. They were tested in *Salmonella typhimurium* TA1535 and TA100 as well as carcinogenicity as lung tumors in strain A mice. Using the concentration necessary to produce 100 revertants above background, $B + 100$, Eq. 5 was obtained, where the single most important variable is π:

$$\log \frac{1}{B + 100} = 0.3\pi - 0.5\sigma + 1.4 \tag{5}$$

The negative coefficient with the electronic term is consistent with what was observed with triazenes. For a high-level mutagenicity, 200 revertants above threshold, $Th + 200$, Eq. 6 was found:

$$\log \frac{1}{Th + 200} = 0.4\,\pi - 0.07\,\pi^2 + 1.5 \tag{6}$$

The electronic term has disappeared and the high-level mutagenicity is accounted for by π alone.

For the carcinogenicity test, the dose needed to exceed the background produced by the tricaprylin control 0.5 tumor per mouse, $B.5$, was used to obtain Eq. 7:

$$\log \frac{1}{B.5} = -1.6I_4 + 3\,\sigma^2 - 1.1\,\sigma + 0.9 \tag{7}$$

where I_4 is an indicator variable equal to 1 for congeners having a 4 substituent and equal to 0 for all others. The higher level of carcinogenicity based on the concentration necessary to produce one tumor per mouse, $B + 1$, gave Eq. 8, which is essentially the same as Eq. 7.

$$\log \frac{1}{B + 1} = -1.7\,I_4 + 3\,\sigma^2 - \sigma + 0.8 \tag{8}$$

Perhaps the most interesting point of this study is the comparison of mutagenicity and carcinogenicity for these compounds as given in Eq. 9:

$$\log \frac{1}{B + 1\,(\text{mice})} = 0.8\log -0.8\log \frac{1}{Th + 200\,(\text{bacteria}) + 4} \tag{9}$$

The *inverse* relationship is marginally significant, $r = 0.64$, but the trend certainly shows that one should not automatically assume that carcinogenicity parallels mutagenicity. Here, the reverse is true.

In the light of the findings of the Hansch group (5–8), it is appropriate to consider the work of Sugiura and co-workers (9, 10) and Harfenist (11). Table 2 gives a summary of compounds studied, the mutagenicity test system, and comments by the authors regarding the electronic effects. All of the

Table 2 Conclusions Regarding Electronic Effects and Mutagenicity

Compounds	Mutagenicity test system	Reference	Conclusion
Styrene oxides	TA100	9	"This suggests that the presence of an electron-withdrawing group in the benzene ring decreases the mutagenicity."
1-(X–Phenyl)-3,3-dialkyltriazenes	TA92	5	". . . increased electron release via through resonance increases mutagenicity."
Aryl amides	TA100	11	". . . mutagenicity can be removed from an otherwise mutagenicity-causing pharmacophore by reducing the electron availability."
(o-Phenylenediamine) platinum dichlorides	TA92	8	". . . electron-withdrawing groups promote mutagenic activity."
Aniline mustards	TA100	Leo et al. (personal communication)	"The negative coefficient with the electronic term in Eq. 4 is consistent with the activity being related to nucleophilic substitution . . ."

observations on these different series of compounds are consistent, with the exception of the platinum compounds. That is, the generalization is that one should look for electron-withdrawing groups on an aromatic ring if the intention is to reduce mutagenicity.

In the area of quantitative structure-mutagenicity relationship studies the work of Kier and associates (12) should be mentioned. They used molecular connectivity indexes to correlate the mutagenicities of 15 nitrosamines evaluated by McCann and co-workers (13). A good correlation was found using two molecular connectivity indexes and the natural log of the number of revertants per nanomole in *Salmonella typhimurium*.

Loew and co-workers conducted molecular orbital calculations on 15 aniline derivatives (14). They found that the mutagenicities of the amino-anilines decrease with decreasing N-superdelocalizabilities. The nitroanilines, however, do not show this qualitative trend.

Along the same lines, Shahin and co-workers demonstrated a qualitative structure-activity relationship with the mutagenicity of a series of *m*-diamino-benzenes (15). Mutagenicity was found to decrease with increasing alkyl chain length substituted on the benzene ring.

EXPECTATIONS AND RESEARCH NEEDS

It is clear that we have scratched the surface with regard to the application of QSAR techniques to the understanding of mutagenicity. Some points can be made at the present state-of-the-art, however:

1   Test should be standardized.

2   It appears that electronic effects play a dominant role in mutagenicity. This should be investigated by selecting a carefully designed series of compounds (16), which would spread the electronic properties. Studies along these lines should shed some light on the mechanistic interpretation of mutagenicity.

3   Correlation or the lack of correlation should be determined between mutagenicity and carcinogenicity. For example, the QSAR study on nitro-samine carcinogenicity reported by Wishnok and co-workers (17) could be investigated by comparing the mutagenicities of these same compounds.

4   As test procedures become standardized, as compounds are designed for testing that have the elements of solid QSAR analysis, and as more becomes known regarding the mechanism of mutagenicity, one should be able to predict mutagenicity from QSAR models.

REFERENCES

1   Purcell, W. P., G. E. Bass, and J. M. Clayton. *Strategy of Drug Design: A Molecular Guide to Biological Activity.* New York: Wiley (1973).

2   Martin, Y. C. *Quantitative Drug Design.* New York: Dekker (1978).

3   Seydel, J. K., and K. J. Schaper. *Chemische Struktur und biologische Aktivitat von Wirkstoffen Methoden der Quantitativen Struktur-Wirkung-Analyse.* New York: Verlag Chemie (1979).

4   Hansch, C., and A. Leo. *Substituent Constants for Correlation Analysis in Chemistry and Biology.* New York: Wiley (1979).

5   Venger, B. H., et al. Ames test of 1-(X-phenyl)-3,3-dialkyltriazenes: A quantitative structure-activity study. *J. Med. Chem.* 22:473–476 (1979).

6   Hatheway, G. J., et al. Antitumor 1-(X-aryl)-3,3-dialkyltriazenes. 1. Quantitative structure-activity relationships vs. L1210 leukemia in mice. *J. Med. Chem.* 21:563–574 (1978).

7   Hansch, C., et al. Antitumor 1-(X-aryl)-3,3-dialkyltriazenes. 2. On the role of correlation analysis in decision making in drug modification. Toxicity quantitative structure-activity relationships of 1-(X-phenyl)-3,3-dialkyl-triazenes in mice. *J. Med. Chem.* 21:574–577 (1978).

8   Hansch, C., et al. Mutagenicity of substituted (o-phenylenediamine)-platinum dichloride in the Ames test. A quantitative structure-activity analysis. *J. Med. Chem.* 23:459–461 (1980).

9 Sugiura, K., et al. Mutagenicities of styrene oxide derivatives on *Salmonella typhimurium* TA100. Relationship between mutagenic potencies and chemical reactivity. *Muta. Res.* 58:159–165 (1978).

10 Sugiura, K., et al. The mutagenicity of substituted and unsubstituted styrene oxides in *E. coli:* Relationship between mutagenic potencies and physicochemical properties. *Chemosphere* 9:737–742 (1978).

11 Harfenist, M. Prevention of Ames test mutagenicity by chemical modification in a series of monoamine oxidase inhibitors. *J. Med. Chem.* 23:825–827 (1980).

12 Kier, L. B., et al. Structure-activity studies on mutagenicity of nitrosamines using molecular connectivity. *J. Pharm. Sci.* 67:725–726 (1978).

13 McCann, J., et al. Detection of carcinogens as mutagens in the *Salmonella*/microsome test. *Proc. Natl. Acad. Sci. USA* 72:5135–5139 (1975).

14 Loew, G. H., et al. Correlation of calculated electronic parameters of fifteen aniline derivatives with their mutagenic potencies. *J. Environ. Pathol. Toxicol.* 2:1069–1078 (1979).

15 Shahin, M. M., et al. Structure-activity relationship within a series of *m*-diaminobenzene derivatives. *Mutat. Res.* 78:25–31 (1980).

16 Wooldridge, K. R. H. A rational substituent set for structure-activity studies. *Eur. J. Med. Chem.* 15:63–67 (1980).

17 Wishnok, J. S., et al. Nitrosamine carcinogenicity: A quantitative Hansch-Taft structure-activity relationship. *Chem.-Biol. Interact.* 20:43–54 (1978).

Chapter 15

Short-Term Tests for Carcinogens and Mutagens: A Data Base Designed for Comparative Quantitative Analysis

Joyce McCann, Laura Horn, Gerry Litton,
John Kaldor, Renae Magaw, Leslie Bernstein,
and Malcolm Pike

INTRODUCTION

The use of short-term tests, such as the *Salmonella* (Ames) test (1), for predicting the carcinogenic potential of chemicals has expanded so rapidly that development of a systematic, quantitative approach for analyzing and interpreting results has become essential. In a recent review of the literature (2) we identified over 100 different short-term testing methods. It is now generally agreed that for thorough evaluation, a chemical should be tested in more than one of these short-term tests; however, it is not clear which tests should be used nor how conflicting results from the different tests should be interpreted. Since different short-term tests appear to detect carcinogens with varying degrees of sensitivity and specificity (2, 3), the analysis and interpretation of results can be complex. For further discussion on analysis and interpretation the reader is referred to Golberg (4) and McCann (5).

We thank L. Gold and T. Tenforde for helpful comments and P. Lal for typing the manuscript. We also gratefully acknowledge the invaluable contribution of P. Presentation.

The potential of short-term tests to provide quantitative information about carcinogenicity is much less certain than their potential to provide qualitative information (6). There is, however, suggestive evidence that some quantitative correlation in potency between short-term tests and animal cancer tests may exist (7-9). It is important to thoroughly explore this possibility for practical as well as scientific reasons. Application of short-term tests to evaluation of thousands of synthetic and natural chemicals has resulted in the identification of far more potential carcinogens than can reasonably undergo confirmatory testing in conventional animal cancer tests. It is known that the carcinogenic potency of different chemicals can vary by more than 1 million-fold (7, 10). Clearly, if potency in short-term tests could be used to make rough predictions of potency in animal cancer tests, further risk evaluation could be more easily focused on chemicals with the greatest potential hazard.

We are constructing a data base of short-term test results, which will provide a powerful resource for resolving issues of comparability, between short-term tests and between short-term tests and animal cancer tests, by allowing quantitative comparisons to be made. We describe below the design of this data base, including methods used to extract and analyze short-term test data from the published literature, statistical methods for analyzing these data, and some applications of the data base.

OVERALL DATA BASE DESIGN

We use the general purpose data base management system, SPIRES, that was developed at Stanford University (11). This system can operate on a variety of IBM computer systems and is now used extensively throughout the United States as well as abroad. It has powerful searching, updating, and display capabilities and may be used in either interactive or batch mode. Also, data input to the SPIRES system can be in a variety of input formats, which permits the analysis of data from other data bases with minimal conversion problems.

Information on each short-term test is contained in a series of separate data bases (Fig. 1). We have completed the design of data bases for the *Salmonella* test and for mammalian cell mutagenesis assays. We are in the process of adding two additional data bases for *in vitro* transformation assays and sister chromatid exchange assays.

Each data base consists of a collection of records, each of which contains data from one dose-response experiment. Figure 2 shows a typical short-term test record structure. Each element within a record represents a different parameter of the experiment. For example, in addition to the numeric dose-response data, there are 53 other possible elements in each *Salmonella*

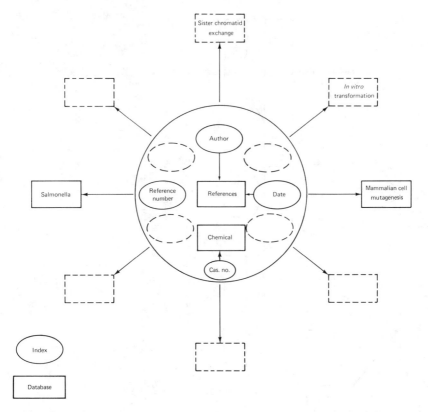

Figure 1 Overall data base design. Dotted figures indicate sections of the data base not yet implemented.

record, such as "amount of S-9* added per petri plate" and the "tissue used as the source of the S-9." The selection of test parameters to include in the data base and the method of extraction of data from the published literature are described below.

Also shown in Fig. 1 are a bibliographic data base and chemical name and CAS number data base, which are linked to the short-term test data bases.

Data input routines have been developed to facilitate entry and correction of data. These routines automatically prompt for specific data elements so that with minimal instruction, one can rapidly and accurately enter data into the system.

---

*Most chemical carcinogens are metabolized to their active forms by enzymes in mammalian tissues. In the *Salmonella* test a tissue homogenate (S-9), usually from rat liver, is added directly to the mutagen test system.

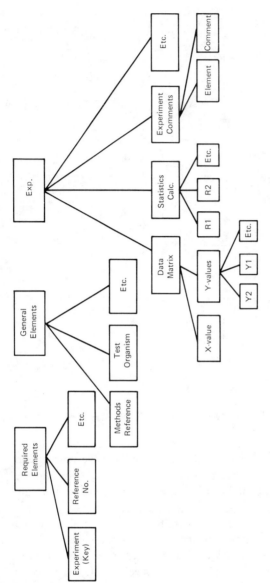

Figure 2 Typical structure of a short-term test data base record. All elements in the Required Elements structure must be present in each record; other elements may or may not be present. Elements in the EXP structure contain dose-response data, results of statistical calculations, and other related infromation.

ACCOMPANYING PROGRAM PACKAGES

In addition to the overall system of data bases, there are several accompanying program packages for manipulation of information in the data bases. The statistical analysis package consists of a set of FORTRAN routines for analysis of the dose-response data. The routines are completely independent of the data base structure, thus permitting independent development and refinement of the statistical routines and the data base sections. Interaction between the data base and the FORTRAN programs is carried out using a method that permits one to select records for analysis interactively at the terminal.

A package of output routines has been developed for displaying various parts of the data base. Output routines used to summarize the data and the results of the statistical analysis for the *Salmonella* (Ames) test are in Fig. 3*a* and *b*. This output design is based on a format used by Ames and colleagues (10, 21) to display results of their carcinogenic potency calculations. Each line represents results of a single experiment (one dose-response curve) and has a unique experiment number, which appears in the last column of Fig. 3*a* and the first column of Fig. 3*b*. Various parameters describing the assay protocol, bibliographic information, and results of the statistical analyses are displayed on each line. To facilitate visual comparison of results on different chemicals, results of the potency calculation are also plotted on the printout, on a log scale ranging over seven orders of magnitude.

SOURCES AND EXTRACTION OF DATA
IN THE PUBLISHED LITERATURE

The Environmental Mutagen Information Center (EMIC)[†], which we assess directly through the RECON-DOE information system, has been an invaluable resource in helping to rapidly identify published articles for quantitative analysis. EMIC is a bibliographic data base of the published literature in the field of short-term testing. We have focused our attention on articles in the EMIC data base, which we screen to determine if data meet our minimum criteria for analysis. We require that articles report quantitative results either in tabular or graphical form for at least two non-zero doses or replicate results at a single non-zero dose. For graphical data, we also include an estimate of the error we introduce by estimating results from the graph.

The extraction of data from published articles is a time-consuming and tedious task. We have designed data sheets (Fig. 4), which simplify this task so that parameters that have the same values for different experiments in the same journal article need be recorded only once. Special data-entry programs automatically record these repeated parameters for each experiment entered.

[†]EMIC, Box Y, Oak Ridge, TN 37830. Dr. John Wassom, Director.

Thus, the data sheets are oriented logically around the manner in which data are reported in published articles, and the data base is oriented around individual experiments.

We extract all information relevant to a quantitative analysis of the experiment. For example, for the *Salmonella* assay (Figs. 2 and 4) we extract data on (*a*) the general assay type (e.g., tester strain used, whether the assay was a standard plate test or a preincubation assay); (*b*) the metabolic activation system parameters (e.g., species and strain of animal used as a source of tissue, inducer, the composition of the activation system); (*c*) the units used for the amount of metabolic activation system, chemical dose, and mutagenic response, as well as associated information required to convert the reported units to our "standard units" (i.e., μl S-9/petri plate, μg chemical/ plate, and revertant colonies/plate); (*d*) pertinent information for analysis of the data, such as whether only means are reported, and number of replicates; (*e*) the authors' evaluation of the experiment; and (*f*) the actual dose-response data. The dose-response data are recorded in a data matrix (Fig. 4), designed so that a variety of data may be entered by variously defining the X and Y variables. For example, the X variable is almost always dose of chemical but can also be amount of S-9 per plate. The data matrix also allows us to record values for more than one Y variable (Fig. 4).

STATISTICAL ANALYSIS OF DOSE-RESPONSE DATA

Our primary aim is to develop procedures for estimating "mutagenic potency" from dose-response data. We would like procedures for the different short-term tests to have the same logical basis in order to facilitate comparative studies. Various statistical approaches are being compared using data currently in the data base.

The first short-term test that we have addressed is the *Salmonella* assay (1). Details of our statistical procedure, and comparisons with other models, will be described elsewhere. For most mutagens at low doses in this system, the dose-response curves are approximately linear. Then, as the dose increases, most curves flatten and finally turn downward due primarily to toxicity. Some dose-response curves do not show an initial linear portion; instead they appear to increase initially at a faster than linear rate. Our general approach has been to consider the slope of the initial linear part of the curve as representing the mutagenic potency and to consider those chemicals with curves that increase at a faster than linear rate as special cases needing further investigation.

Two different functions of the slope have been considered as measuring the mutagenic potency of a chemical. One measures strength in terms of the amount of chemical required to increase the background rate a fixed number of times (Fig. 3a shows D5X, the amount required to increase background five

SALMONELLA_POTENCY_PLOT 04/21/81 -1-

100ns....1us........10.......100.......1ms........10.......100........1s

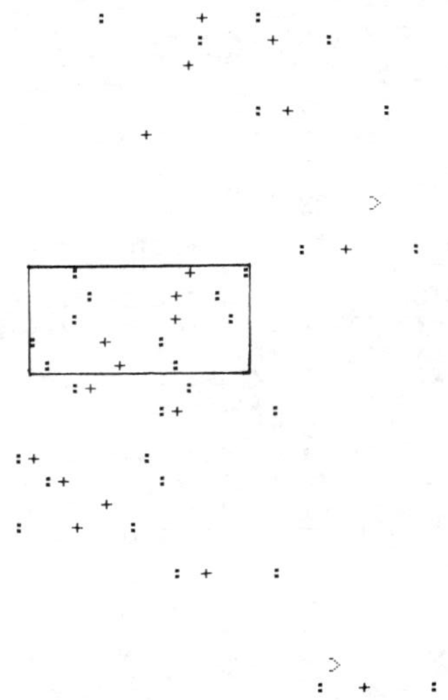

CAPTAN

*REF	ORG	ASS	IND	SPE	STR	TIS	ACT	PRO*	*POT		PVL	QUA	EXP*
[19]	0	S	A	R	NS	LIV	50	NS	17us		0.0000	+	109
[33]	0	S	A	M	NS	LIV	NS	NS	46us		0.0000	+	43
[72]	5	S	P	R	SDA	LIV	NS	NS	12us	B	0.0000	+	711
[7]	5	S	P	M	NMR	LIV	NS	NS		X		+	17
[33]	5	S	A	M	NS	LIV	NS	NS	57us		0.0010	+	45
[72]	7	S	P	R	SDA	LIV	NS	NS	6us	B	0.0000	+	708
[7]	7	S	P	M	NMR	LIV	NS	NS		X		+	18
[33]	7	S	A	M	NS	LIV	NS	NS		A		-	47
[72]	8	S	P	R	SDA	LIV	NS	NS	332us		0.0542	N	705
[7]	8	S	P	M	NMR	LIV	NS	NS		X		-	19
[33]	8	S	A	M	NS	LIV	NS	NS	150us		0.0029	-	49
[233]	0	S							13us		0.0000	N	1321
[6]	0	S							9us		0.0000	+	225
[19]	0	S							10us		0.0000	+	108
[1]	0	S							3us		0.0000	+	15
[33]	0	S							4us		0.0000	+	42
[6]	9	S							3us		0.0000	N	224
[136]	5	S							10us		0.0000	+	723
[5]	5	S								X		+	20
[136]	5	S							905ns		0.0000	+	724
[233]	5	S							1us		0.0000	N	1322
[6]	5	S							3us	B	0.0000	+	226
[72]	5	S							2us		0.0000	+	710
[1]	5	S								V		N	14
[33]	5	S							15us		0.0014	+	44
[72]	7	S								A		+	709
[33]	7	S								A		-	46
[72]	8	S								A		N	707
[33]	8	S							161us		0.1563	-	48
[233]	2	S							217us		0.0034	N	1323

Figure 3(*a*) See page 237 for key.

```
CAPTAN
 109 [ 19] DeFlora,1978.       NATU,271,p455//      0,204.6/ 1.25,223/ 2.5,284/ 5,421/ 10,645/ [5,5]
  43 [ 33] Simmon et al.,1977.       EPA,NS//       0,{98}/ 1,{141}/ 5,{210}/ 10,{285}/ 15,{340}/ 25,{300}/ 50,{704}/ [7,7]
 711 [ 72] Marshall et al.,1976.  JAFC,24,p560//    0,14/ 25,117/ 50,231/ [3,3]
  17 [  7] Herbold, Buselmaier,1976.  MURE,40,p73//[0],[130]/ [1],[2975]/ [10],[17.5]/ [20],[0]/ [4]
  45 [ 33] Simmon et al.,1977.       EPA,NS//       0,{14}/ 1,{20}/ 5,{60}/ 10,{113}/ 15,{55}/ 25,{71}/ 50,{143}/ [7,7]
 708 [ 72] Marshall et al.,1976.  JAFC,24,p560//    0,9/ 25,148/ 50,288/ [3,3]
  18 [  7] Herbold, Buselmaier,1976.  MURE,40,p73//[0],[55]/ [1],[345]/ [10],[0]/ [20],[0]/ [4]
  47 [ 33] Simmon et al.,1977.       EPA,NS//       0,{3}/ 1,{2}/ 5,{2}/ 10,{2}/ 15,{0}/ 25,{0}/ 50,{1}/ [7]
 705 [ 72] Marshall et al.,1976.  JAFC,24,p560//    0,32/ 25,32/ 50,51/ [3,3]
  19 [  7] Herbold, Buselmaier,1976.  MURE,40,p73//[0],[215]/ [1],[302.5]/ [10],[0]/ [20],[0]/ [4]
  49 [ 33] Simmon et al.,1977.       EPA,NS//       0,{25}/ 1,{19}/ 5,{22}/ 10,{26}/ 15,{21}/ 25,{46}/ 50,{44}/ [7,7]
1321 [233] Ames,1976.  //                           0,224/ 5,2973/ 20,4644/ 50,2593/ [4,3]
 225 [  6] McCann et al.,1975.   PNAS,72,p979//     0,154/ 1,302/ 10,972/ 50,1716/ 100,262/ [5,3]
 108 [ 19] DeFlora,1978.       NATU,271,p455//      0,226.3/ 1.25,325/ 2.5,397/ 5,570/ 10,1115/ [5,5]
  15 [  1] Shirasu et al.,1977.  OHCA,A,p267//      0,206/ 1.3,412/ 2.6,882/ 10,2528/ 25,1970/ 50,118/ [6,4]
  42 [ 33] Simmon et al.,1977.       EPA,NS//       0,{72}/ 1,{211}/ 5,{532}/ 10,{822}/ 15,{820}/ 25,{720}/ 50,{T}/ [7,3]
 224 [  6] McCann et al.,1975.   PNAS,72,p979//     0,27/ 5,282/ 10,349/ 50,211/ [4,3]
 723 [136] Hallett et al.,1975.   Chemical Control R0,4/ 1,11/ 10,12/ 25,20/ 50,66/ 100,180/ [6,6]
  20 [  5] Seiler,1975.   PCSt,17,p398//           [0],[1]/ [9.9E-04],[1.24]/ [0.01],[1.83]/ [0.1],[4.32]/ [1],[3.73]/ ***[7]
 724 [136] Hallett et al.,1975.   Chemical Control R0,5/ 1,6/ 10,10/ 25,18/ 50,67/ 100,84/ 250,2000/ [7,7]
1322 [233] Ames,1976.  //                           0,28/ 5,697/ 20,1722/ 50,366/ [4,3]
 226 [  6] McCann et al.,1975.   PNAS,72,p979//     0,16/ 1,35/ 5,106/ 10,163/ 50,275/ [5,3]
 710 [ 72] Marshall et al.,1976.  JAFC,24,p560//    0,10/ 10,248/ 25,320/ 50,596/ [4,3]
  14 [  1] Shirasu et al.,1977.  OHCA,A,p267//      0,NS/ 5,118/ 10,265/ 25,382/ 50,118/ [5]
  44 [ 33] Simmon et al.,1977.       EPA,NS//       0,{18}/ 1,{29}/ 5,{80}/ 10,{76}/ 15,{104}/ 25,{80}/ 50,{0}/ [7]
 709 [ 72] Marshall et al.,1976.  JAFC,24,p560//    0,7/ 10,335/ 25,47/ 50,0/ [4]
  46 [ 33] Simmon et al.,1977.       EPA,NS//       0,{7}/ 1,{2}/ 5,{5}/ 10,{0}/ 15,{0}/ 25,{0}/ 50,{0}/ [7]
 707 [ 72] Marshall et al.,1976.  JAFC,24,p560//    0,32/ 10,19/ 25,11/ 50,0/ [4]
  48 [ 33] Simmon et al.,1977.       EPA,NS//       0,{8}/ 1,{7}/ 5,{14}/ 10,{16}/ 15,{26}/ 25,{6}/ 50,{22}/ [7,7]
1323 [233] Ames,1976.  //                           0,61/ 5,67/ 20,65/ 50,118/ [4,4]
```

Figure 3(b) See page 237 for key.

times). The other measures strength in terms of how much chemical is required to produce a given number of revertants. These measures will be highly correlated, yet they are conceptually quite different. We hope the data base will enable us to determine the most useful measure.

APPLICATIONS OF THE DATA BASE

A number of questions in the short-term testing field are being examined using the data base. The first of these, as discussed above, is to compare different methods of statistical analysis for the *Salmonella* test. The second project is to examine the reproducibility of *Salmonella* test results. Figure 3a and b shows this type of analysis for the fungicide captan. We reviewed 28 of the 30 articles containing original data cited in the EMIC data base on captan (as of Sept. 1980), and 8 of these (13–20) contained data that met minimum criteria for a quantitative analysis. For output, experiments with similar test parameters have been sequenced. For example, the box in Fig. 3a encloses results from different laboratories in which captan was tested in the standard plate test using TA100 (one of several different bacterial tester strains used in

---

Figure 3 Summary output for *Salmonella* test data including results of the statistical analyses. Each line represents a single dose-response experiment. The columns in (a) are, from left to right: REF = a bibliographic number. ORG = the *Salmonella* tester strain used (0 = TA100, 9 = TA98, 5 = TA1535, 7 = TA1537, 8 = TA1538). ASS = the type of assay conducted [S = standard plate test (1), P = preincubation assay (12)]. IND = the inducer, if an external metabolic activation system was used (A = Arochlor, P = phenobarbital, M = 3-methylcholanthrene, O = other, U = uninduced). Brackets around a letter in this column indicate the metabolic activation system used was not S-9. SPE = the animal species used as the source of metabolic activation (R = rat, M = mouse). STR = the strain of animal (a series of three letter codes, or four letter codes for FI hybrid strains). TIS = the tissue used, also indicated by a series of three letter codes (LIV = liver). ACT = microliters S-9 per petri plate. PRO = mg per milliliter of protein in the S-9. Potencies, calculated as the dose to increase the revertant background five times are plotted on a log scale using one of three symbols (+, ±, >) depending on the one-sided p value obtained from the statistical test on the significance of the slope: + = $p < .01$; ± = $0.01 \leqslant p < .05$; $p \geqslant .05$. Associated lower and upper confidence bounds are plotted as ∎. POT = the calculated potency value followed in some cases by qualifying or error codes (A = estimated slope negative; B = confidence intervals could not be calculated; V = spontaneous revertants not specified; X = nonstandard response units). PVL = a one-sided p-value testing whether the slope of the dose-response curve is significantly different from zero. QUA = the opinion of the author as to whether or not the chemical was positive (+), negative (−); N = not specified. EXP = the "experiment number" assigned to the particular dose-response curve.

The information in (b) is, from left to right: the experiment number; the bibliographic reference number (Reference #233 unpublished; Reference #6 dose-response curve not published); the bibliographic reference (4 letter codes are used for journal citations); dose/response data from which the potency was calculated ([] = dose or response units are not μg/plate or revertants/plate); the number of dose-response pairs in the experiment, followed by the number used by the statistical program to estimate the initial slope.

SALMONELLA DATA SHEET

QUANTITATIVE DATA MATRIX

---

49 [EXPERIMENT NO.] _____

50 Varying elements (those that are not the same for all experiments from a particular
journal article).
[VARY ELEMENTS] Chemical name = _____

= _____   = _____

= _____   = _____

= _____   = _____

51 If data unpublished, enter date of experiment.
[DATE] _____

52 Qualitative results (author's opinion, if indicated)
[QUAL. RESULTS] _____   (1) Negative or too (2) Positive (3) Borderline
toxic to test

53 [DATA MATRIX]

	Mutation Response Y_1	Survivors Y_2	Standard Deviation SEM, 95% CI Y_3*	P-Value Y_4	Y_5	Y_6	Y_7 ....
$X_1 = 0$							
$X_2 -$							
$X_3 =$							
$X_4 =$							
$X_5 =$							
$X_6 =$							
$X_7 =$							

54 Was data obtained from personal communication?
(PERS. COMM] _____   (1) Yes   (2) No

*SEM = Standard error of the mean; 95% CI = 95% confidence interval about the mean.

Figure 4 Data matrix used to record *Salmonella* test data. Illustrated is the last page of
five-page data sheet (briefly summarized in text).

the *Salmonella* assay). As illustrated, when the potencies are compared, results from the eight EMIC sources (plus one unpublished source), spanning a 4-year period, are strikingly consistent. In Fig. 3, similar comparisons can also be made for other tester strains and test conditions. Test results from different laboratories on a number of widely tested substances will appear elsewhere. This type of analysis should help us determine if there are parameters not currently controlled for in the *Salmonella* assay that can significantly affect potency. This is an essential first step that must be taken for each short-term test in the data base before we can make valid comparisons between results obtained for different chemicals or between results obtained in different short-term test systems.

REFERENCES

1 Ames, B. N., J. McCann, and E. Yamasaki. Methods for detecting carcinogens and mutagens with the *Salmonella*/mammalian-microsome mutagenicity test. *Mutat. Res.* 31:347–364 (1975).

2 Hollstein, M., J. McCann, F. A. Angelosanto, and W. W. Nichols. Short term tests for carcinogens and mutagens. *Mutat. Res.* 65:133–226 (1979).

3 IARC. Long-term and short-term screening assays for carcinogens: a critical appraisal. LYON: IARC Monographs on the Evaluation of Carcinogenic Risk of Chemicals to Humans, 1980.

4 Golberg, L. Rapid tests in animals and lower organisms as predictors of long-term toxic effects. In *Current Concepts in Cutaneous Toxicity*. New York: Academic Press (1980).

5 McCann, J. Short-term tests and cancer policy. In L. McDonald (ed), *Advances in Occupational Health*, vol. 1. London: Churchill-Livingstone (1981).

6 Ashby, J., and J. A. Styles. Does carcinogenic potency correlate with mutagenic potency in the Ames assay? *Nature* 271:452–455 (1978).

7 Meselson, M., and K. Russell. Comparisons of carcinogenic and mutagenic potency. In H. H. Hiatt J. D. Watson, J. A. Winston (eds.) *Origins of Human Cancer,* Book C. pp. 1473–1481. New York: Cold Spring Harbor Laboratory (1977).

8 Ames, B. N., and K. Hooper. Does carcinogenic potency correlate with mutagenic potency in the Ames assay? *Nature* 274:19–20 (1978).

9 Clive, D., K. O. Johnson, J. F. S. Spector, A. G. Batson, and M. M. M. Brown. Validation and characterization of the L5178Y/TK +/− mouse lymphoma mutagen assay system. *Mutat. Res.* 59:61–108 (1979).

10 Ames, B. N., K. Hooper, C. B. Sawyer, A. D. Friedman, R. Petro, W. Havender, L. S. Gold, T. Haggin, R. H. Harris, and M. Rosenfield. Carcinogenic potency: a progress report. In *Ethylene Dichloride: A Potential Health Risk?* Banbury Report No. 5, pp. 55–63. New York: Cold Spring Harbor Laboratory (1980).

11 *Computing Information Technology: SPIRES Searching and Updating.* Stanford, California: Stanford Univ. Press (1980).

12 Yahagi, T., M. Nagao, Y. Seino, T. Matsushima, T. Sugimura, and M. Okada. Mutagenicities of N-nitrosamines on *Salmonella. Mutat. Res.* 48:121–130 (1977).

13 De Flora, S. D. Metabolic deactivation of mutagens in the *Salmonella*-microsome test. *Nature* 271:455–456 (1978).

14 Simmon, V., A. Mitchell, and T. Jorgenson. *In vivo* and *in vitro* studies of selected pesticides to evaluate their potential as chemical mutagens. Prepared for the Environmental Protection Agency. Contract 68-01-2458 (1977).

15 Marshall, T. C., H. W. Dorough, and H. E. Swim. Screening of pesticides for mutagenic potential using the *Salmonella typhimurium* mutants. *J. Agric. Food Chem.* 24:560–563 (1976).

16 Herbold, B., and W. Buselmaier. Induction of point mutations by different chemical mechanisms in the liver microsomal assay. *Mutat. Res.* 40:73–84 (1976).

17 McCann, J., N. E. Spingarn, J. Kobori, and B. N. Ames. The detection of carcinogens as mutagens: Bacterial tester strains with R factor plasmids. *Proc. Natl. Acad. Sci. USA* 72:979–983 (1975).

18 Shirasu, Y., M. Moriya, K. Kato, F. Lienard, H. Tezuka, S. Teramoto, and T. Kada. Mutagenicity screening on pesticides and modification products: A basis of carcinogenicity evaluation. In: H. H. Hiatt, J. Watson, J. Winston (eds.), *Origins of Human Cancer,* Book A. pp. 267–285. New York: Cold Spring Harbor Laboratory (1977).

19 Seiler, J. P. Evaluation of some pesticides for mutagenicity. *Proc. Curr. Soc. Toxicol.* 17:398–404 (1975).

20. Hallett, D. J., P. Weinberger, R. J. Greenhalgh, and R. Prasad. Comparative uptake and metabolism of fenitrothion by three species of forest tree seedlings and one species of a rodent. Canada Forestry Service, Chem Control Res Inst, Ottawa: INF Rep cc-x (cc-x-107) (1975).

21 Hooper, K., L. S. Gold, and B. N. Ames. The carcinogenic potency of ethylene dichloride in two animal bioassays: A comparison of inhalation and gavage studies. In *Ethylene Dichloride: A Potential Health Risk?* Banbury Report No. 5, pp. 65–81. New York: Cold Spring Harbor Laboratory (1980).

Chapter 16

Structure-Activity Analysis of Propyl and Related Nitrosamines in the Hepatocyte-Mediated V79 Cell Mutagenesis System

Robert Langenbach, Charles Kuszynski, Ralph Gingell,
Terry Lawson, Donald Nagel, Parviz Pour,
and Stephen C. Nesnow

INTRODUCTION

The nitrosamines are a class of chemicals that are of environmental importance, with possible involvement in the etiology of human cancer. These compounds are present in foods, drugs, and pesticides. They can be synthesized by bacteria or formed under certain conditions by the reaction of naturally occurring amines and nitrites. The carcinogenicity of nitrosamines is well documented (1-3), and many of them are organ-specific in the production of tumors (4). Although it is known that metabolic activation is required for manifestation of nitrosamines' carcinogenic activity, the exact mechanisms of activation are not entirely clear at this time. For an excellent review of nitrosamine carcinogenesis see Magee et al. (3).

DMN, dimethylnitrosamine; MOP, methyl-2-oxypropylnitrosamine; MHP, methyl-2-hydroxypropylnitrosamine; BOP, bis(2-oxypropyl)nitrosamine; 2-MOB, methyl-2-oxybutyl-nitrosamine; MP, methylpropylnitrosamine; HPOP, 2-hydroxypropyl-2-oxypropylnitro-samine; POP, propyl-2-oxypropylnitrosamine; 3-MOB, methyl-3-oxybutylnitrosamine; 2-HPP, propyl-2-hydroxypropylnitrosamine; DP, dipropylnitrosamine; BHP, bis(2-hydroxy-propyl)nitrosamine; BAP, bis(2-acetoxypropyl)nitrosamine; 3-HPP, propyl-3-hydroxy-propylnitrosamine.

We have been interested in developing *in vitro* mammalian cell systems for detecting hazardous agents. The technique reported here employs a hepato-cyte-mediated V79 cell mutagenesis system (5) based on the previous report of an embryonic fibroblast-mediated mutagenesis system (6). The rationale behind using intact liver cells from adult animals is that they probably closely simulate the metabolic competency of the differentiated hepatocyte as it exists *in vivo*. Many *in vitro* bioassay systems have used liver homogenates for metabolic activation; however, homogenates differ from intact cells in several known respects (7–12) and therefore are probably not representative of liver tissues or cells *in vivo*. Nitrosamines are one class of chemicals for which the hepatocyte-mediated mutagenesis system is quite sensitive (5, 13, 14). For a limited number of these compounds we have previously published that this assay offers a better correlation with *in vivo* carcinogenicity than does the *Salmonella typhimurium* assay (13). Most of the nitrosamines have been extensively studied by Pour and co-workers for carcinogenicity in the Syrian golden hamster, and a successful animal model for pancreatic carcinogenesis has been developed (15–19). The activity of some of these aliphatic nitrosamines in the Ames system has been previously reported (20, 21). It has also been pro-posed that several of these compounds are metabolically interrelated (22) and that nitrosamine structures closer to the ultimate active form may be identifiable.

Structure-activity relationships for carcinogenic or mutagenic chemicals are receiving increased attention. The structure-activity approach may be useful as one parameter in the selection of chemicals for bioassay as well as in elucidating mechanisms involved in the biological activity. Therefore, in the present study, we have compared the mutagenic activities of several propyl and related nitro-samines with three physicochemical descriptors for predicting structure-activity relationships. Because of the close structural similarities of the nitrosamines studied and their subtle structural differences in alkyl chain length and degree and position of oxygenation, these chemicals lend themselves to very interesting structure-activity anlaysis. Furthermore, on the basis of data elucidating a relationship between mutagenic activity in hamster hepatocyte-mediated V79 cell mutagenesis and the physicochemical descriptors, the nitrosamines' carcino-genic potential can be extrapolated.

MATERIALS AND METHODS

Chemicals

Dimethylnitrosamine was purchased from Eastman Organic Chemicals (Rochester, New York). All other nitrosamines were prepared in the Eppley Institute (Omaha, Nebraska) and were determined to be greater than 98 percent pure. Ouabain purchased from Sigma Chemical Co. (St. Louis, Missouri) was dissolved in boiling water before dissolution in medium. Fetal calf serum and Williams Media E were obtained from GIBCO (Grand Island, New York).

Hepatocyte-Mediated Mutagenesis

Primary hamster hepatocytes prepared from 6- to 10-week-old male Syrian golden hamsters were used in mutagenesis studies, which were carried out as previously described (5). The data are expressed as ouabain-resistant mutants per 10^6 survivors at 0.7 mM concentration of the respective nitrosamine. DMN was run as a positive control in all experiments. All data for the various nitrosamines have been normalized to the average number of mutants induced by 0.7 mM DMN. (For additional information on the hepatocyte-mediated mutagenesis system, see references 5 and 13.)

Calculations

Calculations for molecular connectivity were derived from the connectivity tables of Kier and Hall (23); calculations for molecular refractivity were derived from the summation of individual bond refractions according to Vogel (24). These calculations were accomplished using the ADAPT computer system of Jurs (25) installed on a UNIVAC 1110 computer. Entry of two-dimensional structures was accomplished on a Tektronix 4054 graphics display terminal using the UDRAW subroutine of ADAPT, which generated connection tables for each structure. Calculated log octanol:water partition coefficients were supplied by Dr. Peter Jurs.

RESULTS

Figure 1 shows schematically how the hepatocyte-mediated V79 cell mutagenesis system is performed. The primary liver cells are seeded on the already growing V79 cells. Approximately 3 h after seeding, a monolayer of liver cells will have attached; the medium is then changed to fresh solution containing the appropriate concentration of the chemical. After a 48-h cocultivation in the presence of the chemical, the cells are reseeded to determine toxicity and mutagenesis in the V79 cells. The liver cells do not reattach when reseeded. In this system, the liver cell metabolizes the nitrosamine to a reactive intermediate, which is then transported, presumably by cell-to-cell junctions, to the V79 cells, which are then mutated. This proximity between the activating cell and the target cell has been found an essential prerequisite for the occurrence of mutagenesis with certain chemicals in the cell-mediated system (26).

The cell-to-cell arrangements in the hepatocytes to V79 cells *in vitro* may provide a model for the *in vivo* initiation of transformation or mutation (Fig. 1). A differentiated cell (like the hepatocyte in the cell-mediated system) lacks or has limited replicative capacities, but it does have the metabolic capabilities to carry out the tissues' metabolic function. The less well-differentiated cells,

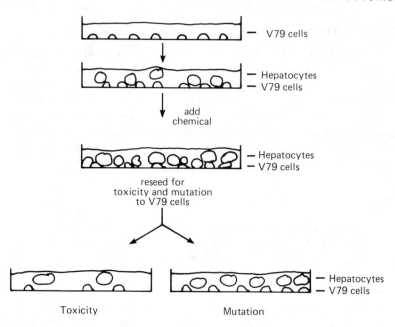

Figure 1 Schematic for the hepatocyte-V79 cell mutagenesis system.

including stem or precursor cells (represented by the V79 cells) that probably have less metabolic capability but can replicate, are arranged below the differentiated cells. *In vivo* the terminally differentiated cells metabolize the xenobiotics and the activated intermediates are transported to the stem cells. At this point, replication of the mutated or transformed stem cell could give rise to the mutant colony or tumor in the animal. Such a phenomenon would explain the difficulty in transforming or mutating differentiated cells in culture. In the hepatocyte-mediated system the production of cytotoxic nitrosamine intermediates by hepatocytes is measured by the reduction in cloning efficiency of the V79 cells (Fig. 2, top panel) and the production of mutagenic nitrosamine intermediates by the increase in ouabain-resistant mutant colonies of V79 cells (Fig. 2, bottom panel).

The structures of the nitrosamines and their abbreviations are shown in Fig. 3. The nitrosamines can be divided into three main classes: dipropylnitrosamines, methylpropylnitrosamines and methylbutylnitrosamines, whose close structural similarities are apparent. Their mutagenic activities in hamster hepatocytes are shown in Table 1. In the absence of hamster hepatocytes, none of the nitrosamines showed appreciable mutagenic activity to V79 cells; but in the presence of hepatocytes, varying mutagenic activities were observed (Table 1).

Several interesting comparisons regarding the nature of alkyl substituent and position and degree of oxidation on mutagenic activity can be made from Table

1. MOP is the most mutagenic nitrosamine studied in the system and, surprisingly, is more mutagenic than DMN. In general, those nitrosamines containing a methyl group were the most active mutagens in the hamster hepatocyte-mediated mutagenesis system. The exception was 3-MOB, being less mutagenic than the other methylated nitrosamines; its activity, however, does demonstrate the effect of oxygenation and its position on activity (see below). The dipropylnitrosamines were somewhat less mutagenic than most methylpropylnitrosamines, although BOP was slightly more mutagenic than would be expected on the basis of alkyl chain length alone.

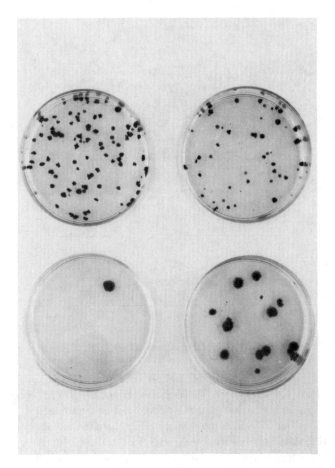

Figure 2 Petri dishes containing colonies showing toxicity and mutagenicity. (Top left) Control colonies of V79 cells. (Top right) Colonies of V79 cells after treatment with nitrosamine in the presence of hepatocytes. (Bottom left) Mutant V79 colony in control dish (usually only 1–2 colonies per 20 dishes are observed). (Bottom right) Mutant V79 colonies from nitrosamine-, V79 cell-, and hepatocyte-treated cultures.

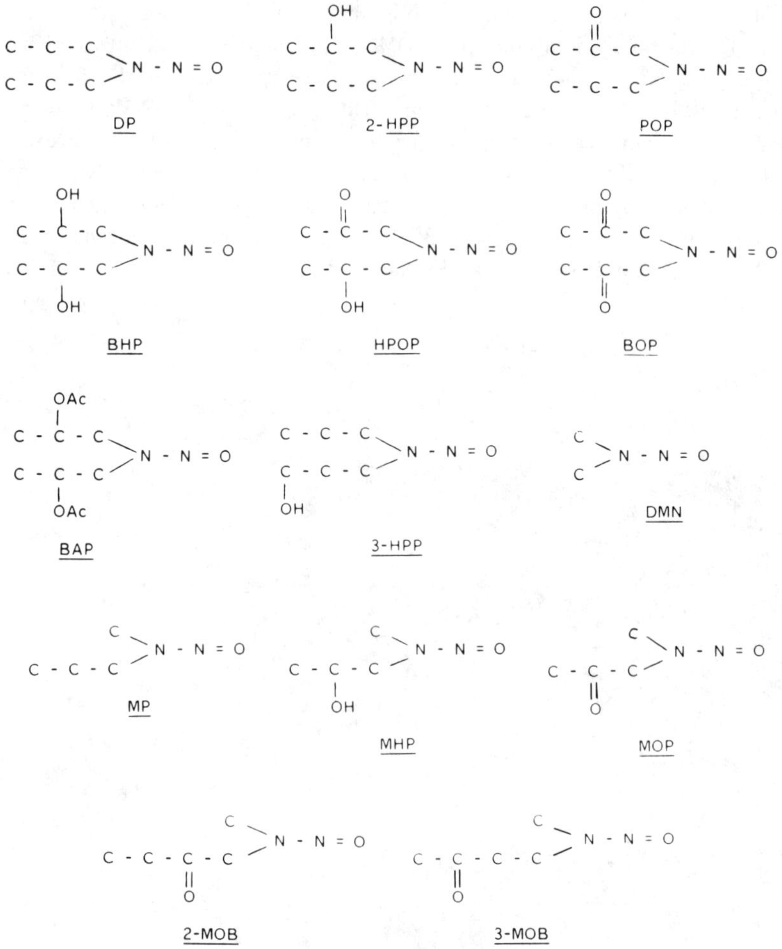

Figure 3 Structures and abbreviations of the nitrosamines studied.

By comparing the mutagenic activity of 2-MOB to 3-MOB (210 vs 30) and of 2-HPP to 3-HPP (25 vs 1) (see Table 1) the effect of position of oxygenation on the mutagenic activity of the molecule can be determined. It is apparent that the position of oxidation can significantly alter mutagenic activity. Similarly, the state of oxidation has an effect on the mutagenic activity; in general, compounds with keto groups are more active than compounds with hydroxyl groups when the same position is compared (MOP > MHP > MP). These observations suggest that pathways of metabolism, nature of activated species, and types of DNA adducts formed, as well as other unknowns, are possible contributors to biological activity.

The data in Fig. 4 show the relationship between mutagenic potency in the hamster hepatocyte-mediated assay and carcinogenic potency *in vivo* in the hamster for several of the nitrosamines. Because of space limitations in Fig. 4, not all nitrosamines are shown; however, the correlation coefficient, 0.97, was calculated based on data for all the compounds except MHP and DMN. Comparable data on the carcinogenicity of MHP and DMN are not yet available using the route of administration used for the other nitrosamines. In Fig. 4, carcinogenic potency is defined quantitatively as the reciprocal of the lowest dose required to produce an overall tumor incidence of at least 60–70 percent in the hamster. The excellent correlations observed with the hamster hepatocyte-mediated assay demonstrate its versatility as a research instrument capable of bioassaying nitrosamines, investigating mechanisms of activation and DNA interaction, and supplying a quantitative data base for structure-activity analysis.

We have previously shown that carcinogenic potency and mutagenic potency do not correlate when the Ames system is used as the assay system

Table 1 Mutagenic Activities of Nitrosamines in the Hamster Hepatocyte-Mediated V79 Cell Mutagenesis System

Chemical	Mutagenic activity[*]
MOP	650
MHP	380
DMN	320
BOP	250
2–MOB	210
MP	105
HPOP	90
POP	75
3–MOB	30
2–HPP	25
DP	20
BHP	10
BAP	10
3–HPP	1
Control	1

[*]Data are reported for each nitrosamine at the 0.7 mM concentration. As the nitrosamines could not all be run in one experiment with a single preparation of liver cells, DMN was run as a positive control in each experiment and all other values normalized to the average DMN activity. The data are expressed as number of ouabain-resistant mutants per 10^6 surviving V79 cells.

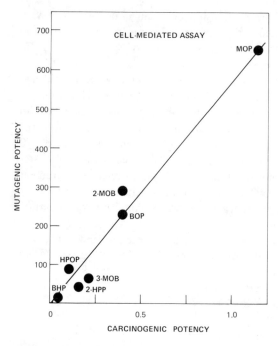

Figure 4 The relationship of carcinogenic and mutagenic potency in the hepatocyte-mediated system. The carcinogenicity of 2–MOB and 3–MOB was estimated from preliminary studies.

for mutagenicity (13). This generalization does not apply to other chemicals studied for mutagenicity in *Salmonella typhimurium*; however, nitrosamines have been a particularly difficult class of chemicals to evaluate in the bacterial system.

For performing structure-activity analysis, we have attempted to correlate the mutagenic activities in the hepatocyte-mediated system with the following descriptors: molecular connectivity, molecular refractivity, and octanol:water partition coefficient. Molecular connectivity or the degree of branching is based on the topology of the molecule. This nonempirical quantitative method groups subgraphs of the molecule into a connectivity index or number that reflects the complexity of the molecule. The relationship between log mutation frequency and molecular connectivity index calculated for path 1 (2-atom fragments) is shown in Fig. 5. The correlation coefficient (R) was −0.64 between the two variables. BAP seems to be an outlier in this correlation, presumably because of its acetyl groups, which do not affect mutation frequency (compared to the nonacetylated BHP) but do increase molecular connectivity.

Molecular refractivity was calculated by summation of the individual bond refractions and is a measure of the ability (of the bonds) of an organic molecule to refract a monochromatic light beam passing through it. The refractivity can also be computed from the Lorentz and Lorentz equation, which requires measurement of the refractivity and density of the substance (24). The relationship between the log of the mutation frequency and the molecular refractivity is found in Fig. 6. The correlation coefficient between these two variables is −0.60. Again, the outlier status of BAP is probably the consequence of its acetyl groups, which increase refractivity but do not decrease the mutation frequency.

The octanol:water partition coefficient, a measure of the lipophilicity or hydrophobicity of molecules, previously has been related to biological activity, chiefly in the work of Dunn and Hansch (27). The partition coefficients of the nitrosamines were calculated based on additivity functions and taking into account hydrogen bonding. The relationship of the log of the octanol:water partition coefficient and the log of the mutation frequency is described in Fig. 7. The correlation coefficient for all nitrosamines was −0.30. HPOP, 3-MOB, 3-HPP, and BHP exhibited negative log octanol:water partition coefficients, but these chemicals are medium to weak mutagens. Exclusion of these substances from the correlation gave a correlation coefficient of −0.90. HPOP and BHP could possibly exist in cyclical forms in solution, an effect not taken into account in the calculation of log P values. The outlier status of 3-MOB and 3-HPP may be attributable to metabolic factors. Also in Fig. 7, calculated

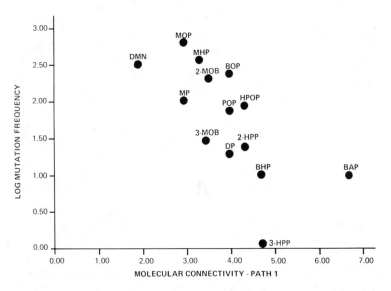

Figure 5 The relationship between log mutation frequency and molecular connectivity. Correlation coefficient, −0.64.

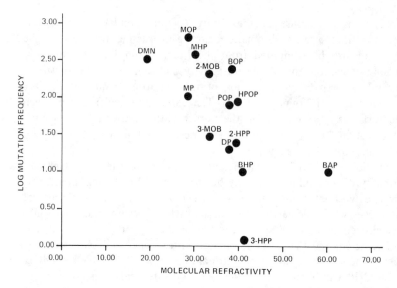

Figure 6 The relationship between molecular refractivity and log mutation frequency. Correlation coefficient, −0.60.

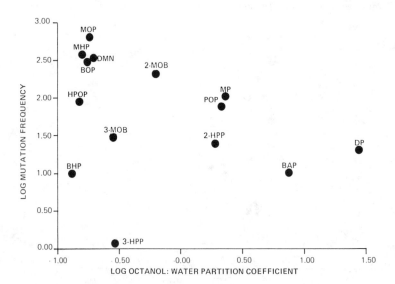

Figure 7 The relationship between log octanol:water partition coefficient and log mutation frequency. Correlation coefficient, −0.30.

log P values were used; a better correlation for some of the chemicals may be obtained with experimentally determined P values.

DISCUSSION

In the present work, possible correlations between nitrosamine mutagenicity in the hamster hepatocyte-mediated V79 cell system and three descriptors used to determine structure-activity relationships were investigated. The nitrosamines chosen for the study were propylnitrosamines or related analogues; therefore, because of the basic structural similarities among the nitrosamines, the effects of subtle changes in nitrosamine structure on mutagenic activity were observed. Several interesting observations can be made about the mutagenesis data. First, oxidation at the β-position increased mutagenic activity, in which the keto group was more active than the hydroxyl group. Second, as carbon number decreased mutagenic activity increased. However, notable exceptions to this effect were MOP and MHP, which proved more mutagenic than DMN. Third, the position of the keto or hydroxyl group had an important effect on mutagenic activity. These latter findings indicate the complexity of nitrosamine-induced mutagenesis or carcinogenesis.

In two of the descriptors (molecular connectivity and molecular refractivity) chosen to be compared with the mutation frequency, BAP was an outlier and substantially decreased the correlation coefficient. Pour et al. (28) has shown that BAP is rapidly hydrolyzed to BHP *in vitro* and *in vivo* and that both have similar *in vivo* carcinogenic potential. The lack of good correlation between log octanol:water partition coefficients may result from the use of calculated rather than experimentally determined log P values or, on the other hand, may reflect the lack of utility of this parameter. Interestingly, Singer et al. (29) found a good correlation between the octanol:water partition coefficient and the carcinogenicity of cyclic nitrosamines, but they found no such correlation with a group of seven acyclic nitrosamines, the chemical type under study in this paper. For the cyclic nitrosamines they observed increased carcinogenicity with decreased log P, the same general result found for the nitrosamines in Fig. 7. The extent of correlation between mutation frequency and the descriptors, molecular connectivity, molecular refractivity, and the log partition coefficient, may relate to the fact that smaller nitrosamines are generally more active than larger ones. Therefore, parameters based on the addition of substructure fragments may, in fact, correlate with mutation frequency solely on the basis of the relationship between size and mutagenic activity. Wishnok and Archer (30) have also reported an inverse relationship between carbon number and nitrosamine carcinogenesis.

The fact that smaller nitrosamines are more carcinogenic and mutagenic than larger ones may relate to their mechanism of action, and particularly their requirement for metabolic activation. Evidence has indicated that

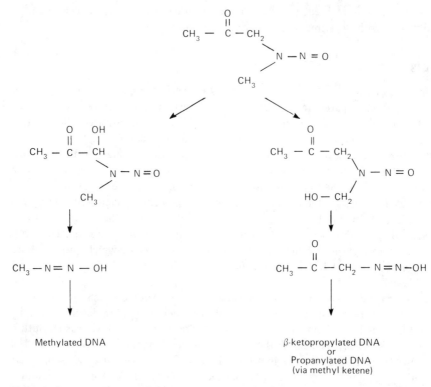

Figure 8 Possible pathways of activation and alkylation of DNA for MOP.

α-oxidation is important in the activation of nitrosamines (23). However, for MOP, even if α-oxidation were considered as the only factor in metabolic activation, it would be sufficient to generate two different species: a methyl group or a β-ketopropyl group, which would interact with the DNA (Fig. 8). A β-ketopropyl group can rearrange to form methyl ketene, which can also acylate DNA. The sites of interaction on the bases, the repair of the different adducts, and other biological effects could be different for the methylated compared to propylated bases. In addition, the presence of a β-keto group could also cause metabolism at a different site on the nitrosamine, prior to its interaction with the DNA, thus producing an alkylating species different from either alkyl group on the parent nitrosamine. In fact, Lawson et al. (31) have shown that after administration of BOP, methylation, and apparently β-ketopropylation, occurs in liver and pancreatic DNA; however, proportionally higher levels of methylation occurred in the pancreas than in the liver. Also, Park and Archer (32) have reported that for DP, approximately 85 percent of the metabolism occurs at the α-position and 15 percent at the β-position, and that oxidation at the β-position may be leading to a species that methylates DNA. These findings are a further indication of the complexity of nitrosamine activation and DNA interaction; they also point out the need to consider electronic factors and metabolism from standpoints other than the α-position of alkyl nitrosamines.

Varying degrees of correlation of structure-activity relationships for nitroso compounds have been reported by other authors. Wishnok and Archer (30) found an inverse relationship between the number of carbon atoms per compound and the carcinogenic activity for approximately 50 nitroso compounds. Wishnok et al. (33) later reported a correlation between both electronic factor (at the β-position) and water:hexane partition coefficients and carcinogenicity for approximately 30 N-nitroso compounds. Certain basic exceptions to their correlations were pointed out, and, as discussed above, metabolism at sites other than the α-carbon, either to reactive intermediates or as a detoxification process, may be involved. Edelman et al. (34) recently proposed a model for determining the organ specificity of nitrosamines, although liver and esophagus were primarily considered. Singer et al. (29) found a correlation between the octanol:water partition coefficient and carcinogenicity for cyclic nitrosamines but could not find a correlation for acyclic nitrosamines. Kier et al. (35) have used molecular connectivity to predict mutagenicity in the Ames test. However, as indicated above, the Ames system may not be the best method of determining nitrosamine biological activity. In a recent comprehensive study, Chou and Jurs (36) used a pattern-recognition approach, involving 15 molecular structure descriptors, to analyze 144 N-nitroso compounds. The predictive ability of this approach was approximately 92 percent for carcinogens and 85 percent for noncarcinogens.

In the present study we have attempted to correlate structure with mutagenic activity. The results are encouraging. From such studies could emerge a computerized approach to predict mutagenic or carcinogenic activity. The data could then be used as part of an initial screening battery to detect potentially hazardous chemicals. However, before implementing such a system, further understanding of the mechanism of the chemicals is needed to improve the data base.

REFERENCES

1 Druckrey, H., R. Preussmann, S. Ivankovis, and D. Schmahl. Organotrope carcinogene Wirkungen bei 65 verschiedenen N-nitroso-Verbindungen an BD-Ratten. *Z. Krebsforsch.* 69:103–201 (1967).

2 Lijinsky, W. Interaction with nucleic acids of carcinogenic and mutagenic N-nitroso compounds. *Progr. Nucleic Acid Res. Mol. Biol.* 17:247–269 (1976).

3 Magee, P. N., R. Montesano, and R. Preussmann. *N-Nitroso Compounds and Related Carcinogens*, ACS Monograph No. 173, pp. 491–625. Washington, D.C.: American Chemical Society (1976).

4   Magee, P. N. Organ specificity of chemical carcinogenesis. In G. P. Margison (ed.), *Carcinogenesis*, vol. 1, pp. 213–221. Oxford: Pergamon Press (1979).

5   Langenbach, R., H. J. Freed, and E. Huberman. Liver cell-mediated mutagenesis of mammalian cells by liver carcinogens. *Proc. Natl. Acad. Sci. USA* 75:2864–2867 (1978).

6   Huberman, E., and L. Sachs. Cell-mediated mutagenesis of mammalian cells with chemical carcinogens. *Int. J. Cancer* 13:326–333 (1974).

7   Brouns, R. E., R. P. Bos, P. J. L. van Gremert, E. W. M. Yig-van de Hurk, and P. T. Henderson. Mutagenic effects of benzo(a)pyrene after metabolic activation by hepatic 9000 g supernatants or intact hepatocytes. *Mutat. Res.* 62:19–26 (1979).

8   Selkirk, J. Benzo(a)pyrene carcinogenesis: A biochemical selection mechanism. *J. Toxicol. Environ. Health* 2:1245–1258 (1977).

9   Decad, G. M., D. P. H. Hsieh, and J. L. Byard. Maintenance of cytochrome P-450 and metabolism of aflatoxin B_1 in primary hepatocyte cultures. *Biochem. Biophys. Res. Commun.* 78:279–287 (1977).

10 Newbold, R. E., C. B. Wigley, M. H. Thompson, and P. Brooks. Cell-mediated mutagenesis in cultured Chinese hamster cells by carcinogenic polycyclic hydrocarbons: Nature and extent of the associated hydrocarbon-DNA reaction. *Mutat. Res.* 43:101–116 (1977).

11 Bigger, C. A. H., J. E. Tomaszewski, and A. Dipple. Differences between products of binding of 7, 12-dimethylbenz(a)anthracene to DNA in mouse skin and in a rat liver microsomal system. *Biochem. Biophys. Res. Commun.* 80:229–235 (1978).

12 Bigger, C. A. H., J. E. Tomaszewski, A. Dipple, and R. S. Lake. Limitations of metabolic activation systems used with *in vitro* tests for carcinogens. *Science* 209:503–505 (1978).

13 Langenbach, R., R. Gingell, D. Nagel, C. Kuszynski, and P. Pour. Mutagenic activities of oxidized derivatives of N-nitrosodipropylamine in the liver cell-mediated and *Salmonella typhimurium* assays. *Cancer Res.* 40:3463–3467 (1980).

14 Jones, C. A., and E. Huberman. A sensitive hepatocyte-mediated assay for the metabolism of nitrosamines to mutagens for mammalian cells. *Cancer Res.* 40:406–411 (1980).

15 Pour, P., J. Althoff, F. W. Kruger, and U. Mohr. A potent pancreatic carcinogen in Syrian hamsters: N-nitroso-bis(2-oxopropyl)amine. *J. Natl. Cancer Inst.* 58:1449–1453 (1977).

16 Pour, P., R. Gingell, R. Langenbach, D. Nagel, C. Grandjean, T. Lawson, and S. Salmasi. N-nitrosomethyl(2-oxopropyl)amine, a potent pancreatic carcinogen in Syrian hamsters. *Cancer Res.* 40:3585–3590 (1980).

17 Pour, P., F. W. Kruger, I. Althoff, A. Cardesa, and U. Mohr. Effect of beta-oxidized nitrosamines on Syrian hamsters. III. 2.2'-Dihydroxy-di-n-propylnitrosamine. *J. Natl. Cancer Inst.* 54:141–146 (1975).

18 Pour, P., L. Wallcave, R. Gingell, D. Nagel, T. Lawson, S. Salmasi, and S. Tines. Carcinogenic effect of N-nitroso(2-hydroxypropyl) (2-oxopropyl)-amine, a postulated proximate pancreatic carcinogen in Syrian hamsters. *Cancer Res.* 39:3828–3833 (1979).

19 Pour, P. M., S. Z. Salmasi, and R. Runge. Selective induction of pancreative ductular tumors by single doses of N-nitroso-bis(2-oxopropyl)amine in Syrian hansters. *Cancer Lett.* 4:317–323 (1978).

20 Rao, T. K., J. A. Young, W. Lijinsky, and J. L. Eppler. Mutagenicity of aliphatic nitrosamines in *Salmonella typhimurium*. *Mutat. Res.* 66:1–7 (1979).

21 Wislocki, P., and R. Gingell. Mutagenicity of several pancreatic carcinogenic derivatives of N-nitrosodipropylamine in the Ames assay. *Mutat. Res.* 77:215–219 (1980).

22 Pour, P., R. Runge, D. Birt, R. Gingell, T. Lawson, D. Nagel, L. Wallcave, and S. Salmasi. Current knowledge of pancreatic carcinogenesis in the hamster and its relevance to the human disease. *Cancer* 47:1573–1587 (1981).

23 Kier, L. B., and L. H. Hall. *Molecular Connectivity in Chemistry and Drug Research*. New York: Academic Press (1976).

24 Vogel, E. *Elementary Practical Organic Chemistry*. 2nd ed. New York: Wiley (1966).

25 Jurs, P. C. Pattern recognition methods. In *Proceedings of the Second FDA Office of Science Summer Symposium*, Department of Health, Education, and Welfare Publication No. 78-1046, pp. 88–94. Rockville, MD: U.S. Department of Health, Education, and Welfare (1978).

26 Kuroki, T., and C. Drevon. Direct or proximate contact between cells and metabolic activation systems is required for mutagenesis. *Nature* 279:368–370 (1978).

27 Dunn, W. J. III, and C. Hansch. Chemico-biological interaction and the use of partition coefficients in their correlation. *Chem.-Biol. Interact.* 9:75–95 (1974).

28 Pour, P., J. Althoff, R. Gingell, R. Kupper, F. W. Kruger, and V. Mohr. N-Nitroso-bis(2-acetoxypropyl)amine as a further pancreatic carcinogen in Syrian golden hamsters. *Cancer Res.* 36:2877–2884 (1976).

29 Singer, G. M., H. W. Taylor, and W. Lijinsky. Liposolubility as an aspect of nitrosamine carcinogenicity: Quantitative correlations and qualitative observations. *Chem.-Biol. Interact.* 19:133–142 (1977).

30 Wishnok, J. S., and M. C. Archer. Structure-activity relationships in nitrosamine carcinogenesis. *Br. J. Cancer* 33:307–311 (1976).

31 Lawson, T. A., R. Gingell, D. Nagel, L. A. Hines, and A. Ross. Methylation of hamster DNA by the carcinogen N-nitroso-bis(2-oxopropyl)amine. *Cancer Lett.* 11:251–255 (1981).

32 Park, K. K., and M. C. Archer. Microsomal metabolism of N-nitrosodi-n-propylamine: Formation of products resulting from α- and β-oxidation. *Chem.-Biol. Interact.* 22:83–90 (1978).

33 Wishnok, J. S., M. C. Archer, A. S. Edelman, and W. M. Rand. Nitrosamine carcinogenicity: A quantitative Hansch-Taft structure-activity relationship. *Chem.-Biol. Interact.* 20:43–54 (1978).

34 Edelman, A. S., P. L. Kraft, W. M. Rand, and J. S. Wishnok. Nitrosamine carcinogenicity: A quantitative relationship between molecular structure and organ selectivity for a series of acyclic N-nitroso compounds. *Chem.-Biol. Interact.* 31:81–92 (1980).

35 Kier, L. B., R. J. Simons, and L. H. Hall. Structure-activity studies on mutagenicity of nitrosamines using molecular connectivity. *J. Pharm. Sci.* 67:725–726 (1978).

36 Chou, J. T., and P. C. Jurs. Computer-assisted structure-activity studies of chemical carcinogens. An N-nitroso compound data set. *J. Med. Chem.* 22:792–797 (1979).

Chapter 17

Development of Statistical Models Relating Structural Parameters, Physical Properties, and Toxicological Activities of Diverse Chemicals

Paul N. Craig
and Kurt Enslein

Since 1976 we have been developing statistical models with the goal of providing reasonable estimates of toxicity for untested chemicals to assist in setting priorities for scheduling toxicity tests. The models have been developed from the following parameters associated with each chemical: log of the n-octanol:water partition coefficient, molar refractivity, molecular connectivity indexes, molecular weight, and various substructural features that are determined by the actual molecular composition of each chemical.

Initial work was centered on 525 chemicals for which rat oral LD_{50} data were available in the literature (1). Computer-assigned substructural keys were obtained from the U.S. Army CIDS files, which included all of the chemicals listed in the 1974 Toxic Substances List.

A model was developed that related the rat oral LD_{50} data to the partition coefficient, molecular weight, and 25 substructural features. A similar model of essentially equivalent statistical utility was constructed using substructural features obtained from the Wiswesser Line Notations (WLN) by use of the CROSSBOW system, for which computer programs were more readily available than the U.S. Army CIDS programs (2). As an example of the application of such a model, Table 1 presents the estimates obtained by

Table 1 Estimation of LD$_{50}$ for 11 Chemicals

Coefficient			−.0095	−.00068	.00022	.000021
					A	
Line no.	CAS no.	Short name	Log P	(Log P)^2	MW	MW × log P
1	50066	Luminal	1.44 (−.0137)	2.07 (−.00141)	232. (.051)	334. (.00700)
2	50215	Lactic acid	−0.62 (.0059)	0.38 (−.00026)	90.1 (.020)	−55.8 (−.0012)
3	50293	Zerdane	5.76 (−.0547)	33.2 (−.0226)	355. (.078)	2042. (.0429)
4	50317	Zobar	3.40 (−.0323)	11.6 (−.00786)	226. (.050)	767. (.0161)
5	50475	Desimipramine	3.65 (−.0347)	13.3 (−.00906)	266. (.059)	972. (.0204)
6	50486	Amitriptyline	5.46 (−.0519)	29.8 (.0203)	277. (.061)	1515. (.0318)
7	50497	Tofranil	4.80 (−.0456)	23.0 (−.0157)	280. (.062)	1346. (.0283)
8	51285	Aldifen	1.51 (−.0143)	2.28 (−.00155)	184. (.041)	278.0 (.0058)
9	51309	Isuprel	−0.47 (.0045)	0.22 (−.00015)	248. (.054)	−116. (−.0024)
10	51649	Amphetamine	1.76 (−.0167)	3.10 (−.00211)	135. (.030)	238.0 (.0050)
11	51683	Acephene	2.62 (−.0249)	6.86 (−.00467)	258. (.057)	675. (.0142)

Table 1 Estimation of LD$_{50}$ for 11 Chemicals (Continued)

B

Co-efficient	.0847	.0390	.0121	.0275	.0144	.0245	.0453	.0297	.0285	−.0268	.0203	.0690	.0538	−.0246	.0423	.0538	−.0357	−.0328	−.0311	.0579	.0835	−.0589	Log 1/c		
Line no.	1	3	8	10	17	18	22	28	30	37	45	46	50	51	65	66	67	73	99	134	135	144	Estimated	Observed	Difference
1																				X			2.46	3.16	−0.70
2					X					X													1.82	1.38	0.44
3					X	X																	2.94	3.50	−0.56
4													X										2.29	2.54	−0.25
5					X			X												X			2.76	2.63	0.13
6			X			X														X			2.57	2.72	−0.15
7			X			X														X			2.64	2.65	−0.01
8		X													X								2.55	3.79	−1.24
9					X	X		X		X						X							2.76	2.05	0.71
10					X				X		X												2.29	3.55	−1.26
11			X			X							X	X									2.51	2.00	0.51

WLN structural keys

use of the WLN-derived model for rat oral LD_{50} values for 11 well-known chemicals. The differences between the estimated and observed log $1/c$ values ranged from −0.01 to −1.26.

We now describe the extension of this approach to the development of a carcinogenesis model, which was constructed from 343 chemicals reported in volumes 1–17 of the International Agency for Research on Cancer (IARC) reviews (3). Those chemicals labeled by IARC as "definite human carcinogens" and "definite animal carcinogens" were combined and called "definite." Those compounds labeled as "noncarcinogens" or "indefinite" were combined and called "indefinite" for purposes of model building. Chemicals that IARC labeled as "suspected carcinogens" were not included in the model. These data were then used to develop a discriminant analysis model by the stepwise regression method (4). This model contained 78 substructural keys (from the CROSSBOW system, as modified and extended for this study) and the molecular weight.

The classification matrix for the discriminant analysis equations is shown in Table 2. The most critical factor, the so-called "negative" category, was assigned incorrectly to approximately 4 percent of the chemicals assigned as "positive" by IARC, whereas the positive label was assigned to approximately 11 percent of the chemicals assigned as indefinite or noncarcinogenic by IARC. Overall, some 84 percent of the chemicals (287/343) were properly classified, approximately 10 percent could not be classified, and approximately 6 percent (21/343) were incorrectly classified by this model. A portion

Table 2   Classification Matrix for Carcinogenesis Model

		Classification by discriminant equation					
		Non or indefinite		Indeterminate		Definite	
		No.	%	No.	%	No.	%
		Indeterminate: .4–.599					
IARC carcinogen classification	Non or indefinite	96	80.0	10	8.33	14	11.7
	Definite	11	4.9	9	4.0	203	91.0
		Indeterminate: .3–.699					
IARC carcinogen classification	Non or indefinite	93	77.5	14	11.7	13	10.8
	Definite	8	3.6	21	9.4	194	87.0

Table 3   A Representative Portion of the Carcinogenesis Model

Key	Frequency Ind.	Def.	Description	Coefficient	F
114	10	12	1 carbo/carbo fusion	11.70	41.0
137	41	21	1 benzene ring	−4.51	38.1
122	0	5	1 hetero/hetero fusion	15.64	31.7
103	10	25	Heterocyclic rings other than 5- and 6-membered	11.62	30.3
86	9	10	Single occurrence of carbonyl	−7.33	21.4
13	2	0	>1 − C = S group	−17.88	20.8
8	18	58	3-branch nitrogen atom	4.82	20.5
246	2	0	Fe	−13.12	19.8
204	5	4	Phenylazo or phenylhydrazono substituent fragment	−11.46	18.0
113	1	1	>1 single carbocyclic ring	−16.24	17.7
321	5	6	Epoxide	−8.01	17.5
79	6	13	1 occurrence of nitrogen in 1 ring	−11.06	17.4
227	4	4	Cr	−8.15	17.1
335	0	8	Combination key	9.10	16.9

of this model is shown as Table 3, to illustrate the format that we use for such models.

An illustration of the difficulty in working with this type of data is shown by further consideration of the classifications made by IARC for several of these 343 chemicals, some of which have been retested since the time of the IARC evaluations by the National Cancer Institute (NCI)/National Toxicology Program (NTP). One chemical, the pesticide heptachlor, was classified as indefinite carcinogen by IARC, and our model was developed with that classification. Recent tests by NCI/NTP have found that chemical to be a positive animal carcinogen, which would change its classification and would modify the model accordingly (5). Such changes may be expected for several other chemicals used in developing this model; this "softness" of the biological test data undoubtedly is the major reason for the incorrect assignments. It is a tribute to the statistical processes used that this model correctly categorizes approximately 84 percent of the chemicals used in its derivation, despite these imperfections in the data.

This example illustrates the need to monitor the raw data used in model development and to revise the models as new data (either additional new data or corrected old data) become available. Such adjustments should become less necessary when large numbers of chemicals are available for model development, but we do not yet know the relationships between the numbers of chemicals, the quality of the test data, and the variety of structural features required for the generation of robust models. These relationships are subjects for future research in this field.

We have also applied this methodology to develop a model that permits extrapolation of the oral LD_{50} in the mouse to the rat (6). Based on only 160 compounds, the model contains eight WLN-derived substructures, the molecular weight, and the square of the log of the n-octanol:water partition coefficient. This model improves the standard error of estimate from ±0.41 log $1/c$ units (when the 160 mouse LD_{50} data are correlated directly to the rat data) to ±0.33 log $1/c$ units (using the full model). The fraction of variance accounted for by the model (R^2) is improved from 0.4–0.79 on application of the full model. We recognize that 160 is not a large enough number of compounds on which to base such a transformation, but this test shows the feasibility of this approach to species-to-species extrapolation.

Models have been prepared by this approach for teratogenic compounds and for chemicals that undergo biotransformation. These preliminary models give encouragement for continuing this approach to the modeling of biological activities and will be reported elsewhere in detail.

REFERENCES

1 Enslein, K., and P. N. Craig. A toxicity estimation model. *J. Environ. Pathol. Toxicol.* 2:115–121 (1978).

2 Eakin, D. L., E. Hyde, and G. Parker. The CROSSBOW System, *Pestic. Sci.* 5:319–326 (1974).

3 International Agency for Research on Cancer. *IARC Monographs on the Evaluation of the Carcinogenic Risk of Chemicals to Humans*, vol. 1–17. Geneva: World Health Organization (1972–1978).

4 Enslein, K., H. S. Wilf, and A. Ralston (eds.). *Statistical Methods for Digital Computers.* New York: Wiley (1977).

5 National Cancer Institute Carcinogenesis Technical Report Series No. 9, *Bioassay of Heptachlor for Possible Carcinogenicity*, NCI-CG-TR-9; DHEW Publication No. (NIH) 77-809 (1977).

6 Craig, P. N., and K. Enslein. Extrapolation of LD_{50}'s between the rat and mouse utilizing chemical structure. *J. Environ. Pathol. Toxicol.* (in press).

Chapter 18

Molecular Basis
for the Structure
Carcinogenicity Relationships
of Polynuclear Aromatic
Hydrocarbons

Edmond J. LaVoie, Stephen S. Hecht,
and Dietrich Hoffmann

Major advances in our understanding of the structure-carcinogenicity relationships of polynuclear aromatic hydrocarbons (PAH) have been achieved in recent years through detailed studies on their metabolism and DNA binding. Benzo[a]pyrene (BaP) was the first PAH for which the metabolic activation pathway to its ultimate carcinogenic form was established. Evidence from several laboratories engaged in binding studies of BaP to DNA *in vitro* and *in vivo*, metabolic experiments, and bioassays for mutagenicity and carcinogenicity revealed that a single enantiomer of 7,8-dihydrodiol-BaP (*2*, Fig. 1) is a major proximate carcinogen of BaP and that the 7,8-dihydrodiol-9,10-epoxide isomer (*3*) is the major ultimate carcinogen of BaP (1-10).

These results on the metabolic activation of BaP led to the formulation of the bay region theory of PAH activation (1, 2, 11-13). The basis of this theory is the relative stability calculated for a benzylic carbonium ion formed at a position in the bay region (Fig. 1). Such a carbonium ion could be formed from an angular ring dihydrodiol epoxide in which one carbon of the epoxide ring is in the bay region. This theory has been tested for a number of hydrocarbons, and the evidence supports the role of bay region dihydrodiol

263

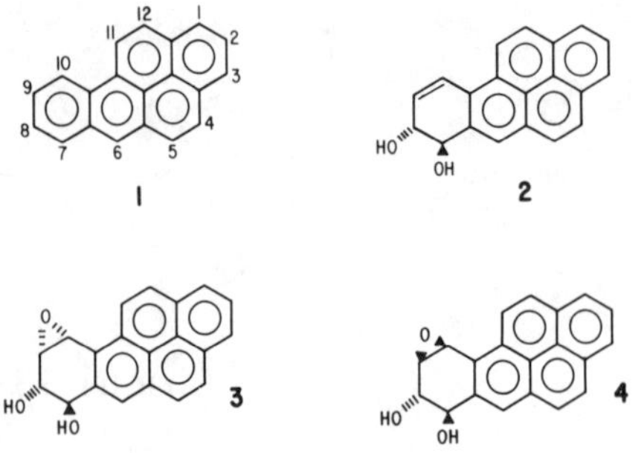

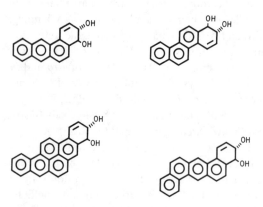

Figure 1 Structure of benzo[a]pyrene and its derivatives.

epoxides as ultimate carcinogens of a number of PAH. In addition to BaP, the bay region theory of PAH activation has been shown to be associated with the metabolic activation of benz[a]anthracene, chrysene, dibenzo[a,i]pyrene, and dibenz[a,h]anthracene, as illustrated in Fig. 2 (14–17).

The bay region theory has significantly advanced our understanding of the molecular basis of the carcinogenicity of PAH. In contrast to the classic three-sided bay region of BaP, benzo[c]phenanthrene and benzo[j]fluoranthene are carcinogenic PAH that contain four-sided bay regions. Studies on the metabolic activation of benzo[c]phenanthrene and benzo[j]fluoranthene have demonstrated that dihydrodiol precursors for the formation of these four-sided bay region diol epoxides are formed *in vitro* (18, 19) (Fig. 3). Studies on the tumorigenicity of the 3,4-dihydrodiol of benzo[c]phenanthrene indicate that its dihydrodiol epoxide is the ultimate carcinogen of benz[c]-phenanthrene. In contrast to these results, the 9,10-dihydrodiol of benzo[j]-fluoranthene was found to be less tumorigenic than its parent hydrocarbon. These data suggest that the pseudo bay region dihydrodiol epoxide of benzo[j]fluoranthene is not its major ultimate carcinogenic metabolite.

Figure 2 Dihydrodiol metabolites of benz[a]anthracene, chrysene, dibenzo[a,i,]pyrene, and dibenz[a,h]anthrancene, which are potent proximate carcinogens.

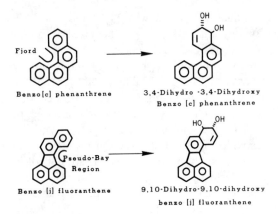

Figure 3 Four-sided bay regions of the chemical carcinogens benzo [c] phenanthrene and benzo [j] fluoranthene.

Understanding the mechanisms by which PAH are ultimately activated to carcinogens can provide a sound basis for advancing structure-activity relationships of PAH. While the bay region theory does not take metabolic factors into account in the prediction of relative carcinogenicity, metabolism is a major determinant of carcinogenic potential among PAH. While benzo[b]-fluoranthene [B(6)F] has a classic bay region within its structure (Fig. 4), it does not appear to be activated to a bay region diol epoxide. Studies on the metabolic activation of B[b]F have shown that the 9,10-dihydrodiol, the requisite precursor for the formation of the bay region dihydrodiol epoxide, is more active than B[b]F as a tumorigenic agent. However, this dihydrodiol has not been identified as a metabolite from *in vitro* metabolism studies using rat liver or mouse skin homogenates (20, 21). The major dihydrodiol metabolite

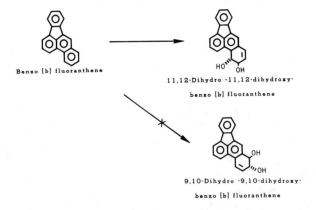

Figure 4 Dihydrodiol derivatives of benzo [b] fluoranthene.

of B[b]F identified in these metabolism studies was 11,12-dihydro-11,12-dihydroxy-B[b]F. These data suggest that B[b]F is metabolized to a bay region epoxide, which may represent its ultimate carcinogenic form.

The lack of carcinogenic activity of benzo[e]pyrene [B(e)P] was initially correlated with its extent of conversion to the 9,10-dihydrodiol (Fig. 5). In addition, metabolism studies using rat liver microsomes demonstrated that negligible amounts of 9,10-dihydro-9,10-dihydroxy-B[e]P were converted to the bay region diol epoxide (22). The weak biological activity of the synthetic diastereomeric bay region diol epoxides of B[e]P as observed on mouse skin and in newborn mice indicate that metabolic factors, however, are not solely responsible for the lack of tumorigenicity of B[e]P (23, 24). The weak tumorigenic activity of these bay region diol epoxides is believed related to the quasidiaxial conformation of the hydroxyl groups (25). In the case of 7,8-dihydro-7,8-dihydroxy-9,10-epoxy-B[a]P, the hydroxyl groups of the dihydrodiol assume a diequatorial conformation. Thus, conformational aspects of active metabolites in addition to metabolic factors themselves can exert considerable influence on the biological activity of PAH.

Several methylated PAH have both mutagenic and carcinogenic activities that would not have been anticipated on the basis of their parent compounds. On the basis of results of carcinogenicity bioassays and metabolic studies, we have proposed that the structural requirements favoring carcinogenicity of methylated PAH are a bay region methyl group and a free peri position, both adjacent to an unsubstituted angular ring, as illustrated in Fig. 6 (26). These structural requirements can best be demonstrated from studies performed on methylchrysenes. The complete carcinogenic activity of each of the six possible isomers of methylchrysene is illustrated in Fig. 7. The most carcinogenic methylchrysene is 5-methylchrysene (5-MeC), with potency comparable to benzo[a]pyrene (27). Among the six possible monomethylchrysene isomers, only 5-MeC possesses a bay region methyl group, position 5

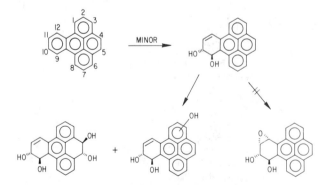

Figure 5 Results on metabolism studies on benzo[e]pyrene.

1. A BAY REGION METHYL GROUP AND

2. A FREE PERI POSITION

*BOTH ADJACENT TO AN UNSUBSTITUTED ANGULAR RING

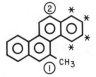

Figure 6 Structural features favoring the carcinogenicity of methylated PAH illustrated for 5-methylchrysene (5-MeC).

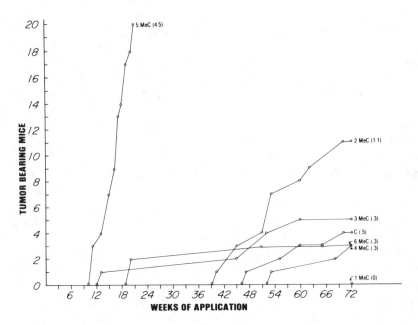

Figure 7 Comparison of the complete carcinogenicity of methylchrysenes when applied at a dose of 100 μg three times weekly.

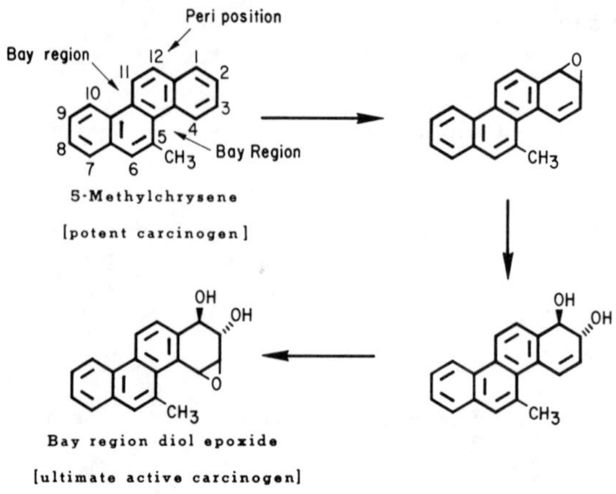

Figure 8   Metabolic activation pathway for 5-methylchrysene.

(Fig. 8), and a free peri position, position 12, adjacent to an unsubstituted angular ring, positions 1–4. Substitution of an additional methyl group or fluorine atom at position 12 reduces activity significantly; thus, 5,12-diMeC and 12-fluoro-5-MeC are only weak carcinogens or inactive (28, 29). In contrast, 5,11-diMeC, which satisfies the above structural requirements, is a potent tumor initiator with activity comparable to 5-MeC. The mechanistic basis for these structural rules appears to be the activation of 5-MeC through formation of the 1,2-dihydrodiol-3,4-epoxide, in which the epoxide ring and the methyl group are in the same bay region (Fig. 6) (30). In a comparison of the tumor-initiating activity of the 1,2- and 7,8-dihydrodiols of 5-MeC as isolated from *in vitro* metabolism studies, we found only the 1,2-dihydrodiol of 5-MeC to be more active than the parent hydrocarbon (Fig. 9) (31). This specific activation pathway, involving the 1–4 positions, was supported by previous results obtained with a series of fluorinated 5-meC derivatives (Table 1) (28, 29). Substitution of fluorine at the 1- or 3-positions of 5-MeC either diminished or abolished tumorigenic activity. Substitution of fluorine in either the 7- or 9-position of 5-MeC did not significantly affect tumorigenic activity. These data not only support the involvement of the 1–4 positions of 5-MeC in its ultimate activation to a tumorigen but also indicate that positions 7–10, which comprise the other angular ring, are not involved.

These structural requirements favoring the carcinogenicity of methylated PAH derivatives are evident from assays of a number of exceptionally carcinogenic methylated PAH derivatives, such as 7,12-dimethylbenz[a]anthracene, 11-methylbenzo[a]pyrene, 7,14-dimethyldibenz[a,h]anthracene, and 15,16-dihydro-11-methylcyclopenta[a]phenanthrene-17-one (Fig. 10) (16, 32–36). These specific methylated derivatives are all more carcinogenic than related isomers in the same series.

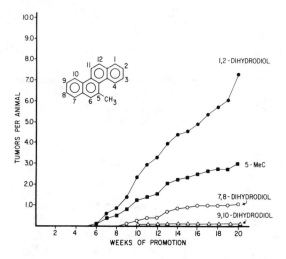

Figure 9 Tumorigenic activity of the 1,2-, 7,8-, and 9,10-dihydrodiols of 5-methylchrysene.

TABLE 1   Tumor-Initiating Activity*

	Tumor initiation		Complete carcinogenicity		
	% TBA	T/A	% TBA	T/A	Blanding index
5-Methylchrysene	68	2.0	80	1.0	31
1–F	10	.1	5	0	(0)
3–F	0	0	0	0	(0)
6–F	80	4.1	100	3.2	32
7–F	60	0.9	70	1.0	30
9–F	45	0.8	75	1.0	26
11–F	45	0.8	80	1.0	33
12–F	18	0.2	25	0.2	(17)
Acetone control (100 μl)	0	0	0	0	(0)

% TBA = the percentage of tumor-bearing animals; T/A = average number of tumors per animal.

*Tumor-initiating activity was determined with a total initiation dose of 30 μg with promotion thrice weekly of 2.5 μg tetradecanoylphorbol acetate. Complete carcinogenicity results were obtained at a dose of 5 μg applied thrice weekly for 72 weeks.

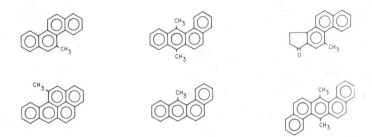

Figure 10 Carcinogenic methylated PAH with a bay region methyl group and a free peri position adjacent to an unsubstituted angular ring.

Studies performed on methylated phenanthrenes have demonstrated that a further structural requirement is necessary to elicit tumorigenic activity. While 4-methylphenanthrene satisfies the structural requirements that would favor carcinogenicity, it was inactive as a tumorigen (37). Studies on the metabolism of 4-methylphenanthrene have shown that 9,10-dihydro-9,10-dihydroxy-4-methylphenanthrene is its principal metabolite. This major detoxification pathway had been previously observed in metabolism studies with phenanthrene (38, 39). In the case of methylated phenanthrene derivatives, inhibition of 9,10-dihydrodiol formation was found to be an additional structural requirement for tumorigenicity. Thus, 1,4-dimethylphenanthrene and 4,10-dimethylphenanthrene were found to be active as tumor initiators on mouse skin (Fig. 11). Metabolism studies performed with 1,4-dimethylphenanthrene confirmed that the major dihydrodiol metabolite was 7,8-dihydro-7,8-dihydroxy-1,4-dimethylphenanthrene. 4,9-Dimethylphenanthrene, which has a

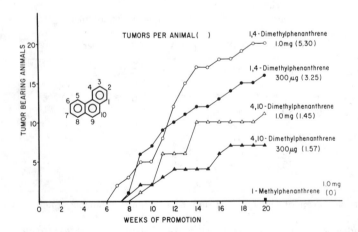

Figure 11 Tumor initiating activity of 1-methylphenanthrene, 1,4-dimethylphenanthrene, and 4,10-dimethylphenanthrene.

peri methyl substituent adjacent to the free angular ring, was inactive as a tumor initiator on mouse skin.

The bay region theory of PAH activation and the structural rules favoring carcinogenicity of methylated PAH provide a clearer understanding of the molecular basis for the structure-activity relationship of PAH. These concepts were formulated primarily through detailed studies on metabolic activation pathways. While these principles are limited only to carcinogenic bay region PAH, they appear to be valid for a majority of the more potent carcinogenic PAH. Further studies are needed to elucidate the mechanism(s) by which carcinogenic PAH that do not contain a bay region are ultimately activated. As additional insight develops into the mechanisms by which these PAH are activated, the molecular basis for the structure-activity relationships of these additional carcinogenic PAH will be determined.

REFERENCES

1 Conney, A. H., W. Levin, A. W. Wood, H. Yagi, R. E. Lehr, and D. M. Jerina. Biological activity of polycyclic hydrocarbon metabolites and the bay-region theory. In Y. Cohen (ed.), *Advances in Pharmacology and Therapeutics*, pp. 43–52. Oxford: Pergamon Press (1978).

2 Nordquist, M., D. R. Thakker, H. Yagi, R. E. Lehr, A. W. Wood, W. Levin, A. H. Conney, and D. M. Jerina. Evidence in support of the bay-region theory as a basis for the carcinogenic activity of polycyclic aromatic hydrocarbons. In R. S. Bhatnager (ed.), *Molecular Basis of Environmental Toxicity*, pp. 329–357. Ann Arbor, Michigan: Ann Arbor Science Publishers (1980).

3 Lehr, R. E., H. Yagi, D. R. Thakker, W. Levin, A. W. Wood, A. H. Conney, and D. M. Jerina. The bay-region theory of polycyclic aromatic hydrocarbon-induced carcinogenicity. In P. W. Jones and R. I. Freudenthal (eds.), *Carcinogenesis, vol. 3, Polynuclear Aromatic Hydrocarbons*, pp. 231–241. New York: Raven Press (1978).

4 Buening, M. K., P. G. Wislocki, W. Levin, H. Yagi, D. R. Thakker, H. Akagi, M. Koreeda, D. M. Jerina, and A. H. Conney. Tumorigenicity of optical enantiomers of the diastereomeric benzo(a)pyrene 7,8-diol-9,10-epoxides in newborn mice: Exceptional activity of (+)-7β,8α-dihydroxy-9α,10α-epoxy-7,8,9,10-tetrahydrobenzo(a)pyrene. *Proc. Natl. Acad. Sci. USA* 75:5358–5361 (1978).

5 Kapitulnik, J., P. G. Wislocki, W. Levin, H. Yagi, D. R. Thakker, H. Akagi, M. Koreeda, D. M. Jerina, and A. H. Conney. Marked differences in the carcinogenic activity of optically pure (+)- and (−)-7,8-dihydrobenzo(a)pyrene in newborn mouse. *Cancer Res.* 38:7661–7665 (1976).

6 Borgen, A., H. Darvey, N. Castegnoli, J. J. Crocker, R. E. Rasmussen, and I. Y. Wang. Metabolic conversion of benzo(a)pyrene by Syrian hamster liver microsomes and binding of metabolites to deoxyribonucleic acid. *J. Med. Chem.* 16:502–506 (1973).

7   Koreeda, M., P. D. Moore, P. G. Wislocki, W. Levin, A. H. Conney, H. Yagi, and D. M. Jerina. Binding of benzo(a)pyrene 7,8-diol-9,10-epoxides to DNA, RNA and protein of mouse skin occurs with high stereoselectivity. *Science* 199:778–781 (1978).

8   Sims, P., P. L. Grover, A. Swaisland, K. Pal, and A. Hewer. Metabolic activation of benzo(a)pyrene proceeds by a diol-epoxide. *Nature* 252:326–327 (1974).

9   Weinstein, I. B., A. M. Jeffrey, K. W. Jennette, S. H. Blobstein, R. G. Harvey, C. Harris, H. Autrup, H. Kasai, and K. Nakanishi. Benzo(a)pyrene diol epoxide as intermediate in nuclei acid binding *in vitro* and *in vivo*. *Science* 193:592–595 (1976).

10 Yang, S. K., D. W. McCourt, J. C. Leutz, and H. V. Gelboin. Benzo(a)pyrene diol epoxides: Mechanism of enzymatic formation and optically active intermediates. *Science* 196:1199–1201 (1977).

11 Jerina, D. M., and J. W. Daly. Oxidation at carbon. In. D. V. Parke and R. L. Smith (eds.), *Drug Metabolism—from Microbes to Man*, pp. 13–32. London: Taylor and Francis (1966).

12 Jerina, D. M., R. E. Lehr, M. Schaefer-Ridder, H. Yagi, J. M. Karle, D. R. Thakker, A. W. Wood, A. Y. H. Lu, D. Ryan, S. West, W. Levin, and A. H. Conney. Bay-region epoxides of dihydrodiols: A concept which explains mutagenic and carcinogenic activity of benzo(a)pyrene and benzo(a)anthracene. In H. Hiatt, J. D. Watson, and I. Winsten (eds.), *Origins of Human Cancer*, pp. 639–658. Cold Spring Harbor, New York: Cold Spring Harbor Laboratory (1977).

13 Jerina, D. M., R. E. Lehr, H. Yagi, O. Hernandez, P. M. Dansette, P. G. Wislocki, A. W. Wood, R. L. Chang, W. Levin, and A. H. Conney. Mutagenicity of benzo(a)pyrene and the description of a quantum mechanical model which predicts the ease of carbonium ion formation from diol epoxides. In F. J. deSerres, J. R. Fouts, J. R. Bend, and R. M. Philpot (eds.), *In Vitro Metabolic Activation in Mutagenesis Testing*, pp. 159–177. Amsterdam: Elsevier/North Holland (1976).

14 Levin, W., D. R. Thakker, A. W. Wood, R. L. Chang, R. E. Lehr, D. M. Jerina, and A. H. Conney. Evidence that benzo(a)anthracene 3,4-diol-1,2-epoxide is an ultimate carcinogen on mouse skin. *Cancer Res.* 38:1705–1710 (1978).

15 Levin, W., A. W. Wood, R. L. Chang, H. Yagi, H. D. Mah, D. M. Jerina, and A. H. Conney. Evidence for bay region activation of chrysene 1,2-dihydrodiol to an ultimate carcinogen. *Cancer Res.* 38:1831–1834 (1978).

16 Slaga, T. J., R. P. Iyer, W. Lyza, A. Secrist III, G. H. Daub, and R. G. Harvey. Comparison of the skin tumor-initiating activities of dihydrodiols, diol-epoxides, and methylated derivatives of various polycyclic aromatic hydrocarbons. In A. Bjørseth and A. J. Dennis (eds.), *Polynuclear Aromatic Hydrocarbons: Chemistry and Biological Effects*, pp. 753–769. Columbus, Ohio: Battelle Press (1980).

17 Hecht, S. S., E. J. LaVoie, V. Bedenko, D. Hoffmann, D. J. Sardella,

E. Boger, and R. E. Lehr. On the metabolic activation of dibenzo[a,i] pyrene and dibenzo[a,h] pyrene. In M. Cooke and A. J. Dennis (eds.), *Polynuclear Aromatic Hydrocarbons: Chemical Analysis and Biological Fate*, pp. 43–54. Columbus, Ohio: Battelle Press (1981).

18 Levin, W., A. W. Wood, R. L. Chang, Y. Ittah, M. Croisey-Delcey, H. Yagi, D. M. Jerina, and A. H. Conney. Exceptionally high tumor initiating activity of benzo(c)phenanthrene bay-region diol-epoxides on mouse skin. *Cancer Res.* 40:3910–3914 (1980).

19 LaVoie, E. J., S. S. Hecht, S. Amin, V. Bedenko, and D. Hoffmann. Identification of mutagenic dihydrodiols as metabolites of benzo(j)-fluoranthene and benzo(k)fluoranthene. *Cancer Res.* 40:4528–4532 (1980).

20 LaVoie, E. J., S. S. Hecht, V. Bedenko, S. Amin, R. Mazzarese, and D. Hoffmann. On the metabolic activation of the environmental carcinogens benzo(j)fluoranthene and benzo(b)fluoranthene. *Proc. Am. Assoc. Cancer Res.* 20:81 (1979).

21 Hecht, S. S., E. J. LaVoie, S. Amin, V. Bedenko, and D. Hoffmann. On the metabolic activation of the benzofluoranthenes. In A. Bjørseth and A. J. Dennis (eds.), *Polynuclear Aromatic Hydrocarbons: Chemistry and Biological Effects*, pp. 417–433. Columbus, Ohio: Battelle Press (1980).

22 Wood, A. W., W. Levin, D. R. Thakker, H. Yagi, R. L. Chang, D. E. Ryan, P. E. Thomas, P. M. Dansette, N. Wittaker, S. Tarujman, R. E. Lehr, S. Kuman, D. M. Jerina, and A. H. Conney. Biological activity of benzo(e)pyrene: An assessment based on mutagenic activities and metabolic profiles of the polycyclic hydrocarbon and its derivatives. *J. Biol. Chem.* 254:4408–4415 (1979).

23 Chang, R. L., W. Levin, A. W. Wood, R. E. Lehr, S. Kuman, H. Yagi, D. M. Jerina, and A. H. Conney. Tumorigenicity of the diasteromeric bay-region benzo(a)pyrene 9,10-diol-11,12-epoxide in newborn mice. *Cancer Res.* 41:915–918 (1981).

24 Slaga, T. J., G. L. Gleason, G. Mills, L. Ewald, P. P. Fu, H. M. Lee, and R. G. Harvey. Comparison of the skin tumor-initiating activities of dihydrodiols and diol-epoxides of various polycyclic aromatic hydrocarbons. *Cancer Res.* 40:1981–1984 (1980).

25 Wood, A. W., R. L. Chang, M-T Huang, W. Levin, R. E. Lehr, S. Kumar, D. R. Thakker, H. Yagi, D. M. Jerina, and A. H. Conney. Mutagenicity of benzo(e)pyrene and triphenylene tetrahydroepoxides and diol-epoxides in bacterial and mammalian cells. *Cancer Res.* 40:1985–1989 (1980).

26 Hecht, S. S., A. Amin, A. Rivenson, and D. Hoffmann. Tumor initiating activity of 5,11-dimethylchrysene and the structural requirements favoring carcinogenicity of methylated polynuclear aromatic hydrocarbons. *Cancer Lett.* 8:65–70 (1979).

27 Hecht, S. S., W. E. Bondinell, and D. Hoffmann. Chrysene and methylchrysenes: Presence in tobacco smoke and carcinogenicity. *J. Natl. Cancer Inst.* 52:1121–1133 (1974).

28 Hecht, S. S., N. Hirota, M. Loy, and D. Hoffmann. Tumor-initiating activity of fluorinated 5-methylchrysenes. *Cancer Res.* 38:1694–1698 (1978).

29 Hecht, S. S., E. J. LaVoie, R. Mazzarese, N. Hirota, T. Ohmori, and D. Hoff-
    mann. Comparative mutagenicity, tumor-initiating activity, carcino-
    genicity, and *in vitro* metabolism of fluorinated 5-methylchrysenes. *J.
    Natl. Cancer Inst.* 63:855–861 (1979).
30 Hecht, S. S., E. J. LaVoie, R. Mazzarese, S. Amin, V. Bedenko, and D. Hoff-
    mann. 1,2-Dihydro-1,2-dihydroxy-5-methylchrysene, a major activated
    metabolite of the environmental carcinogen, 5-methylchrysene. *Cancer
    Res.* 38:2191–2194 (1978).
31 Hecht, S. S., A. Rivenson, and D. Hoffmann. Tumor-initiating activity of
    dihydrodiols formed metabolically from 5-methylchrysene. *Cancer Res.*
    40:1396–1399 (1980).
32 Iyer, R. P., J. W. Lyza, J. A. Secrist, G. H. Daub, and T. J. Slaga.
    Comparative tumor initiating activity of methylated benzo(a)pyrene
    derivatives in mouse skin. *Cancer Res.* 40:1073–1076 (1980).
33 Coombs, M. M., T. S. Bhatt, and C. J. Croft. Correlation between
    carcinogenicity and chemical structure in cyclopenta(a)phenanthrenes.
    Cancer Res. 33:823–837 (1973).
34 Coombs, M. M., and C. J. Croft. Carcinogenic cyclopenta(a)phenan-
    threnes. In *Progress in Experimental Tumor Research*, vol. 11, p. 69–85,
    New York: Karger (1969).
35 Heidelberger, C., M. E. Baumann, L. Greisbach, A. Ghobar, and T. M.
    Vaughan. The carcinogenic activities of various derivatives of dibenzan-
    thracene. *Cancer Res.* 22:78–83 (1962).
36 Dipple, A. Polynuclear aromatic carcinogens. In *Chemical Carcinogens*,
    ACS Monograph No. 173, pp. 245–314. Washington, D.C.: American
    Chemical Society (1976).
37 LaVoie, E., L. Tulley, V. Bedenko, and D. Hoffmann. Mutagenicity,
    tumor initiating activity, and metabolism of tricyclic polynuclear aromatic
    hydrocarbons. In A. Bjørseth and A. J. Dennis (ed.), *Polynuclear
    Aromatic Hydrocarbons: Chemistry and Biological Effects*, pp. 1041–
    1057. Columbus, Ohio: Battelle Press (1980).
38 Boyland, E., and P. Sims. Metabolism of polynuclear compounds. The
    metabolism of phenanthrene in rabbits and rats: Dihydro-dihydroxy
    compounds and related glucosiduronic acids. *Biochem. J.* 84:571–582
    (1962).
39 Sims, P. Qualitative and quantitative studies on the metabolism of a series
    of aromatic hydrocarbons by rat-liver preparations. *Biochem. Pharmacol.*
    19:795–818 (1970).

Chapter 19

Quantum Chemical
and Theoretical Predictions
of Toxicity

Joyce J. Kaufman

INTRODUCTION

The ultimate objective is to formulate and implement a global approach to quantum chemical and theoretical predictions of toxicity. This is a rational and attainable goal based on our closely related experience with a wide variety of molecules with diverse biological and pharmacological effects.

The pharmacological (toxicological) effects of any exogenous compounds are governed by a combination of several factors:

1 Topological, topographical, and substructure analyses of the exogenous molecules (and when appropriate those of the relevant biomolecules into whose pathways these molecules intrude)

2 Electronic structure of the exogenous molecules (and also when appropriate those of the relevant biomolecules into whose pathways these molecules intrude)

3 Physicochemical properties of the exogenous molecules, primarily its lipophilicity, i.e., its tendency to partition from aqueous to lipid phase

(appropriately defined), which influences its ability to reach the site of action

4 Systems analyses and control theory of just how exogenous molecules intrude into the pathways of normal biomolecules and the various influences these exogenous molecules exert on the normal biomolecules, on their synthesizing and metabolizing enzymes and processes, on their release and reuptake, and on other physiological processes

One must be meticulous to distinguish between the extremes of inherent activity (the pharmacological or toxicological activity of a drug or other exogenous molecule once it reaches its locus of action, which is presumably due to the interaction of the vital pharmacophoric or toxicophoric portion of the exogenous molecule with its receptor site or place of action) as opposed to whole animal or human *in vivo* potency, which is influenced by transport, metabolism, and excretion in addition to inherent activity. In the context of this paper, toxic is taken to mean causing any undesirable physiological effects, not merely lethal toxicity (acute or chronic).

In our interdisciplinary group at Johns Hopkins we have been devoting considerable care to delineating as precisely as possible how best to calculate or to measure the various factors that contribute to quantitative structure-potency relations (QSPR). Our studies encompass the gamut from (*a*) quantum chemical calculations, in which we have given major attention to developing new effective techniques for carrying out *ab initio* quality wave functions especially aimed at being efficient for large drug and biomolecules; to (*b*) theoretical approaches such as systems analysis and control theory and catastrophe theory aimed at codifying and predicting the influence of endogenous diseases and exogenous drugs or other molecules (such as toxicants) on the dynamic balance of neurotransmitters and thus shedding light on the mechanisms of action of CNS agents; to (*c*) physicochemical studies, including development of a novel microelectrometric titration procedure that enables us to deconvolute overlapping pK_a's and to determine accurately the pH dependence of lipophilicities; to (*d*) experimental pharmacology studies and teratology studies, in which we were able to find a correlation between the lipophilicities of lipophilic acids and their ability to induce birth defects, as well as a close interaction with physicians in the clinical use of various types of CNS agents. Under ONR Biophysics sponsorship we have just initiated extending our quantum chemical and theoretical studies to the understanding and prediction of toxicity.

STRATEGY

For codification and prediction of toxicity we have recently derived a new strategy for data base searching based on topological, topographical, and substructure analyses, combined with systems analyses and control theory, which is the reverse of what is usually done. While there have been about 6 million different molecules listed in Chemical Abstracts (and thus it would be a gargantuan task to do a compound by compound search for toxicity and that still would not lead to predictive capacity) there are only a few dozen (less than 100) "triggering events" that lead to toxicity. These triggering events, which may themselves cause a cascade of other physiological events, are related to the physiologically observed signs and symptoms on exposure to or administration of drugs or toxicants or any exogenous molecules. The drugs, toxicants, or other exogenous molecules that cause any observed physiological effect must be coded so they are retrievable by name, structural formula, chemical family, *and* all reasonable substructural fragments, both topological and topographical, especially ones identifiable as pharmacophores or toxicophores. Thus, by being able to computer query "signs and symptoms," this will lead back both to the triggering events, as well as to the subsequent physiological events these triggering events cause, and to the pertinent substructural fragments and especially to the toxicophores. Also, when it is desired to try *to predict* if a certain compound will be toxic, the computer can compare the topological, topographical and substructural characteristics of all identified toxicophores to those of the compounds to be investigated, and output what matches it finds to previously identified toxicophores and also the triggering events, subsequent physiological events, and the physiologically observed signs and symptoms these toxicophores cause.

When metabolism plays an important role, this information on possible metabolic pathways must be included appropriately along with the computer coding of the parent molecule. This can be done by tracing possible pathways of metabolism relevant to substructural fragments known to undergo metabolism. Metabolism can enter in several ways. In the case of carcinogens, the parent carcinogens (precarcinogens) must be activated metabolically to proximate carcinogens and then to ultimate carcinogens, which then attack DNA (or RNA or the relevant enzymes) and lead to improper replication of the DNA and thence to cancer. For drugs (or toxicants), metabolism may either activate them, if a metabolite is the physiologically active species, or deactivate them.

Such a theoretical approach appropriately formulated can form one of the most sophisticated and cogent examples of what has been called the use of "artificial intelligence in medicine" (AIM). Even more, while "artificial intelligence" programs usually refer to programs for semantic information processing that are designed to emulate human performance in problem-solving activities in using the reasoning processes of scientists in proceeding from data to conclusions based on the data, theoretical pharmacology and toxicology employ the computer also to generate some of the fundamental data needed for rationalization of the problem not obtainable from any experimental data, namely, the *electronic structures* of the exogenous and endogenous molecules involved.

The electronic structure of a drug, toxicant, or biomolecule is closely related to its intrinsic activity. Several various electronic properties of a drug, toxicant, or biomolecule may relate to its pharmacology or toxicology and to its structure-activity relationships. Charges on crucial atoms, geometrical conformations, occupied or virtual molecular orbital energies, electrostatic molecular potential contour maps in three dimensions around the molecule, and intermolecular interactions may all play key roles in relating structure to activity.

Recent quantum chemical advances have made it possible to carry out such quantum chemical calculations for large drugs and biomolecules rapidly and reliably, and these will be mentioned briefly later in this section. Quantum chemical methods to characterize electronic structure of molecules, including large drugs and biomolecules, span a variety of techniques ranging from *ab initio* through semirigorous to semiempirical. Once one can identify the theoretical requisites necessary for effective drug (or toxic) action, it then becomes possible to screen new drugs (or suspected toxicants) quantum chemically even prior to their syntheses.

In this regard the electrostatic molecular potential contour maps are particularly valuable. A drug that is a direct agonist of an endogenous biomolecule at the biomolecule's receptor site or two drugs topographically, or perhaps topologically, related that act by the same mechanism generate similar electrostatic molecular potential maps around their pharmacologically significant pharmacophores. This concept can be extended to toxicity and toxicophores.

We have also been able to demonstrate the application of these electrostatic molecular potential contour maps in tracing the metabolic activation of polycyclic aromatic hydrocarbons (PAH) carcinogens from precarcinogens (PAH) through proximate carcinogens (PAH oxides and dihydrodiols) to ultimate carcinogens (PAH dihydrodiolepoxides), for the opening of the epoxide ring of ultimate carcinogen, and for a new electrophilicity index for the ultimate carcinogens.

These electrostatic molecular potential contour maps can be used in several ways in understanding and in predicting toxicity. There must be a great similarity in shape between toxicophores that act in the same manner at the same receptor. The shape of the map is probably determining of the activity; the magnitude of the map may well relate more to the strength of the specific binding. Also, for a substance whose toxicity one would like to predict, the strategy would be, in addition to topological, topographical, and substructure searching, calculation of the *ab initio* wave function of the molecule, from the wave function generation of the electrostatic molecular potential contour map around the molecule and then computer matching of that map to those for known toxic compounds. This could enable one to identify similar toxicophores in chemically dissimilar compounds.

Each of these methods has its historical place in the chronology of quantum chemical calculations on large drugs and biomolecules. However, semiempirical methods are procedures whose time has long since past and even semirigorous procedures should no longer be considered adequate in themselves but only appropriate to give approximate molecular geometries for more rigorous (*ab initio* or *ab initio* effective core model potential) calculations.

This is because the difficulty and time of the quantum chemical calculations go up as more than N^4, where N is the number of atoms in the molecule. Our major attention for the past several years has been devoted to the development and implementation of procedures for calculating nonempirical *ab initio* quality wave functions for the valence electrons of a molecule by incorporating into our own new fast *ab initio* computer programs a number of desirable options for quantum chemical calculations on large drugs and biomolecules.

Most importantly our methods save computer time compared to conventional *ab initio* methods. Thus rapid and reliable quantum chemical calculations on large drugs, toxicants, and biomolecules are more than possible at present, even on this generation's computers. However, on this generation's computers, computer core size and speed are still limiting factors for quantum chemical calculations on very large molecules. However, there are supercomputers available now and super-super computers being designed which will be orders of magnitude larger and faster than the computers in common usage today.

Hence, the future of computational quantum chemistry in the field of biology and medicine can only be even brighter. The greatest drawback to date has been the almost total lack of support and even interest from NIH in development and implementation of new strategies for *ab initio* computations on large molecules and the application of *ab initio* quantum chemical methods to molecules of biomedical significance. It is hoped that a strong recommendation will emerge from this workshop that NIH support be forthcoming for fundamental breakthroughs in the area of *ab initio* quantum chemical calculations on large molecules, which will be commensurate with the stunning pace at which the new supercomputers and super-super computers are being developed. Our preliminary analysis for *ab initio* calculations using even presently available supercomputers has already indicated that completely new theoretical strategies will make *ab initio* calculations on large molecules much more tractable and faster. *Ab initio* quantum chemistry, which deals with the electronic structure of molecules, is a discipline that transcends "specific diseases" and is applicable to all fields of biology and medicine. It deserves support as a discipline itself for the insight it can give to all fields of biology and medicine.

Chapter 20

Concept of the Integrated Approach

Michael D. Waters

INTRODUCTION

This report considers aspects of developing and applying SAR models in conjunction with genetic bioassay data as part of an integrated approach to the assessment of human health hazard. Our principal objective, to develop valid SAR models, requires high-quality data bases of evaluated biological research results. The EPA GENE-TOX Program is offered as an example of the development of such a data base. A second objective, to apply SAR models in an integrated assessment of human health hazard, may be best achieved in concert with appropriate mutagenicity-carcinogenicity testing schemes. EPA's recent application of a *phased approach* in evaluating 38 pesticides is reviewed.

BUILDING THE BIOLOGICAL DATA BASE

The assessment of human health hazard from exposure to an environmental chemical requires knowledge of:

1   Physical/chemical properties of the chemical
2   Extent and route of human exposure
3   Distribution and metabolism of the chemical
4   Targets of the active metabolites
5   Immediate and long-term effects as a function of exposure (i.e., dose-response relationships)

The requirement for dose-response information encompasses both short- and long-term toxic effects. To possess all of this information for a given compound constitutes major progress in our health hazard assessment of that compound as well as a potentially important building block for SAR theorists and experimentalists.

Short-Term Tests for Mutagenicity
and Presumptive Carcinogenicity

Assessing acute toxicity is a relatively straightforward task. To definitively assess chronic toxicity, however, requires expensive and time-consuming whole-animal testing. In the field of genetic toxicology, short-term tests for mutagenicity and presumptive carcinogenicity were developed as a rapid and relatively inexpensive alternative to initial whole-animal testing, both for purposes of detection and also to understand the underlying biological phenomena. At present, these short-term bioassays represent the only practical means to quickly build a genetic toxicological data base that adequately considers the range and diversity of chemicals with which we must be concerned.

Five types of biological activity can be detected using short-term *in vitro* tests: gene (point) mutations, chromosomal effects, primary DNA damage and repair, oncogenic transformation, and related toxic effects. Because of similarities in the basic molecular mechanisms by which chemical mutagens and most carcinogens appear to induce their effects (i.e., molecular alterations of DNA), it has been postulated that knowledge of mutagenic effects can be used to predict carcinogenicity (1). As shown in Fig. 1, the proposed relationship between mutagenicity and carcinogenicity is not simple and includes mechanisms not fully understood. We believe that many carcinogens act through mutational mechanisms, but clearly other physiological processes may be involved as well.

Mutations can occur at either the gene or chromosomal level. Gene mutations include base-pair substitutions, frameshifts, and small deletions. Chromosomal mutations include changes in chromosome number or alterations in chromosome or chromatid structure. Among the available short-term tests, *in vitro* microbial systems are highly sensitive to point mutations; mammalian cell systems in culture are sensitive to gene mutations and chromosomal

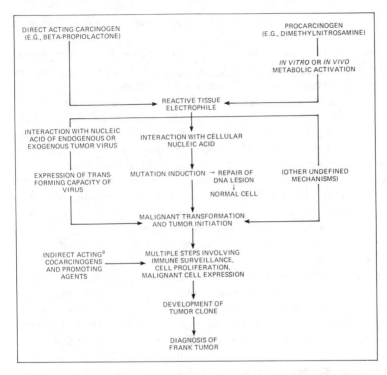

Figure 1 Proposed relationship between carcinogenicity and mutagenicity. The model shown accounts for many facets of what is known about tumor production in mammals. While there is significant indirect support for this model, formal proof is not yet available. [a]There are a number of agents known to influence the expression of malignancy in cells once the initiation process has occurred. However, these agents are not capable of producing the initiation event. *From Brusick (1). Used by permission of the publisher.*

damage. Genetic toxicologists usually recommend that the initial evaluation of any compound include tests that measure, either individually or in concert, both types of damage (2). Vogel's work in *Drosophila* (3) suggests that point or gene mutations are observed at lower test concentrations than are chromosomal aberrations.

The short-term point mutation assay that has been most extensively used, of course, is the *Salmonella typhimurium*/microsome mutagenicity bioassay or "Ames test" (4). Ames test results have demonstrated good *qualitative* correlations with whole-animal carcinogenicity results for most compound classes (5, 6). This concordance appears to be largely due to the incorporation in the Ames test of a presumptive mammalian metabolic activation system that employs a mammalian liver homogenate with necessary cofactors ("S-9" activation). McCann et al. describes recent efforts to improve Ames test *quantitative* correlations for purposes of relative potency analysis (see Chap. 15, this volume).

The nature and degree of correlation between short-term (mutagenesis) and long-term (carcinogenesis) results is an important issue both for bioassay development and for SAR modeling. Improved correlations between short- and long-term test results would have important implications for the ways in which we approach future assessments of human health hazard. The available human data (i.e., epidemiological data) and most of the long-term experimental data are for carcinogenesis, which is only in part simulated in short-term tests. Increased reliance on mutagenesis bioassays as *predictors* of carcinogenic potency or levels of carcinogenic effect will hinge on the demonstration of quantitative correlations between the two types of assays. However, it must be expected, based on present knowledge, that quantitative correlations will not be good for all classes of compounds.

From a qualitative point of view, reducing the potential for false-negative or false-positive results in either the long- or short-term bioassay system remains a major priority. With short-term systems, false-negatives can result from any of several factors: insensitive indicator cells or organisms, an incomplete test system (e.g., a system that detects point mutations but not chromosomal alterations), the masking of mutagenic effect by overall toxic effect, or inadequate metabolic activation. False-positives can be due to the high sensitivity of a short-term test or to the statistical limitations of a long-term test (i.e., too few animals may be treated).

One of the critical factors in obtaining good qualitative and quantitative correlations between short- and long-term results is the appropriateness and effectiveness of the method of *metabolic activation*. At present, three basic types of activation are available. The first of these, *in vitro* S-9 activation, involves the centrifugal separation of enzymatic components from cell fragments of mammalian liver (or other organ); these extracted enzymatic compounds together with suitable cofactors are added to an indicator cell system. A second basic type of metabolic activation involves the cocultivation of metabolically active primary whole liver (or other organ) cells with appropriate indicator cells. The third type, *in vivo* activation, has several forms. In one technique, the active metabolites of a test chemical are extracted from the body fluids of a treated animal and then added to an indicator cell system. In another technique, indicator organisms (e.g., bacteria or mammalian cells) are injected into an exposed animal and subsequently recovered and cultured using appropriate techniques to demonstrate any genetic change that may have occurred.

The importance of the method of metabolic activation has become increasingly apparent as investigators have sought quantitative correlations between mutagenic potency as measured in short-term tests and carcinogenic potency as measured in long-term tests. For example, the early results of

Langenbach et al. (7) suggest that the cell-mediated mutagenesis test [primary Syrian hamster whole liver cells cultured with Chinese hamster lung (V79) indicator cells] produces a more linear correlation with *in vivo* carcinogenesis data than does the Ames assay provided with hamster liver S-9. This improved correlation may be largely due to the fact that metabolic activation by whole liver cells, in comparison to S-9 activation, more closely simulates the activation that occurs in the intact mammal.

More than 100 short-term tests now exist. As illustrated in Fig. 2, these tests may be categorized with respect to their ability to provide information about a particular biological endpoint and by the test organism employed. From an inspection of the range of biological activity detected by any short-term test, it is immediately apparent that a battery of *in vitro* tests would be required to evaluate the full range of genetic effects seen in mammals.

Because certain theoretical and methodological advantages and limitations and resource considerations are inherent in each test system, each is generally best applied as a particular stage of the evaluative process. In Fig. 2, the tests are grouped according to perceived principal utility (detection, confirmation, or risk assessment).

A *detection* bioassay should represent a relevant type of biological activity that is genetically well defined. The test should be selective for that activity (i.e., should display few false-positive results) and sensitive to compounds that display the activity under evaluation (i.e., few false-negative results). The power of the test should be great (i.e., there should be a large number of potential respondents per total number of indicator cells or organisms treated). The test should be reproducible and available as a routine procedure in testing laboratories. And, if possible, a detection system should be simple, rapid, and inexpensive. Probably the best example of a detection system is the Ames test. Figure 3 lists some specific advantages and limitations of this bioassay.

A *confirmatory* bioassay, in turn, should display greater complexity in terms of genetic organization and increased relevance to the mammalian (human) response. A confirmatory test is usually more selective for a specific biological activity. The test may be less sensitive, reproducible, and available and is typically not simple, rapid, or inexpensive. An example of a confirmatory bioassay would be a test for gene mutation in mammalian cells. Figure 4 lists some advantages and limitations of this system.

At present, *risk assessment* procedures rely principally on the use of whole-animal methods. Carcinogenesis risk assessment is accomplished by combining the results of conventional long-term whole-animal carcinogenesis bioassays and, if available, epidemiological information with environmental exposure data. In mutagenesis risk assessment, the results of *in vivo* bioassays for heritable genetic damage are integrated with environmental exposure

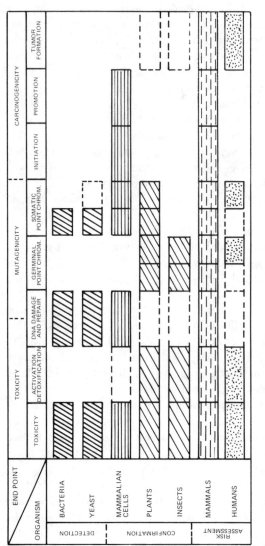

Figure 2 Available short-term tests categorized by endpoint and test organism.

SALMONELLA TYPHIMURIUM (AMES TEST)

ADVANTAGES
1. RELIABLE. IN TESTING KNOWN CARCINOGENS AND NONCARCINOGENS: FALSE POSITIVES, ≤ 10%; FALSE NEGATIVES, ≤ 10%.
2. HAS EXTENSIVE DATA BASE.
3. TESTER STRAINS ARE EXTENSIVELY ENGINEERED TO ENHANCE SENSITIVITY.
4. RESULTS IN DIFFERENT TESTER STRAINS PROVIDE INFORMATION ABOUT THE MECHANISM OF MUTATION (E.G., FRAMESHIFT VS. BASE-PAIR SUBSTITUTION.
5. KNOWN HUMAN PURE CHEMICAL CARCINOGENS ARE POSITIVE. THESE INCLUDE β-NAPHTHYLAMINE, BENZIDINE, BIS-CHLOROMETHYLETHER, AFLATOXIN-B, VINYL CHLORIDE, 4-AMINO-BIPHENYL.
6. USEFUL AS A TOOL IN RAPIDLY OBTAINING INFORMATION ABOUT THE POTENTIAL MUTAGENIC/CARCINOGENIC ACTIVITY OF UNCHARACTERIZED COMPOUNDS IN COMPLEX MIXTURES. HAS BEEN APPLIED TO CIGARETTE SMOKE CONDENSATE AND FRACTIONS, HAIR DYES, SOOT FROM CITY AIR, ETC.
7. VALUABLE AS A BIOASSAY TO DIRECT THE CHEMICAL FRACTIONATION AND IDENTIFICATION OF MUTAGENIC COMPONENTS IN COMPLEX MIXTURES.

LIMITATIONS
1. CONSIDERED QUALITATIVE IN NATURE.
2. NOT RESPONSIVE TO METALS, CHLORINATED HYDROCARBONS (LONG CHAIN), ASBESTOS AND LIKE PARTICLES.
3. SAMPLE MUST BE STERILE. (PROBLEMS IN SAMPLE STERILIZATION.)
4. HIGHLY TOXIC COMPONENTS OF COMPLEX SAMPLES MAY MASK MUTAGENIC PROPERTIES OF OTHER CHEMICALS.
5. ORGANIC SOLVENTS USED IN CHEMICAL FRACTIONATION (E.G., METHYLENE CHLORIDE) MAY BE MUTAGENIC AND THEREFORE MAY REQUIRE REMOVAL (E.G., BY SOLVENT EXCHANGE) PRIOR TO BIOASSAY.

Figure 3 Specific advantages and limitations of the Ames test.

MAMMALIAN CELL MUTAGENESIS IN VITRO

ADVANTAGES
1. ALLOWS OBSERVATION OF THE FULL RANGE OF MUTATION RESPONSES OF SOMATIC CELLS, NOT JUST POINT MUTATIONS.
2. FASTER AND LESS EXPENSIVE THAN IN VIVO ASSAYS.
3. CAN BE COUPLED WITH IN VITRO METABOLIC ACTIVATION SYSTEMS FROM VARIOUS SOURCES.
4. MUTATIONS MEASURED IN CULTURED MAMMALIAN CELLS ARE MORE RELEVANT TO THE INTACT MAMMAL THAN ARE MUTATIONS MEASURED IN BACTERIAL SYSTEMS.
5. RESPONDS TO PARTICULATES (CLASTOGENIC EFFECT).
6. MAY OFFER BETTER QUANTITATIVE CORRELATION WITH CARCINOGENICITY THAN DOES THE AMES TEST (PRELIMINARY RESULTS).

LIMITATIONS
1. THE CELL LINES USED FOR EXPERIMENTATION ARE TRANSFORMED LINES AND THEREFORE DO NOT REPRESENT "NORMAL" CELLS.
2. THESE CELLS DO NOT UNDERGO MEIOSIS.
3. ONLY ONE OR TWO LOCI FROM THE ENTIRE GENOME ARE MONITORED.
4. CELLS HAVE LIMITED ENDOGENOUS METABOLIC ACTIVATION CAPABILITY.
5. THERE ARE SOME DOUBTS ABOUT THE GENETIC NATURE OF THE EVENTS OBSERVED AT CERTAIN LOCI.

Figure 4 Specific advantages and limitations of a test for mammalian cell mutagenesis *in vitro*.

information. There are no documented cases of induced mutation in the human population. However, there is reason to believe that man is subject to the same kinds of genetic effects as other animal species, and there is a large genetic component in human disease.

Mutagenesis risk assessment has two basic approaches. The first considers induced germinal mutations in intact animals. Using bioassays such as the specific locus test, the offspring of mutagen-treated mammals are examined for evidence of heritable genetic damage. The treatment dose is correlated with effects observed in the offspring, and these effects are extrapolated to environmental levels of exposure for humans. Mutagenesis risk assessment is also accomplished through the study of germ cell dosimetry. First, the offspring of mutagen-treated animals (e.g., *Drosophila melanogaster*) are examined for evidence of heritable genetic damage. Then the treatment/germinal dose in the insect, in this case, is correlated with a treatment/germinal dose in a mammal. The effects in the insect are then extrapolated to environmental levels of exposure for humans.

The *Drosophila* sex-linked recessive lethal test can serve either as a confirmatory bioassay (see Fig. 2) or as part of a mutagenesis risk assessment protocol (as suggested above). Figure 5 details the advantages and limitations of this system.

These examples (Figs. 3–5) of tests that are appropriate to the stages of detection, confirmation, and risk assessment represent just 3 of the more than 100 available bioassays. Which of these tests or combinations of tests would be most useful in building the data base needed for SAR modeling and for the larger goal of assessing human health risk? To address this question, a reasonable and informed approach would be to carefully examine the toxicological tools that are presently available and to ascertain what each can or cannot do. Such an evaluation would seek to identify the advantages, limitations, and principal utility of each existing bioassay.

SEX-LINKED RECESSIVE LETHAL TEST IN *DROSOPHILA MELANOGASTER*

ADVANTAGES
1. A LARGE NUMBER OF THE TEST ORGANISMS CAN BE RAISED EASILY AND ECONOMICALLY.
2. METABOLIC ACTIVATION IS ENDOGENOUS.
3. GENOTOXIC EFFECTS ARE EVALUATED IN THE GERM CELLS.
4. MANY LOCI IN THE GENOME ARE MONITORED AT THE SAME TIME.
5. HAS LARGE DATA BASE ON CHEMICAL MUTAGENS.

LIMITATIONS
1. RESPONDS POORLY TO MUTAGENIC POLYCYCLIC AROMATIC HYDROCARBONS.
2. INSECTICIDES CANNOT BE EVALUATED.

Figure 5 Specific advantages and limitations of the *Drosophila melanogaster* sex-linked recessive lethal test.

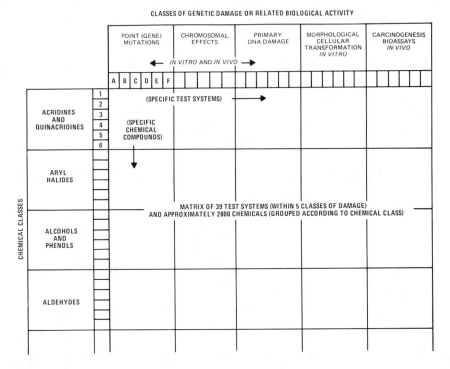

Figure 6   GENE-TOX data matrix.

The GENE-TOX Program

EPA's GENE-TOX Program (evaluation of current status of bioassays in GENEtic TOXicology) (8, 9) is the first major, systematic assessment of this kind. Sponsored and directed by the Office of Testing and Evaluation within the Office of Pesticides and Toxic Substances, GENE-TOX evaluates the current utility of selected mutagenicity and related bioassays by means of a thorough and methodical examination of the open literature. Conceptually, this exercise involves first the construction of a two-dimensional matrix (9) that plots the results of specific bioassays versus specific test compounds (Fig. 6). Then the performance of each bioassay is compared, on a chemical-by-chemical basis, to that of the others.

GENE-TOX is basically a two-phased effort (Fig. 7). In the first phase (now essentially complete), work groups of scientists evaluated the available literature on selected bioassays. There were 24 work groups (Table 1), each consisting of 5–10 scientists chosen for knowledge of and familiarity with the bioassay to be evaluated. Approximately 39 major bioassay systems were examined under this first phase of the GENE-TOX Program.

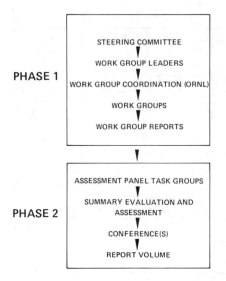

Figure 7 Phases of the GENE-TOX Program.

Table 1   GENE-TOX Work Groups

Endpoint	Assay	Group leader
Gene mutation	*Salmonella typhimurium*	V. Simmon
	Escherichia coli WP2	D. Brusick
	Mouse lymphoma (L5178Y) cells	D. Clive
	Chinese hamster lung (V79) cells	E. Huberman
	Chinese hamster ovary (CHO) cells	A. Hsie
	Neurospora crassa	H. Brockman
	Aspergillus nidulans	B. Scott
	Tradescantia	M. Constantin
	Drosophila melanogaster	W. Lee
	Mouse specific locus (including spot test)	L. Russell
Chromosomal effects	*Drosophila melanogaster*	R. Valencia
	Plant cytogenetics	M. Constantin
	Saccharomyces cerevisiae	F. Zimmerman
	Schizosaccharomyces pombe	
	Mammalian cytogenetics	J. Preston
	Sister chromatid exchange	S. Latt
	Micronucleus test	J. Heddle
	Dominant lethal test	S. Green
	Heritable translocation test	W. Generoso
Primary DNA damage	*Escherichia coli* Pol A	H. Rosenkranz
	Bacillus subtilus rec	
	Unscheduled DNA synthesis	A. Mitchell
	DNA repair	R. Painter
Oncogenic transformation	C3H10T1/2 mouse fibroblasts	
	BALB/c 3T3 mouse fibroblasts	C. Heidelberger
	Syrian hamster embryo cells	
Ancillary tests	Host-mediated assay	M. Legator
	Sperm morphology	A. Wyrobeck

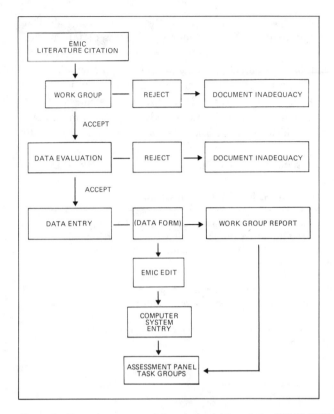

Figure 8 Flow chart summarizing the activities of the GENE-TOX work groups.

As shown in Fig. 8, each work group began with a list of citations on the bioassay provided by the Environmental Mutagen Information Center (EMIC) at Oak Ridge National Laboratory. The work group's first task was to screen and reduce this literature pool. The "first cut" was based on general GENE-TOX guidelines and requirements for the evaluative process. The "second cut" considered the adequacy of each experimental protocol, including proper experimental design; proper use of positive and negative controls; proper selection of solvents and vehicles; acceptable spontaneous background frequency or rate; provision of metabolic activation systems, if necessary; appropriate criteria for positive, negative, and inconclusive results; and provision of dose-response information (not critical if all other criteria were met). When a final literature pool had been obtained, the experimental data were extracted from each report and entered, by EMIC, into the GENE-TOX computer system. (Akland and Waters present a complete list of the elements of the GENE-TOX data base in Chap. 3, this volume.) EMIC edited and processed the data to categorize the results of each study as positive/negative/inconclusive and to indicate whether or not the published report contains dose-response data. These standardized items of information are now retrievable by CAS chemical number, chemical class, organism, specific test system, endpoint, obtained results, and bibliographic details.

The final and most important task of each work group was to utilize the extracted data in compiling a report (Table 2) on the test system. The work group reports were submitted for review by the GENE-TOX Assessment Panel and are currently being published in *Mutation Research—Reviews in Genetic Toxicology*.

One very important ramification of the computerized GENE-TOX data

Table 2 Outline of Reports by GENE-TOX Work Groups

  I. Introduction (general description and brief historical review of the assay system, including key references and the criteria for literature selection and rejection)
 II. Test description (a detailed discussion of the system including but not necessarily limited to the following)
    A. Genetic basis of effect detected
    B. Description of strains and uses (with procedures for genotype confirmation)
    C. Suggested protocol for testing (with modifications required for specific chemical classes or physical states)
       1. Standard treatment conditions (e.g., time, temperature, pH, buffer)
       2. Controls (positive, negative)
       3. Vehicles or solvents
       4. Acceptable spontaneous background frequencies or rates
       5. Dosage selection and numbers of doses
       6. Proper collection of raw data
III. Interpretation of data
    A. Presentation of data
       1. Dose-response curves
       2. Data transformations
       3. Various units of expression
    B. Criteria for acceptability of data
    C. Statistical evaluation
    D. Criteria for positive/negative conclusions
    E. Applicability of results to hazard evaluation
 IV. Test performance
    A. Number of chemicals and chemical classes tested
    B. Chemicals or chemical classes that give anomalous results and reasons or speculations as to cause
    C. Chemicals or chemical classes for which the test is particularly well suited
    D. Correlation with mammalian mutagenicity and carcinogenicity data
  V. Conclusions
    A. Strengths and weaknesses of the assay
    B. Role of the assay in a mutagenicity testing program and in a carcinogenicity testing program
    C. Recommendations for research, development, and validation of the system
 VI. Bibliography (references evaluated by the work group)

```
     CHEMICAL CLASS:    POLYCYCLIC AROMATIC HYDROCARBONS
 ASSAY SYSTEM CLASS:    PROKARYOTES
METABOLIC ACTIVATION:   +


                        B(a)P    DMBA    BA     3-MC   7-MeBA
         SALMONELLA     5 +      12 +    1 +    3 +    4 +
                        3−       3−      8−     1−     0−
                        2 ?      1 ?     0 ?    0 ?    0 ?
         E. COLI WP2    4 +      3 +     1 +    1 +    4 +
                        0−       0−      0−     0−     0−
                        0 ?      0 ?     0 ?    0 ?    0 ?
```

```
COMPOUND:   BENZO (a) PYRENE
   ASSAY:   E. COLI WP2
```

EMIC #	METABOLIC ACTIVATION (S9) STRAIN	PROTOCOL	RESULTS
11133	CHARLES RIVER	AGAR INCORPORATION	+
23133	CHARLES RIVER	SUSPENSION	+
51170	WISTAR	SUSPENSION	+
81120	SPRAGUE-DAWLEY	SPOT TEST	+

Figure 9 Examples of matrices that can be compiled using the GENE–TOX data base. (Data are hypothetical.)

base will be the ability to select and display portions of the base to permit direct comparison of the experimental results obtained with different compounds or compound classes, with different assay systems, with different types of metabolic activation, and so on. By way of example, Fig. 9 (upper portion) summarizes hypothetical results reported for polycyclic aromatic hydrocarbons using prokaryotic assay systems. The next matrix (Fig. 9, lower portion) further narrows this focus by listing, on a study-by-study basis, the hypothetical results for benzo[a]pyrene in the *Escherichia coli* WP2 assay.

Matrices such as these are presently receiving extensive use by the task groups of the GENE–TOX Coordinating Committee (Table 3), which replaced the Assessment Panel. The Coordinating Committee's efforts comprise the second phase of the program; this phase is approximately 1 year from completion. The membership of these relatively small task groups represents a considerable breadth of expertise in the field of genetic toxicology. The task groups' role is to address the most fundamental goals of the program (Table 3). The groups will individually publish reports in *Environmental Mutagenesis* and will participate in discussions of their findings at one or more

Table 3   Goals of the GENE-TOX Coordinating Committee Task Groups

Goal	Group leader
To identify those genetic and related endpoints that are of concern to human health	F. de Serres
To distinguish those systems that are ready for extensive use in testing from those that should be regarded as developmental	D. Brusick
To determine the sensitivity of each bioassay to respond to specific classes of chemicals and to identify major strengths and weaknesses	V. Ray
To examine qualitative correlations between mutagenesis and carcinogenesis	S. Nesnow
To devise specialized batteries of bioassays that detect the various types of genetic damage induced by specific classes of chemicals	V. Ray
To devise and recommend a general battery of bioassays that is capable of detecting with high probability relevant genetic and related damage induced by various classes of chemicals	M. Waters
To consider the potential utility of *in vitro* mutagenesis and carcinogenesis bioassays for quantitative estimation of effect	J. Springer
To identify information gaps and future research needs and to establish a mechanism for evaluating the status of test systems on a continuing basis	A. Hollaender
To determine the status and utility of existing mutagenesis bioassays for purposes of genetic risk assessment	L. Russell

conferences. [An initial "Conference on Current Status of Bioassays in Genetic Toxicology (GENE-TOX)" was held December 3-5, 1980; at this meeting, the individual work group reports were discussed in detail.] Phase 2 of the GENE-TOX Program will conclude with the publication of a final summary report based on an assessment of the task group reports. However, it is anticipated that the evaluation of scientific literature and the computerization of abstracted data will continue through the efforts of the GENE-TOX Coordinating Committee and EMIC.

The results of the GENE-TOX Program will have immediate and direct utility for workers in the field of SAR analysis. First and foremost, the computerized data base will represent a primary, accessible, versatile information resource on the genotoxic and related biological effects of over 2800 specific chemicals. And it is important to reemphasize that this information resource will consist not of raw laboratory data but of published results that were prescreened according to strict criteria, systematically evaluated by panels of experts, and finally summarized and standardized for computer retrieval. While a number of other existing and planned data bases are of potential utility in SAR analysis (see Chap. 3, this volume), for the near future GENE-TOX is expected to be the most comprehensive source of evaluated results from a variety of short-term tests.

On a broader scale, GENE-TOX might well serve as an example for the evaluation and integration of scientific data in other fields—including other fields relevant to SAR analysis. Additional efforts similar to GENE-TOX would strengthen the overall scientific data base and the quality of scientific papers and certainly improve our ability to perform integrated assessments of biological activity (specifically, assessments of human health risk).

From another perspective, the evaluative component of GENE-TOX is expected to communicate an explicit warning to SAR workers (indeed, to all who consider and use genetic bioassay data) of the need, in attempting to predict the hazard associated with any compound or class, to consider the full *spectrum* of biological activity that is measurable with these tests. For example, many SAR models have been and continue to be based exclusively on Ames test results. As noted earlier, the Ames test offers several advantages, not the least of which is an overall record of good qualitative correlation with carcinogenicity assessed *in vivo* and with known human pure chemical carcinogens. But results from one kind of bioassay may tell us little about how the compound would fare in tests that measure other types of genetic damage, that employ other types of metabolic activation, and so on. Also, bioassay results that are essentially qualitative in nature may not be useful in calculating relative potency. To base SAR models solely on results from one type of bioassay, then, can reduce the SAR models' ability to perform what is potentially their most important role: the identification, among numerous untested compounds, of those most likely to display biological activity that suggests a threat to human health (i.e., the most appropriate candidates for initial short-term screening).

THE APPROACH TO MUTAGENICITY AND CARCINOGENICITY TESTING

In addition to supporting SAR studies, the GENE-TOX Program is also expected to contribute importantly to the overall mutagenesis-carcinogenesis testing strategies of EPA and other regulatory agencies responsible for assessing chemical risk to human health. Just in terms of the numbers of unevaluated compounds, these agencies are faced with a task of immense magnitude: By 1978, over 4 million chemicals had been registered with ACS. Of these, over 40,000 were in U.S. commercial production. Approximately 1000 new chemicals were being produced annually. For at least 50 chemicals, production was in excess of 1.3 billion pounds per year (10). Obviously, our available resources of time, facilities, staff, and funds will simply not permit definitive whole-animal testing of the vast majority of chemicals to which humans may be exposed. Thus, scientists and regulatory officials have increasingly adopted testing strategies that rely heavily on the relatively fast and inexpensive short-term bioassays as indicators of mutagenicity and predictors of carcinogenicity.

Current Strategies

In mutagenesis testing, the fundamental concern is the risk of genetic effects in future generations. To be classified as a mutagen, a chemical must be shown to possess mutagenic activity and to reach the germinal tissues. The current consensus (2, 11, 13) is that a battery of tests is required to operationally define a nonmutagen using these criteria. Such a battery should include, at a minimum, tests for point mutations, chromosomal aberrations, and primary DNA damage (ideally including effects in germinal tissues of intact organisms).

In carcinogenesis testing, our increasing understanding of the ways and degrees in which mutagenesis bioassays may predict carcinogenicity has encouraged their use as screening tools. As noted earlier, tests for point mutations in microorganisms have been found to be highly predictive of carcinogenic potential. Still, the intrinsic limitations of all bioassays suggest that no single screening test is 100 percent predictive of carcinogenicity. Thus, most of the carcinogenicity testing schemes that have been proposed (14, 19) prescribe "tiers" of tests following the detection-confirmation-risk assessment progression discussed above.

SAR analysis has found an obvious role as tier 0 in these schemes (Fig. 10). Due to the numbers of untested chemicals, even simple microbial screening is impossible in most cases. SAR models assist investigators in making "educated guesses" as to which compounds are most likely to carry genetic hazard and should therefore be screened in tier 1.

Tier 1 (detection) tests are chosen for sensitivity, sometimes at the expense of selectivity. That is, detection systems tend to return higher positive fractions when known carcinogens are tested but also to return a higher overall fraction of false-positive results. Tier 2 (confirmation) systems measure endpoints (such as oncogenic transformation *in vitro*) that are considered to be directly relevant to the process of tumor formation in the intact animal. Tier 3 (risk assessment) entails conventional whole-animal carcinogenesis bioassays—still considered the only definitive means, other than human epidemiology, to establish a chemical's carcinogenicity or noncarcinogenicity.

In recommending batteries and tiers of tests for mutagenesis and carcinogenesis, respectively, investigators in both the public and private sectors have argued for the inclusion of numerous specific bioassays. As suggested earlier, each bioassay has intrinsic strengths and weaknesses, is likely to be

TIER 0: STRUCTURE – ACTIVITY CORRELATIONS

TIER 1: DETECTION SYSTEMS

TIER 2: CONFIRMATORY BIOASSAYS

TIER 3: SYSTEMS WHICH PROVIDE DATA SUIT-
        ABLE FOR RISK ASSESSMENT

Figure 10 The tier approach to carcinogenicity testing.

most (or least) effective with certain classes of compounds, and is likely to be most useful at a particular stage in the evaluation process. And, as discussed, the primary goal of the GENE-TOX Program is precisely to explore these factors. In the absence of the final report from GENE-TOX, however, there is little to be gained in restating the relative merits of various testing schemes that have been proposed. Instead, it may be useful to describe a framework or approach to testing—the "phased approach"—that has been advocated by this author in recent years (20, 22).

The Phased Approach

The phased approach (Fig. 11) seeks to *combine* the tier approach to carcinogenicity testing with the battery approach to mutagenicity testing. Overall, three levels or phases of actual testing observe the general tier testing strategy of detection-confirmation-risk assessment. Obviously, SAR analysis may play an important role in the initial selection of compounds for biological evaluation.

Phase 1 (detection) relies on inexpensive, sensitive, and rapid broad-range tests for point mutations, primary DNA damage, and chromosomal effects. Such test systems permit the screening of large numbers of chemicals in an effective manner. Positive phase 1 results are confirmed and more fully evaluated in phase 2 (confirmation). Phase 2 test systems are selected for the capacity to measure the same types of biological activity detected in phase 1 but in ways that are more relevant to the intact mammal and to humans. Positive phase 2 results are pursued in phase 3 (risk assessment). Risk assessment entails the integration of conventional mutagenesis and/or long-term carcinogenesis bioassays in whole animals with appropriate epidemiological information (in the case of carcinogenesis) and human exposure data.

In addition to observing the tier testing philosophy, the phased approach explicitly recognizes that a number of kinds of biological activity are measurable in short-term tests, that short-term tests vary in their ability to detect these different kinds of damage, and that, given our present state of knowledge, a battery of tests having limited redundancy is desirable in determining that a substance is provisionally negative for genetic activity. This battery—the "core battery"—consists of tests selected from phases 1 and 2. (In Fig. 11, suggested components of a core battery are highlighted in boxes.) The core battery tests are considered to be the most essential components of the evaluation, and short-term testing ceases only if the complete core battery returns negative results. Extensive human exposure, high production volume, or other factors of concern may require a more extensive evaluation.

The GENE-TOX Program is expected to provide much information that will be directly relevant to the selection of specific tests and test batteries for the evaluation of genetic activity. In the meantime, we can draw on present

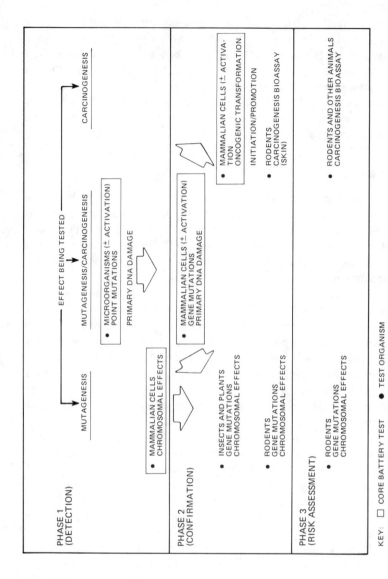

KEY: □ CORE BATTERY TEST ● TEST ORGANISM

Figure 11 The phased approach.

knowledge to suggest some combinations of available test systems or system types. In terms of a core battery of short-term tests, this author would propose tests for the following kinds of genetic activity:

1 Point mutations in microorganisms
2 Gene mutations in mammalian cells
3 Chromosomal effects in mammalian cells and in mammals
4 Primary DNA damage in mammalian cells
5 Oncogenic transformation in mammalian cells

Each of these tests should be performed using metabolic activation methods appropriate to the class of chemical under evaluation. Ray (23) has also considered the types of tests that might comprise an adequate core battery. His recommendations are similar to the above, except that the test for primary DNA damage is seen as a possible augmentation rather than as a standard component of the core battery. In terms of specific tests, Ray proposes the following:

1 Bacterial point mutation assay with five strains of *Salmonella typhimurium* (Ames)
1a Assay of urine from mice treated with test chemical on *Salmonella* strains
2 Mammalian cell point mutation assay with either the mouse lymphoma (L5178Y) or the Chinese hamster ovary cell model
3 Cytogenetic analysis *in vivo* with rat or mouse bone marrow cells
4 A cytogenetic assay in human lymphocytes *in vitro* with mitotic indexes as an indicator for dose selection
5 Transformation in hamster embryo cells *in vitro* or other suitable assays

Ray reports that an ongoing literature review "shows that very few substances with mutagenic or direct-acting carcinogenic potential would be missed by [this] core battery."

An Evaluation of Pesticides
Using the Phased Approach

The first application of the phased approach was a recent evaluation (24, 25) of 38 pesticides (insecticides, herbicides, and fungicides) carried out under the EPA Substitute Chemical Program. In terms of the program suggested above, this pesticide assessment should be viewed as a *partial* trial: a full core battery was not completed and only one phase 3 assay was performed. Complete details of the 38 pesticides tested, the testing protocol, and the quantitative and qualitative results are available elsewhere (26–29). What is important for the present discussion are some general conclusions that may be drawn regarding the feasibility of this approach to testing.

The positive findings are summarized in Table 4. Of 38 pesticides screened, only 6 (acephate, captan, demeton, folpet, monocrotophos, and trichlorfon) were found to be positive in three or more of the *in vitro* tests of phases 1 and 2. All six were positive in the Ames test; four were also positive as point mutagens in *Escherichia coli*. All six caused primary DNA damage in the form of enhanced mitotic recombination in yeast and (except for captan and folpet) increased unscheduled DNA synthesis in mammalian cells in culture. Under the guidelines of the phased approach, then, only these six pesticides would have been considered sufficiently active to warrant further investigation, with the following caveat: a complete core battery (as recommended above) was not performed. (Omitted were phase 1 tests for chromosomal effects *in vitro* and phase 2 tests for gene mutations in cultured mammalian cells.) Thus, while this exercise clearly shows that strategic application of a battery of detection assays can dramatically reduce the number of samples requiring further evaluation (in this case, a field of 38 narrowed to 6), it is certainly possible that completion of a full core battery would have left a somewhat larger field.

Overall, phase 2 testing confirmed the adequacy of the phase 1 microbial detection systems. The six compounds evaluated as positive in two to five of the phase 1 tests were also positive in the phase 2 *in vitro* test or in one of the phase 2 *in vivo* tests. In the case of three additional compounds (disulfoton, bromacil, and simazine), however, phase 2 results indicated mutagenic activity that was *not* detected in phase 1. Disulfoton returned a positive response in the test for unscheduled DNA synthesis in WI38 cells. Bromacil and simazine were positive in the *Drosophila* sex-linked recessive lethal test. These three compounds were tested in phase 2 only because an ancillary goal of this pesticide project was to compare the performance of the different assays; under normal conditions, the three would not have been tested. These findings raise the possibility of false-negatives in the results from phase 1; if additional testing yields further evidence of false-negatives, modification of the phase 1 battery may be necessary. This issue reemphasizes the real need for GENE-TOX and similar efforts: the effectiveness of any testing program begins with and is largely dependent on our understanding of the applicability and limits of each component test.

Only one phase 3 whole-animal test was performed in this study. Captan was evaluated in the mouse heritable translocation test. The result was considered positive in light of historical controls but was treated as negative by the GENE-TOX work group in that a translocation was observed in the concurrent controls.

To the extent that whole-animal carcinogenicity data for these com-

Table 4 Positive Results in an Evaluation of 38 Pesticides by the Phases Approach

	Results*								
	Phase 1					Phase 2			Phase 3
Compound	Ames (38)	WP2 (38)	D3 (38)	POL A (38)	REC (38)	UDS (38)	DRL (30)	MDL (10)	MHT (1)
Positive for point/gene mutation and DNA damage in pro- and eukaryotic systems									
Acephate	+	—	+	N	N	+	—	NT	NT
Captan	+	+	+	+	+	—	+	—	+?[†]
Demeton	+	+	+	—	+	+	—	NT	NT
Folpet	+	+	+	+	+	—	+	—	NT
Monocrotophos	+	—	+	N	N	+	—	—	NT
Trichlorfon	+	+	+	N	N	+	—	NT	NT
Positive only for DNA damage in prokaryotic systems									
Chlorpyrifos	—	—	—	+	+	—	—	NT	NT
2,4-D acid	—	—	—	—	+	—	NT	NT	NT
2,4-DB acid	—	—	—	+	—	—	NT	NT	NT
Dicamba	—	—	—	+	+	—	—	NT	NT
Dinoseb	—	—	—	+	+	—	—	NT	NT
Propanil	—	—	—	—	+	—	NT	NT	NT
Positive only for DNA damage in eukaryotic systems									
Azinphos-methyl	—	—	+	N	N	—	—	—	NT
Cacodylic acid	—	—	+	N	N	—	—	NT	NT
Crotoxyphos	—	—	+	N	N	—	—	NT	NT
Disulfoton	—	—	—	N	N	+	—	NT	NT
Parathion-methyl	—	—	(+)	N	N	—	—	—	NT
Positive only for gene mutation in insects									
Bromocil	—	—	—	—	—	—	+	—	NT
Simazine	—	—	—	—	—	—	+	NT	NT

Data from Waters et al. (24). With changes resulting from Gene-Tox evaluation of original data and additional testing (25).

*Definitions of abbreviations: Ames = reverse mutation in *Salmonella typhimurium* strains TA1535, TA1537, TA1538, and TA100; WP2 = Reverse mutation in *Escherichia coli* WP2 (uvrA); D3 = mitotic recombination in *Saccharomyces cerevisiae* D3; POL A = differential toxicity in DNA repair proficient (W3110) and deficient (P3478) strains of *Escherichia coli*; REC = differential toxicity in DNA repair proficient (H17) and deficient (M45) strains of *Bacillus subtilis*; UDS = unscheduled DNA synthesis in human fetal lung fibroblasts (WI-38 cells); DRL = sex-linked recessive lethal test in *Drosophila melanogaster*; MDL = mouse dominant lethal test; MHT = mouse heritable translocation test. Number of pesticides tested (out of a total 38) is given in parentheses. + = positive; (+) = weak positive; — = negative; NT = not tested; N = no test.

†Positive in light of historical controls.

pounds are available from other sources, the mutagenicity results show a reasonably good overall correlation. Still, it should be noted that positive results from rodent carcinogenesis bioassays have been reported for three compounds (monuron, parathion, and trifluralin) evaluated as negative in the present study. Pending further evaluation, these discrepanices may be resolved. (See reference 24 and 25 for a further discussion of the relationship to the available carcinogenicity data.)

This evaluation of 38 pesticides demonstrated the feasibility of the phased approach in evaluating large numbers of chemicals in a rapid and efficient manner. The major area of concern is the limited occurrence of apparent false-negatives in results from the phase 1 battery. Further testing and an evaluation of the relationships between pesticide structure and observed genetic activity are in progress. Adjustments of the matrix will reflect this SAR evaluation and will receive major guidance form the results of the GENE-TOX Program.

CONCLUSIONS

An important role is foreseen for SAR analysis (*a*) in the selection of compounds for toxicological evaluation, (*b*) in the proper testing of these compounds, and (*c*) in the interpretation of the results obtained. At present, however, the utility of SAR models is limited, primarily by the inadequacy of the biological data on which SAR correlations must be based. A major effort to improve this situation within the area of genetic toxicology—the EPA GENE-TOX Program—has been described in some detail. Also, a limited data base on pesticide chemicals has been discussed as an example of a phased approach to testing. The results of the GENE-TOX Program and data such as those described for pesticide chemicals should provide useful biological activity information to be integrated into the SAR models described in this volume. Refinements in SAR modeling depend on the ability to obtain high-quality biological data in a readily available form. This is an important goal in genetic toxicology—one that should make an integrated approach feasible.

REFERENCES

1 Brusick, D. *Principles of Genetic Toxicology*. New York: Plenum Press (1980).
2 Committee 17 of the Environmental Mutagen Society: Environmental mutagenic hazards. *Science* 187:503–514 (1975).
3 Vogel, E. Identification of carcinogens by mutagen testing in *Drosophila:* The relative reliability for the kinds of genetic damage measured. In H. Hiatt, J. D. Watson, and J. A. Winsten (eds.), *Origins of Human Cancer,*

vol. 4, pp. 1483–1497. Cold Spring Harbor, NY: Cold Spring Harbor Laboratory (1977).

4   Ames, B. N., J. McCann, and E. Yamasaki. Methods for detecting carcinogens and mutagens with the Salmonella/mammalian-microsome mutagenicity test. *Mutat. Res.* 31:347–364 (1975).

5   McCann, J., E. Chai, E. Yamasaki, and B. N. Ames. Detection of carcinogens as mutagens in the Salmonella/microsome test: Assay of 300 chemicals. *Proc. Natl. Acad. Sci. USA* 72:5135–5139 (1975).

6   McCann, J., and B. N. Ames. Detection of carcinogens as mutagens in the Salmonella/microsome test: Assay of 300 chemicals. Discussion. *Proc. Natl. Acad. Sci. USA* 73:950–954 (1976).

7   Langenbach, R., R. Gingell, C. Kuszynski, B. Walker, D. Nagel, and P. Pour. Mutagenic activities of oxidized derivatives of N-nitrosodipropylamine in the liver cell-mediated and *Salmonella typhimurium* assays. *Cancer Res.* 40:3463–3467 (1980).

8   Waters, M. D. The GENE-TOX program. In A. W. Hsie, J. P. O'Neill, and V. K. McElheny (eds.), *Mammalian Cell Mutagenesis: The Maturation of Test Systems*, pp. 449–457. Banbury Report 2. Cold Spring Harbor, NY: Cold Spring Harbor Laboratory (1979).

9   Waters, M. D., and A. Auletta. The GENE-TOX program: Genetic activity evaluation. *J. Chem. Inf. Comput. Sci.* 21(1):35–38 (1980).

10 Maugh, T. H. Chemicals: How many are there? *Science* 199:162 (1978).

11 U.S. Environmental Protection Agency (Office of Pesticides Programs): Mutagenicity testing requirements. In *FIFRA Registration Guidelines for Hazard Evaluation of Humans and Domestic Animals* (draft, July 12). Washington, DC: U.S. Environmental Protection Agency (1977).

12 National Academy of Sciences: *Principles and Procedures for Evaluating the Toxicity of Household Substances.* Prepared for the Consumer Product Safety Commission by the Committee for the Revision of NAS Publication 1138. Washington, DC: National Academy of Science (1977).

13 DHEW Working Group of the Subcommittee on Mutagenicity Testing: Approaches to determining the mutagenic properties of chemicals: Risk to future generations. *J. Environ. Pathol. Toxicol.* 1(2):301–352 (1977).

14 Flamm, W. G. A tier system approach to mutagen testing. *Mutat. Res.* 26:329–333 (1974).

15 Bridges, B. A. Use of a three-tier protocol for evaluation of long-term toxic hazards, particularly mutagenicity and carcinogenicity. In R. Montesano H. Bartsch, and L. Tomatis (eds.), *Screening Tests in Chemical Carcinogenesis,* pp. 549–568. World Health Organization/International Agency for Research on Cancer Publication 12. Lyon, France: International Agency for Research on Cancer (1976).

16 Dean, B. J. A predictive testing scheme for carcinogenicity and mutagenicity of industrial chemicals. *Mutat. Res.* 41:83–88 (1976).

17 Mayer, V. W., and W. G. Flamm. Legislative and technical aspects of mutagenicity testing. *Mutat. Res.* 29:295–300 (1975).

18 Green, S. Present and future uses of mutagenicity tests for assessment of

the safety of food additives. *J. Environ. Pathol. Toxicol.* 1(2):49–54 (1977).

19 Sobels, F. H. Some problems associated with the testing for environmental mutagens and a perspective for studies in "comparative mutagenesis." *Mutat. Res.* 46:245–260 (1978).

20 Waters, M. D., and J. L. Epler. Status of bioscreening of emissions and effluents from energy technologies. In *Energy/Environment. III. Proceedings of the Third National Conference on the Interagency Energy/Environment Research and Development Program,* Washington, D.C. June 1–2, 1978. EPA 600/9-78-022. Springfield, VA: National Technical Information Center (1978).

21 Waters, M. D. A phased approach to the bioscreening of emissions and effluents from energy technologies. In *Proceedings of the Life Sciences Symposium on Potential Health and Environmental Effects of Synthetic Fuel Technologies,* Gatlinburg, Tennessee (September 25–28, 1978).

22 Waters, M. D. Monitoring the environment. In R. M. Nardone (ed.), *Toxicity Testing In Vitro.* New York: Academic Press (in press).

23 Ray, V. Application of microbial and mammalian cells to the assessment of mutagenicity. *Pharmacol. Rev.* 30(4):537–546 (1979).

25 Waters, M. D., S. S. Sandhu, V. F. Simmon, K. E. Mortelmans, A. D. Mitchell, T. A. Jorgenson, D. C. L. Jones, R. Valencia and N. E. Garrett. Study of Pesticide Genotoxicity. In R. Fleck and A. Hollaender (eds), *Genetic Toxicology–An Agricultural Perspective,* New York, NY: Plenum Press (1982). In press.

26 Simmon, V. F. *In vivo* and *in vitro* mutagenicity assays of selected pesticides. In *Proceedings of the Conference: A Rational Evaluation of Pesticidal vs. Mutagenic/Carcinogenic Action.* DHEW Publication (NIH) 78-1306. Bethesda, MD: U.S. Department of Health, Education, and Welfare (1978).

27 Simmon, V. F., A. D. Mitchell, and T. A. Jorgenson. *Evaluation of Selected Pesticides as Chemical Mutagens, In Vitro and In Vivo Studies.* EPA-600/1-77-028. Springfield, VA: National Technical Information Center (1977).

28 Valencia, R. *Mutagenesis Screening of Pesticides Using Drosophila.* Final Report, U.S. Environmental Protection Agency Contract 68-01-2474. Madison, WI: WARF Institute (1977).

29 Jones, D. C. L., V. F. Simmon, K. E. Mortelmans, A. D. Mitchell, E. L. Evans, M. M. Jotz, E. S. Riccio, D. E. Robinson and B. A. Kirkhardt, *In Vitro and In Vivo Studies of Environmental Chemicals,* Final Report, U.S. Environmental Protection Agency Contract 68-02-2947, Menlo Park, CA: SRI International (1981).

Summary

Leon Golberg

Since both toxicology and QSAR techniques are dealt with in this volume, we began with a brief description of basic concepts concerning toxic response. In addressing this topic, Popp (Chap. 1) stressed the variety of criteria that are used in the course of toxicity studies to identify and describe responses that can be regarded as adverse in nature. Scientific advances make possible the application of increasingly sensitive indexes of toxic effect; in fact, the closer we approach an understanding of the mechanism of toxic action of a particular compound, or a group of compounds, the more directly targeted such criteria of toxicity will become.

The target in question may involve specific cells within a particular organ, or the entire organ, or a multiplicity of sites in various organs of the body. By virtue of actions that are still not fully understood, toxic effects may be localized within certain areas, such as the centrilobular zones of liver lobules. It is important to distinguish primary toxic consequences in one organ from secondary effects that may arise elsewhere in the body.

Dose-time relationships play a key role in toxicology. High doses administered over a brief span of time elicit acute responses. The characteristics of such acute poisonings may be radically different from the effects of lower doses that permit survival of the test animals for long periods of time; specifically, repeated administration of the test material leads to subtle forms of subchronic toxicity that may evolve into full-blown chronic lesions under the influence of cumulative dosage and prolonged exposure. During this interval, repair and restoration of structure and/or function may also be in progress, and when such processes prove unsuccessful or inadequate, they may themselves serve to accentuate, distort, or radically transform the pathological effects of the compound under investigation. Cancer is only one of many long-term manifestations of toxic response. As a consequence of intensive investigation devoted to various forms of neoplasia, some understanding has been developed of the biochemical and morphological basis of this particular effect at the cellular, subcellular, and molecular levels. Analyses of these aspects by Bus (Chap. 4) and Chignell (Chap. 5) are described below.

Anderson and colleagues (Chap. 2) discussed the role of inhibitors of carcinogenesis as an illustration of modifying factors that can influence this process. This presentation also served to emphasize the complexities of the "dose" of a compound to which an animal or human is exposed, in contrast to the "dose" at the target organ, or the "dose" of a specific reactive intermediate (formed by metabolic activation) covalently bound to the target macromolecule, DNA. An illustration was thus provided of the way in which increasingly sensitive criteria of effect at earlier and earlier stages of toxic action shed light on mechanisms and afford more accurate measures of response.

Modifying factors can alter the outcome of exposures to a toxicant by a great variety of mechanisms. One of these is alteration of the balance between metabolic activation and detoxification; a tilt in the direction of detoxification serves to prevent or reduce the development of adverse effects such as neoplasia. Among the enzyme systems involved, aryl hydrocarbon hydroxylase (AHH) plays a major role in the case of polynuclear aromatic hydrocarbons such as benzo[a]pyrene (BP), which induces tumors in mouse lung, skin, and forestomach. One of the key reactive intermediates formed is BP diol epoxide (BPDE), and the amount of BPDE-DNA adduct in target organs is an index of ultimate carcinogenic effect. Modification of the activities of enzymes responsible for formation of BPDE is achieved by inducers of AHH and by antioxidants, such as butylated hydroxyanisole, which inhibit neoplasia resulting from administration of BP. Thus, for the particular class of chemicals—polynuclear aromatic hydrocarbons—the possibility of identifying and measuring a quintessential DNA adduct affords a means of assessing carcinogenic activity at doses far below those that are practical in the standard bioassay procedure.

A more general discussion of biochemical mechanisms underlying toxic actions of chemicals was presented by Bus (Chap. 4). He drew a distinction between nonspecific organ toxicity and action limited to one, or a few, specific target organs. Tissue-specific distribution, i.e., localization in the target organ, may be an essential element, as exemplified by the herbicide paraquat. What happens to compounds once they are distributed to the tissues may be of crucial importance. Often, metabolic activation by microsomal mixed function oxidases to electrophilic products such as epoxides (see BPDE, referred to above), or free radicals, creates the potential for attack on nucleophilic centers in cellular macromolecules or other components, with consequent toxic effects. Cellular defense mechanisms come into play, producing detoxification by enzymatic or other means.

An important source of toxic effects arising from xenobiotic metabolism is the production of various forms of activated oxygen, including superoxide anion, hydroxyl radical, and hydrogen peroxide. The corresponding defense mechanisms involve the enzymes superoxide dismutase, catalase, and peroxidases. The consequences of lipid peroxidation by activated oxygen are checked by vitamin E and glutathione peroxidase.

In addition to nonselective attack on tissue components by reactive intermediates, more specific disruption of cellular metabolism and function often occurs. Important examples include phosphorylation of the esteratic site of acetylcholinesterase by organophosphate metabolites, leading to an accumulation of acetylcholine in the nerve synapses, and inhibition of mitochondrial energy production by a variety of mechanisms.

The chapters by Anderson (Chap. 2) and Bus (Chap. 4) serve to emphasize the importance of taking into account the factor of metabolism, and especially metabolic activation, in any approach to QSAR. Relatively little has been done along these lines to date, and the contributions by Loew (Chap. 8) and Wipke (Chap. 10), summarized below, thus assume particular significance.

Akland and Waters (Chap. 3) dealt with the all-important question of data bases for assessment of structure-activity relationships. Several types of data bases, both automated and manual, contain information that can be used for analyzing chemical structure, physicochemical properties, and the relationship of these to biological effects. The first kind of data base contains citations, and in some cases abstracts, from the published literature. Examples of these data bases include Chemical Abstracts, Biological Abstracts, the Environmental Mutagen Information System (EMIC), the Environmental Teratogen Information System (ETIC), MEDLINE (Index Medicus), Excerpta Medica, SCISEARCH, and CANCERLINE & CANCERPROJ.

Secondly, there are data bases that contain information about chemicals, such as synonyms, structural image, chemical and physical properties, molecular formulas, Chemical Abstracts Service Registry number, toxicity values, metabolism, environmental pollution potential, manufacturing information, and occupational exposure limits. Examples of such information systems include the NIH–EPA Chemical Information Systems (CIS) and NLM–ORNL Toxicology Data Bank and the Chemical Abstracts Service's CAS On-Line.

The third type of data base discussed includes actual results of biological experiments, both qualitative as well as, in many instances, quantitative data. Examples of such data bases include EPA's GENE--TOX evaluated data on mutagenicity, data stemming from NCI's carcinogenesis bioassays, and the chemical evaluations carried out by the International Agency for Research on Cancer. A review of existing data bases reveals a pressing need for additional sources of chemical and biological information, especially evaluated qualitative and quantitative experimental data.

Efforts to develop a quantitatively analyzed data base were described by McCann and colleagues (Chap. 15). The results are derived from the major short-term tests for carcinogens and mutagens. Currently available are extensive results of the *Salmonella* (Ames) assay. In the coming year, data from mammalian cell mutagenesis assays, *in vitro* transformation assays, and tests for sister chromatid exchange will be incorporated into the data base. The emphasis throughout is on quantitative measures of potency, for ultimate comparison, in the case of carcinogens, with the results of animal cancer bioassays.

Chignell (Chap. 5) discussed the origins of modern approaches to QSAR, in which both physical and chemical properties of molecules are used to predict their biological activities. The first of the molecular parameters in QSAR is hydrophobicity (lipophilicity), which involves various properties including partition coefficients, chromatographic coefficients, molar refractivity, and parachor. The role of water in hydrophobic interactions is far from being a passive one. The fact was stressed that there are limits to the partition coefficient that permit a molecule to reach its site of action and exert its biological effect.

Among polar or electronic parameters, pride of place must be given to Hammett sigma values, later modified by Taft, who also developed the steric parameter that bears his name. As a quantitative measure of the overall shapes of molecules and their substituents, Verloop and colleagues invented "sterimol" constants. Molar refractivity and parachor can also serve as steric parameters. Among molecular parameters cited are reduction potential (as in the case of aromatic and heterocyclic nitro compounds), bond dissociation energies, hydrogen bonding, polarizability, and molecular symmetry. Together with molecular orbital calculations of electron densities, discussed below, the armamentarium of molecular parameters that relate to toxic potentialities is an impressive one.

The principles and practice of Hansch analysis were outlined by Martin (Chap. 6). The semiempirical linear free energy model elaborated by Hansch and others is typically used in the examination of a series of analogs that have a common parent molecule and variable substituents. The first step in the analysis is the description of the molecules, in quantitative terms, by their physical properties. One would typically consider the octanol:water log P and

pK_a of the whole molecule as well as the physical properties of the substituents at each site of substitution. For the latter one would include the Hansch π value for hydrophobicity, the Hammett σ constant for electronic effects, the Taft E_s value for steric effects, and the molar refractivity, which models the ability to participate in dispersion bonding.

The next step in the analysis is the examination, typically by regression analysis, of the statistical relationship between the physical properties and the biological potency of the molecule. One or several physical properties acting in concert may correlate with potency. These QSAR may be linear or nonlinear, and particular computer programs are recommended for these purposes.

QSAR have correctly predicted the potency of new analogs in many series, provided methods for the efficient design and criteria for when to stop synthesis in a series, been used in mapping receptors, and shown that some of the relationships between physical properties and pharmacokinetics are not so universal as once thought. The current limitations of QSAR are the difficulty of describing the three-dimensionality of the chemical properties of molecules and of translating biological data into a relevant number.

Among the recently developed procedures for QSAR, pattern recognition analysis (PRA) is a promising entry in the field. One of its foremost exponents, Jurs (Chap. 7), views it as somewhat of a combination of art and science. An interactive computer software system, ADAPT, is used to assist in the investigation of QSAR for large sets of structurally diverse compounds. The art of PRA lies in the selection of descriptors to represent important geometrical, topological, and other molecular structural features of the compounds under study. The objective is to use the sets of descriptors to generate a unique point for each compound in a multidimensional space. A measure of the success of the art is its ability to choose, or develop, descriptors so effectively as to segregate the points representing active compounds into one cluster within that space, while the inactive compounds cluster in another region. To the extent that this separation is achieved, the probability of activity can be foretold for an untested compound that has a similar structural type as the rest of the set: for example, is an aromatic amine, an N-nitroso compound, or a polycyclic aromatic hydrocarbon.

In addition to using the various parameters described in other chapters, PRA builds a three-dimensional model of the molecule to provide spatial information that acts as a source of the following topological and geometrical descriptors: atom and bond fragments, substructure environment, molecular connectivity (extent of branching), path and path environment, and molecular volume, shape, surface area, substructure shape, and moment of inertia. All these descriptors may be manipulated in various ways to generate new descriptors, after which PRA is carried out using parametric and nonparametric techniques. PRA has been applied in this way to a wide range of biological activities, by Jurs and his colleagues using ADAPT PRA and by Dunn, Wold and their co-workers using SIMCA PRA methodology (Chap. 9).

Loew and colleagues (Chap 8) described quantum mechanical methods for mechanistic studies of QSAR in the field of polycyclic aromatic hydrocarbons (PAH). The PAH are known to require multiple transformations to active carcinogens, and addition of methyl groups can dramatically enhance parent compound activity. In the context of the hypothesis that bay region diol epoxides are the active forms of PAH, specific electronic properties related to metabolite transformation and stability of the putative carbocation ultimate carcinogens were calculated for 17 parent PAH and 29 methyl derivatives of benz[a]anthracene and chrysene. All-valence electron semiempirical quantum mechanical methods were used, with the aim of identifying molecular properties that could serve as reliable indicators of relative carcinogenic activity. The calculated substrate reactivities were found to predict major metabolites successfully, supporting the validity of their use in attempted correlations with observed carcinogenic potencies. Positive correlations were found between observed carcinogenic potencies and the reactivities of the parent PAH with respect to the initial bay region epoxidation, as well as the stabilities of the diol epoxide carbocations. These findings indicate the potential usefulness of these attributes as screening parameters for carcinogenic activity in this class of compounds.

The prediction of a variety of biological properties–both desirable and undesirable–was discussed by Kaufman (Chap. 19). The combination of *ab initio* quantum chemical calculations with electrostatic molecular potential contour maps generated from the *ab initio* wave functions not only allows correlation of biological activities with structures but also facilitates uniquely correct predictions of such activities. The electrostatic molecular potential contour maps generated around a common pharmacophore or toxicophore (even in chemically dissimilar molecules) are always similar in shape and often even in magnitude. Moreover, for polycyclic aromatic hydrocarbon carcinogens the electrostatic molecular potential contour maps have been able to predict correctly the bonds across which initial arene oxides form, the stereochemical preferences for opening the oxide ring, for formation of dihydrodiols, for formation of dihydrodiol epoxides, and for opening the epoxide ring. It was also shown that these maps could be used to define a new measure of electrophilicity–an important concept in initial events in induction of carcinogenicity.

Kaufman and colleagues have combined these theoretical approaches with appropriate physicochemical approaches–with graph theory and with concepts of systems analyses and control theory for the dynamic balance of endogenous biomolecules–into an overall strategy for correlation and prediction of biological structure-activity relationships in a wide range of diverse areas of biomedical significance.

A number of recent examples of the application of SIMCA pattern recognition analysis (PRA) were reviewed by Dunn and Wold (Chap. 9). The object was to predict carcinogenic activity of potential environmental pollutants. After describing the principles underlying SIMCA PRA, the authors illustrated applications to polycyclic aromatic hydrocarbons, *N*-nitroso compounds, and compounds related to 4-nitroquinoline-1-oxide. In all three categories, data are available, derived from extensive and reliable carcinogenesis bioassays. An important aspect stressed by the authors was the unique property of SIMCA PRA, in comparison with other forms of PRA used in QSAR, namely its two-way powers of prediction. Not only can structural data be used to predict pharmacological or other biological activity, but, using SIMCA, a molecule can be constructed theoretically that will have a particular defined biological action.

As mentioned above, in many cases the biological activity observed after administering a xenobiotic compound results from the action of one or more metabolites and not directly from the original compound. Rather than attempting to correlate activity indirectly with the structure of the original parent compound, Wipke and colleagues (Chap. 10) have sought to predict the metabolite structures and then base structure-activity studies on these metabolite structures directly. To attempt such predictions by manual metabolic analysis is to court the biases and errors inherent in human frailty; intelligently programmed, the computer is not subject to these limitations.

The *in calculo* model assumes the presence of all metabolic enzyme systems in a single container, acting on the substrate compound. The model does not predict the quantitative production of metabolites, but it assesses the relative prominence of various biotransformations. The authors have developed an interactive computer-graphics program called XENO, which accepts a drawing of the xenobiotic compound and then generates plausible metabolites and displays their structures on a CRT terminal together with a rating of plausible biological activity. XENO's metabolism knowledge base is mechanistically oriented rather than rote-memory oriented; consequently, it is not limited to molecules whose metabolism is known. XENO uses a unique knowledge-based scheme for evaluating plausible activity of each metabolite.

XENO may be viewed as a tool that can assist chemists, biochemists, and pharmacologists not only in predicting biological activity but also in evaluating and studying metabolism itself. The use of ALCHEM transforms to describe each reaction has many advantages, not the least of which has been the creation of a biotransform library. Such important characteristics of metabolic reactions as stereoselectivity, electronic effects, and species specificity can be taken care of by XENO.

Smith and collaborators (Chap. 11) discussed results of their recent research in two areas that represent key components of computer-based QSAR techniques. The first concerns methods for canonical (unique) representation of substructures with conformational designations. This representation is necessary in research efforts to correlate such substructures with observed activities across a wide variety of structural types. The assumption is made that one is characterizing the local substructural environment of an atom (or functionality), wherein atom connectivities play a crucial role in the associated activity. Because local substructural configuration and conformation have been adequately taken into account, this method also serves to build a data base of structures, their component substructures, and their activities.

A related second area under investigation concerns the problem of three-dimensional common substructures. Under the hypothesis that molecules displaying similar activities share a common pharmacophore in their biologically active conformations, the authors have sought to determine the identity of such pharmacophores. A method was described for solving the following, narrowly defined problem: given a set of structures displaying similar biological activity, each in a prescribed conformation (determined by other methods), ascertain common substructural features (in three-dimensional space) of the set. These common features then represent candidates for the pharmacophore.

The development of a structure-activity tree was reported by Sigman, Johnson, and their colleagues (Chap. 12). The tree is the primary component of a systematic method for evaluating the potential carcinogenicity of untested chemicals. The activity tree is developed, maintained, and applied to the evaluation of chemicals via the chemical structure analysis and data management capabilities of the PROPHET computer system.

The activity tree is a framework for identifying structural features of chemicals associated with carcinogenicity; assignments to it are based on expert evaluation of carcinogenicity test data. The major classifications on the tree are chemical structure classes containing known carcinogens (e.g., aromatic amines). The chemical classes are subdivided by additional structural features (nodes) that are judged to reflect differences in the expected carcinogenic behavior of chemicals belonging to the class. Associated with each class and node are estimates of the strength of evidence implicating chemicals having appropriate structural features as carcinogens and data on well-tested chemicals belonging to the structural group (i.e., CAS No., name, structure, species tested, sex, route of administration, and major tumor sites).

In PROPHET, the various processes of applying and developing the activity tree include (a) substructure analysis of untested chemicals in order to classify them on the tree and, hence, to evaluate their potential carcinogenicity; (b) analysis of carcinogens by parameters in addition to structure (e.g., identifying carcinogen classes associated with specific tumor sites); and (c) refining and updating the tree as new carcinogenicity data are added.

Two examples were chosen to illustrate the application of PROPHET software for QSAR analysis in environmental toxicology. The first was concerned with the prediction of reproductive toxicity in fish. The second very clearly illustrated the approaches and problems in anticipating the degree of hazard of environmental chemicals in relation to potential carcinogenic effects in human beings.

Craig and Enslein (Chap. 17) reported on their efforts to develop statistical models relating structural parameters, physical properties and toxicological activities of a variety of chemical agents.

Tinker (Chap. 13) described a computerized program for relating bacterial mutagenesis activity to chemical structure. The program employs a substructure recognition process based on the procedure of Hodes. Structural information is accepted from connection tables (Chemical Abstracts Registry II or III) or MCC–TSS ciphers of Lefkowitz. Typically in this program the basic substructure unit (ganglion) is an atom triplet. Data for correlation are provided by over 1800 results from mutagenesis tests run in the Ames *Salmonella typhimurium* test, obtained from the literature. Statistical weights for ganglia are calculated from the program of Hodes. The program calculates the level of activity to be expected of an unknown structure, with an estimate of confidence.

The operation of the program over several years was described. The results have revealed the dependence of biological data on chemical structure and the self-consistency of the data. Factors and decisions affecting the acceptance of results were discussed. New program facilities—list processing, similarity index, and listing—have become available. The rationale for including a reliability factor related to the test protocol and the purity of the substance, and the manner in which the factor is employed, was made clear by the author. It seeks to compensate for incompleteness of the protocol and thus utilizes many of the existing data that, despite experimental shortcomings, cannot be ignored. Progress in this important area will be followed with great interest by many in this field.

The subject of QSAR in the field of mutagenesis was also addressed by Purcell (Chap. 14), drawing on published and unpublished examples. Some suggestions were made concerning a future course in this field.

Langenbach and colleagues (Chap. 16) described the study of a series of 10 propylnitrosamines for mutagenic activity in the hamster hepatocyte-mediated V79 cell mutagenesis system. Previous work has demonstrated that this liver cell-mediated system is particularly well suited for determining the mutagenic activity of nitrosamines. The compounds studied were: dipropyl-nitrosamine (DP), bis-(2-hydroxypropyl)-nitrosamine (BHP), bis-(2-oxypropyl)-nitrosamine (BOP), 2-hydroxypropyl-2-oxypropylnitrosamine (HPOP), 2-oxypropylpropylnitrosamine (OPP), 2-hydroxypropylpropylnitrosamine (HPP), methylpropylnitrosamine (MP), methyl-2-hydroxypropylnitrosamine (MHP), methyl-2-oxypropylnitrosamine (MOP), and bis-(acetoxypropyl)-nitrosamine (BAP). Dimethylnitrosamine (DMN) served as a positive control in all studies.

in the presence of hamster hepatocytes, the nitrosamines showed varying degrees of mutagenic activity to V79 cells; however, in the absence of hepatocytes the nitrosamines were not mutagenic.

The relative mutagenic activity of the nitrosamines in the cell-mediated system was MOP > MHP > DMN > BOP > MP > OPP, HPOP > DP, HPP > BHP, BAP, which is in relative agreement with the carcinogenic potencies of several of these nitrosamines. Structure-activity relationships correlated with the degree of oxygenation, type of oxygen functionality, and total carbon number. In general, increased β-carbon oxygenation favors increased mutagenic activity as does decrease in total carbon number. These results suggest that metabolism of DP to mutagenic intermediates is rate limiting; however, factors other than metabolism may also participate in determining the mutagenic and carcinogenic potential of these nitrosamines. Clarification of these issues is needed to improve the data base before applying computerized QSAR techniques.

LaVoie, Hecht, and Hoffman (Chap. 18) again discussed the polynuclear aromatic hydrocarbons (PAH), wherein major advances in QSAR with respect to carcinogenicity have been achieved through a more complete understanding of the mechanism of action of PAH [see Loew (Chap. 8)]. The bay region theory of PAH activation has been shown to be applicable to the metabolic activation of benzo[a]pyrene, benz[a]anthracene, chrysene, dibenzo[a,i]-pyrene, and 3-methylcholanthrene. Studies on the metabolic activation of benzo[c]phenanthrene and benzo[j]fluoranthene have also indicated that nonclassic bay region diol epoxides are associated with their metabolic activation. The mechanisms of activation of weak tumorigenic agents, which do not contain within their structures a bay region, have also been investigated in recent years. As mechanisms of PAH activation are elucidated, the molecular basis for the established structure-carcinogenicity relationships for these PAH will be determined.

The authors have proposed that the structural requirements favoring carcinogenicity of methylated PAH are a bay region methyl group and a free peri position, both adjacent to an unsubstituted angular ring. Among the six possible monomethylchrysenes, 5-methylchrysene is by far the most carcinogenic, with potency comparable to benzo[a]pyrene. Consistent with these structural requirements, studies on the metabolic activation of 5-methylchrysene have indicated that the 1,2-dihydrodiol-3,4-epoxide is ultimately associated with its carcinogenic potential. Studies performed on the methylated derivatives of other ring systems such as benz[a]anthracene, dibenz[a,h]-anthracene, cyclopenta[a]phenanthrene, and phenanthrene support these structure-carcinogenicity relationships for methylated PAH.

I realize all too clearly how difficult it is to do full justice to the wealth of information presented in this volume. I have tried to illustrate the interaction of QSAR techniques with problems in toxicology. Perhaps we have overemphasized carcinogenicity and mutagenicity to the detriment of the remainder of the vast domain over which general toxicology pertains. Alas, in many areas of toxic action wherein data bases may be sought, the experience would be akin to Mother Hubbard's. In others, the cupboard may not be quite bare but only sparsely stocked. A concerted effort is needed, on the part of all of us, to produce the necessary information—from unpublished records as well as new systematic approaches—that will permit QSAR studies in toxicology to flourish as never before. Then, and only then, will the application of QSAR assume its rightful place in the hierarchy of hazard evaluation.

Index

317